Immunology Laboratory Testing

Editor

VINAY S. MAHAJAN

CLINICS IN LABORATORY MEDICINE

www.labmed.theclinics.com

Editor-in-Chief

MILENKO JOVAN TANASIJEVIC

December 2019 • Volume 39 • Number 4

ELSEVIER

1600 John F. Kennedy Boulevard • Suite 1800 • Philadelphia, Pennsylvania, 19103-2899

http://www.theclinics.com

CLINICS IN LABORATORY MEDICINE Volume 39, Number 4
December 2019 ISSN 0272-2712, ISBN-13: 978-0-323-71157-9

Editor: Stacy Eastman
Developmental Editor: Laura Fisher

Reprints. For copies of 100 or more, of articles in this publication, please contact the Commercial Reprints Department, Elsevier Inc., 360 Park Avenue South, New York, New York 10010-1710. Tel. 212-633-3874, Fax: 212-633-3820, E-mail: reprints@elsevier.com.

Clinics in Laboratory Medicine (ISSN 0272-2712) is published quarterly by Elsevier Inc., 360 Park Avenue South, New York, NY 10010-1710. Months of issue are March, June, September, and December. Business and Editorial offices: 1600 John F. Kennedy Blvd., Suite 1800, Philadelphia, PA 19103-2899. Periodicals postage paid at NewYork, NY and additional mailing offices. Subscription prices are $274.00 per year (US individuals), $541.00 per year (US institutions), $100.00 per year (US students), $349.00 per year (Canadian individuals), $657.00 per year (Canadian institutions), $185.00 per year (Canadian students), $404.00 per year (international individuals), $657.00 per year (international institutions), $185.00 (international students). Foreign air speed delivery is included in all Clinics subscription prices. All prices are subject to change without notice. POSTMASTER: Send address changes to *Clinics in Laboratory Medicine*, Elsevier Health Sciences Division, Subscription Customer Service, 3251 Riverport Lane, Maryland Heights, MO 63043. **Customer Service: 1-800-654-2452 (US). From outside of the US and Canada, call 1-314-447-8871. Fax: 1-314-447-8029. E-mail: journalscustomerservice-usa@elsevier.com (for print support) or journalsonlinesupport-usa@elsevier.com (for online support).**

Clinics in Laboratory Medicine is covered in *EMBASE/Exerpta Medica, MEDLINE/PubMed (Index Medicus), Cinahl, Current Contents/Clinical Medicine, BIOSIS* and *ISI/BIOMED.*

Contributors

EDITOR-IN-CHIEF

MILENKO JOVAN TANASIJEVIC, MD, MBA
Vice Chair for Clinical Pathology and Quality, Department of Pathology, Director of Clinical Laboratories, Brigham and Women's Hospital, Dana-Farber Cancer Institute, Associate Professor of Pathology, Harvard Medical School, Boston, Massachusetts, USA

EDITOR

VINAY S. MAHAJAN, MD, PhD
Associate Pathologist, Department of Pathology, Center for Advanced Molecular Diagnostics, Brigham and Women's Hospital, Instructor of Pathology, Harvard Medical School, Boston, Massachusetts, USA; Instructor, Ragon Institute of MGH, MIT and Harvard, Cambridge, Massachusetts, USA

AUTHORS

HUGUES ALLARD-CHAMARD, MD, PhD, FRCPC
Visiting Scientist, Ragon Institute of MGH, MIT and Harvard, Cambridge, Massachusetts, USA; Assistant Professor of Medicine, Division of Rheumatology, Faculty of Medicine and Health Sciences, Université de Sherbrooke, Centre de Recherche Clinique du Centre Hospitalier Universitaire de Sherbrooke, Division of Rheumatology, Centre intégré universitaire de santé et de service sociaux de l'Estrie – Centre hospitalier universitaire de Sherbrooke (CIUSSS de l'Estrie-CHUS), Sherbrooke, Québec, Canada

SARA BARMETTLER, MD
Instructor in Medicine, Allergy and Immunology Unit, Division of Rheumatology, Allergy and Immunology, Massachusetts General Hospital, Boston, Massachusetts, USA

GILLES BOIRE, MD, MSc, FRCPC
Professor of Medicine, Division of Rheumatology, Faculty of Medicine and Health Sciences, Université de Sherbrooke; Centre de Recherche Clinique du Centre Hospitalier Universitaire de Sherbrooke; Division of Rheumatology, Centre intégré universitaire de santé et de service sociaux de l'Estrie – Centre hospitalier universitaire de Sherbrooke (CIUSSS de l'Estrie-CHUS), Sherbrooke, Québec, Canada

ANIL CHANDRAKER, MD, FASN
Associate Professor, Department of Medicine, Medical Director, Kidney and Pancreas Transplantation, Director, Transplantation Research Center, Renal Division, Brigham and Women's Hospital, Harvard Medical School, Boston, Massachusetts, USA

JOHN CHOI, MD
Transplantation Research Center, Renal Division, Brigham and Women's Hospital, Harvard Medical School, Boston, Massachusetts, USA

MICHELLE DeLELYS, MLA
Laboratory Manager, Cellular Therapeutics and Transplantation/Flow Cytometry, Departments of Pathology and Cancer Center, Massachusetts General Hospital, Boston, Massachusetts, USA

JOCELYN R. FARMER, MD, PhD
Instructor, Division of Rheumatology, Allergy and Immunology, Massachusetts General Hospital, Boston, Massachusetts, USA; Instructor, Ragon Institute of MGH, MIT and Harvard, Cambridge, Massachusetts, USA

NICOLE A. LaHOOD, MD
Clinical and Research Fellow, Allergy and Immunology, Department of Medicine, Division of Rheumatology, Allergy, and Immunology, Massachusetts General Hospital, Boston, Massachusetts, USA

PATRICK LIANG, MD, FRCPC
Associate Professor of Medicine, Division of Rheumatology, Faculty of Medicine and Health Sciences, Université de Sherbrooke, Centre de Recherche Clinique du Centre Hospitalier Universitaire de Sherbrooke, Division of Rheumatology, Centre intégré universitaire de santé et de service sociaux de l'Estrie – Centre hospitalier universitaire de Sherbrooke (CIUSSS de l'Estrie-CHUS), Sherbrooke, Québec, Canada

MORRIS LING, MD
Division of Rheumatology, Allergy and Immunology, Department of Medicine, Center for Immunology and Inflammatory Diseases, Department of Pathology, Massachusetts General Hospital, Department of Medicine, Harvard Medical School, Boston, Massachusetts, USA

VINAY S. MAHAJAN, MD, PhD
Associate Pathologist, Department of Pathology, Center for Advanced Molecular Diagnostics, Brigham and Women's Hospital, Instructor of Pathology, Harvard Medical School, Boston, Massachusetts, USA; Instructor, Ragon Institute of MGH, MIT and Harvard, Cambridge, Massachusetts, USA

LEWENA MAHER, MD
Internal Medicine, Beth Israel Lahey Health, Burlington, Massachusetts, USA

MANDAKOLATHUR MURALI, MD
Division of Rheumatology, Allergy and Immunology, Department of Medicine, Department of Pathology, Massachusetts General Hospital, Department of Medicine, Harvard Medical School, Boston, Massachusetts, USA

SARITA U. PATIL, MD
Instructor, Department of Medicine, Division of Rheumatology, Allergy, and Immunology, Massachusetts General Hospital, Food Allergy Center, Massachusetts General Hospital for Children, Harvard Medical School, Boston, Massachusetts, USA

CORY PERUGINO, DO
Division of Rheumatology, Allergy and Immunology, Massachusetts General Hospital, Boston, Massachusetts, USA; Ragon Institute of MGH, MIT and Harvard, Cambridge, Massachusetts, USA

ANNE E. TEBO, PhD, D(ABMLI)
Professor (clinical) of Pathology, Department of Pathology, University of Utah School of Medicine and Medical Director of Immunology, ARUP Laboratories, Salt Lake City, Utah, USA

Contents

The presence of antinuclear antibodies (ANAs), which include autoanti-bodies to extractable nuclear antigens (ENAs), in the sera of patients with connective tissue diseases provides useful immunologic and patho-physiologic insight into the nature of their disease. This article discusses the most commonly used diagnostic modalities for detecting and quanti-tating the presence of ANA: indirect immunofluorescence assay, enzyme-linked immunosorbent assay, and multiplex bead technology, which serve as useful screening tests. We also review testing for autoan-tibodies to ENAs, which are often helpful to confirm the diagnosis of a spe-cific connective tissue disease.

Accurate diagnosis of inflammatory arthritides remains a challenge because of substantial clinical overlap. To achieve a granular classifica-tion for informing clinical decisions, numerous potential serologic bio-markers have been identified. Rheumatologists have settled on rheumatoid factor and anti–citrullinated protein antibodies for the diag-nosis of rheumatoid arthritis (RA) based on specificity and sensitivity and their ability to be integrated into clinical algorithms. These biomarkers should be interpreted in their specific clinical context. This article dis-cusses the serologic basis for the diagnosis of RA, how these biomarkers have framed conceptualization of the pathogenesis of RA, and the inherent limitations in their use.

The discovery of antineutrophil cytoplasmic antibodies (ANCA) helped establish ANCA-associated vasculitis as a separate and well-defined clin-ical entity. Its progressive incorporation into the clinical diagnosis algo-rithms has made ANCA testing a cornerstone immunoassay embedded in the management of ANCA-associated vasculitis. After its description by indirect immunofluorescence, proteinase-3 and myeloperoxidase were identified as principal ANCA targets. ANCA, and proteinase-3 and myeloperoxidase immunoassessment, have undergone iterative rounds of improvement in sensitivity and specificity. This article traces landmarks in the development of ANCA tests, describes common pitfalls arising dur-ing ANCA interpretation, and discusses new technologies to improve the future of ANCA testing.

Antiphospholipid syndrome (APS) is as an autoimmune disease character-ized by thrombosis and/or specific pregnancy-related morbidity associ-ated with persistent antiphospholipid antibodies, namely, lupus anticoagulant and IgG and IgM antibodies to cardiolipin and beta2 glyco-protein I. Optimal antibody detection plays a central role in diagnosis and classification. This review discusses antiphospholipid antibodies helpful for diagnosing APS. It includes the criteria and noncriteria antiphospholipid antibodies, methods for their detection, and challenges for clinical report-ing and interpretation. The significance of using specific noncriteria anti-phospholipid tests in an integrated diagnostic approach with criteria antiphospholipid makers for the diagnosis and management of APS is also reviewed.

Immunology testing is relevant for the diagnosis of many autoimmune con-ditions. However, diagnostic pitfalls arise owing to incorrect interpretation of results and incomplete understanding of the underlying technique or immune-mediated condition. Here, we review the diagnostic consider-ations related to commonly used immunology tests. Specifically, we sum-marize the caveats pertinent to the interpretation of rheumatoid factor, antinuclear antibodies, antiphospholipid antibodies, antineutrophil cyto-plasmic antibodies, and serum IgG4 testing.

The complement system is a critical component of both the innate and adaptive immune systems that augments the function of antibodies and phagocytes. Antigen-antibody immune complexes, lectin binding, and accelerated C3 tick-over can activate this well-coordinated and carefully regulated process. The importance of this system is highlighted by the dis-orders that arise when complement components or regulators are defi-cient or dysregulated. This article describes the pathways involved in complement activation and function, the regulation of these various path-ways, and the interpretation of laboratory testing performed for the diag-nosis of diseases of complement deficiency, exuberant complement activation, and complement dysregulation.

Flow cytometry is an incredibly powerful diagnostic tool in the evaluation of primary and secondary immune deficiencies. Assay design and setup in-volves a methodological consideration of specimen collection, marker and fluorochrome selection, antibody titration, instrumentation, compen-sation, gating, reference range development, and cross validation.

Commonly used analyses for lymphocytes are the lymphocyte subset, T-cell subset, B-cell and T-cell naive/memory, double-negative T-cell, and plasmablast panels. Flow cytometry has direct clinical applicability to the workup of severe forms of primary immune deficiency disorders and is used diagnostically and for therapeutic monitoring in the context of secondary immune deficiency disorders.

Laboratory assays of immune cell function are essential for understanding the type and function of immune defects. These assessments should be performed in conjunction with a detailed history and physical examination, which should guide the evaluation of patients with a suspected immune deficiency. Laboratory assays of immune cell function are critical for assessing and demonstrating the functional impact of genetic mutations. Advances in diagnostic techniques continue to expand the ability of clinicians and researchers to understand the complex immune pathophysiology that underlies these disorders.

Although the gold standard for diagnosis of immunoglobulin E (IgE)-mediated food allergy is an oral food challenge, clinically relevant biomarkers of IgE sensitization, including serum-specific IgE and skin prick testing, can aid in diagnosis. Clinically useful values have been defined for individual foods. More recently, specific IgE to particular protein components has provided additional diagnostic value. In summary, food allergy diagnostics to evaluate IgE sensitization are clinically useful and continue to evolve to improve evaluation of IgE-mediated food allergies.

The outcomes of kidney transplantation show a steady improvement with an increasing number of transplantations and decreasing incidence of acute rejection episodes. Successful transplantation begins with a comprehensive immunologic risk assessment and judicious choice of therapeutic agents. In this review, we discuss the trends in transplant immunosuppression practices and outcomes in the United States. We discuss practical testing algorithms for clinical decision making in induction therapy and fine-tuning maintenance immunosuppression. We introduce assessment tools for immune monitoring after transplantation and speculate on future directions in management.

With the increasing application of biotechnology to the realm of pharmacology and therapeutics, the types of biological treatments available have significantly expanded. Currently, recombinant proteins, humanized antibodies, or rationally engineered monoclonal antibodies are used on a regular basis in the clinical setting. Moreover, cell-based therapeutics with molecularly rewired antigenic specificities are becoming increasingly common in oncology and are actively being developed for a broad range of diseases. Nonetheless, there has been a significant lag between the development of these technologies and the emergence of assays that can monitor these novel interventions.

Immune-targeted therapeutics are being used in cancer. Immune "checkpoint inhibition" provides promise for prolonged disease-free patient survival. Use of immune checkpoint inhibitors in cancer has coincided with the onset of immune-related adverse events (irAEs). irAEs are caused by a break in host self-tolerance, which can be deadly. Acute management of irAEs is complicated by difficulty making a prompt clinical diagnosis. The goal is to maximize anticancer benefit while minimizing irAE risk. We currently lack diagnostic tools to assess pretreatment irAE risk and facilitate diagnosis. Current immunologic understanding of irAEs is discussed with an emphasis on how patients with congenital syndromes of T-cell activation may inform this understanding. The prospects of improving diagnostics for and treatment of irAEs are discussed.

Primary immunodeficiency diseases are a heterogeneous group of rare inherited disorders of innate or adaptive immune system function. Patients with primary immunodeficiencies typically present with recurrent and severe infections in infancy or young adulthood. More recently, the co-occurrence of autoimmune, benign lymphoproliferative, atopic, and malignant complications has been described. The diagnosis of a primary immunodeficiency disorder requires a thorough assessment of a patient's underlying immune system function. Historically, this has been accomplished at the time of symptomatic presentation by measuring immunoglobulins, complement components, protective antibody titers, or immune cell counts in the peripheral blood. Although these data can be used to critically assess the degree of immune dysregulation in the patient, this approach fall short in at least 2 regards. First, this assessment often occurs after the patient has suffered life-threatening infectious or autoinflammatory complications. Second, these data fail to uncover an underlying molecular cause of the patient's primary immune dysfunction, prohibiting the use of molecularly targeted therapeutic interventions. Within the last decade, the field of primary immunodeficiency diagnostics has been revolutionized by 2 major molecular advancements: (1) the onset of newborn screening in 2008, and (2) the onset of next-generation sequencing in 2010. In this article, the techniques of newborn screening and next-generation sequencing are reviewed and their respective impacts on the field of primary immunodeficiency disorders are discussed with a specific emphasis on severe combined immune deficiency and common variable immune deficiency.

For decades, autoantibody detection has comprised the bulk of clinical laboratory immunology. However, most immune disorders are caused by imbalances in both humoral and cellular immunity. Our knowledge of the immune system has grown exponentially, resulting in new treatment paradigms in immunology. Extensive functional characterization of lymphocyte subsets is routinely carried out in a research laboratories, facilitated by the emergence of high-dimensional analysis technologies for low cell numbers. It will not be long before these approaches enter the diagnostic realm. This chapter outlines emerging trends in laboratory immunology testing with a focus on deep immune profiling or high-dimensional testing modalities.

CLINICS IN LABORATORY MEDICINE

SERIES OF RELATED INTEREST

Surgical Pathology Clinics
Available at: https://www.surgpath.theclinics.com/

THE CLINICS ARE NOW AVAILABLE ONLINE!
Access your subscription at:
www.theclinics.com

Preface

Update on Clinical Immunology Laboratory Testing

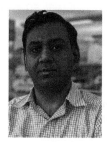

Vinay S. Mahajan, MD, PhD
Editor

The recent explosion in our knowledge of the molecular basis of immune regulatory mechanisms has paved the way for rapid developments in immunosuppression, immunotherapy, allergy, autoimmunity, and immunodeficiencies, all of which have impacted the practice of clinical laboratory immunology. The advent of immune checkpoint inhibitors and cell therapies in recent years has led to a surge of interest in clinical immunology. Advancements in lasers, microfluidics, and advanced electronics have resulted in the proliferation of robust and affordable flow cytometry or cell-sorting instruments that can withstand the demands of a clinical lab. Novel technological advances, enabled in part by the application of deep sequencing as well as high-dimensional analysis techniques to human immunology research, have arrived at the doorstep of clinical immunology diagnostics. Deep sequencing technologies are already widely used in the diagnosis of inherited immunodeficiencies. Indeed, the field of clinical laboratory immunology lies at a technological crossroads, which could take us into a new era of novel immune biomarkers derived from genetic or epigenetic signatures, immune repertoire analysis, as well as a greatly expanded range of functional immunology testing. Therefore, we have assembled a group of expert authors, from clinical as well as laboratory backgrounds, to review widely used immunology laboratory tests and practice contexts, in addition to providing an update on emerging trends in this field. I am extremely grateful to all the authors who have contributed to this issue, as well as the editorial team at Elsevier, led by Laura Fisher and Stacy Eastman. We

Clin Lab Med 39 (2019) xi–xii
https://doi.org/10.1016/j.cll.2019.09.001
0272-2712/19/© 2019 Published by Elsevier Inc.

labmed.theclinics.com

hope that this issue will be a useful resource for practitioners as well as trainees in clinical immunology.

Vinay S. Mahajan, MD, PhD
Ragon Institute of MGH, MIT and Harvard
400 Technology Square, Room 8-890
Cambridge, MA 02139, USA

E-mail address:
vinay.mahajan@mgh.harvard.edu

Antinuclear Antibody Tests

Morris Ling, MD[a,b,c,d],*, Mandakolathur Murali, MD[a,c,d]

KEYWORDS

- Antinuclear antibodies • ANA • SS-A • SS-B • RNP • Sm • Jo-1 • Scl70

KEY POINTS

- Assays for the detection and quantitation of antinuclear antibodies include the indirect immunofluorescence assay, enzyme-linked immunosorbent assay, and multiplex bead technology.
- Serum from patients with autoimmune diseases may contain antibodies to nuclear antigens, some of which are insoluble in saline (for example, double-stranded DNA, deoxyribonucleoprotein, and histones), whereas others are soluble or "extracted" in saline, so-called extractable nuclear antigens (ENAs) (eg, SS-A, SS-B, RNP, Sm, Jo-1, Scl70).
- Testing for autoantibodies to ENAs is often helpful to confirm the diagnosis of a specific connective tissue disease.
- The expanded identification of myositis-specific autoantibodies and a greater understanding of their clinical correlates has facilitated improvement in the diagnosis and management of patients with various forms of inflammatory myositis.

HISTORY

The use of assays for the diagnosis of systemic lupus erythematosus (SLE) originated after the initial description of lupus erythematosus cell (LE cell) in 1948 by Hargraves.[1] LE cells are leukocytes (usually neutrophils or macrophages) that have phagocytosed nuclear debris from dead or dying cells that have been opsonized by autoantibodies and complement. This finding provided the insight that the pathophysiology of SLE may be related to autoimmune and inflammatory responses involving nuclear proteins. LE cell detection, being somewhat cumbersome to prepare and standardize, and being less sensitive and specific than current assays, is not often used today. Nevertheless, its early utility helped set the stage for the subsequent application of more

Disclosure Statement: The authors have nothing to disclose.
[a] Division of Rheumatology, Allergy and Immunology, Department of Medicine, Massachusetts General Hospital, 55 Fruit Street, Cox 201, Boston, MA 02114, USA; [b] Center for Immunology and Inflammatory Diseases, Massachusetts General Hospital, 55 Fruit Street, Cox 201, Boston, MA 02114, USA; [c] Department of Pathology, Massachusetts General Hospital, 55 Fruit Street, Cox 201, Boston, MA 02114, USA; [d] Department of Medicine, Harvard Medical School, 55 Fruit Street, Cox 201, Boston, MA 02114, USA
* Corresponding author. Division of Rheumatology, Allergy and Immunology, Department of Medicine, Massachusetts General Hospital, 55 Fruit Street, Cox 201, Boston, MA 02114.
E-mail address: mling@mgh.harvard.edu

Clin Lab Med 39 (2019) 513–524
https://doi.org/10.1016/j.cll.2019.07.001
0272-2712/19/© 2019 Elsevier Inc. All rights reserved.

labmed.theclinics.com

modern techniques to optimized cell lines (eg, HEp-2 and HEp-2000) for the discovery of antinuclear antibodies (ANAs). Indirect immunofluorescence (IIF) to detect ANAs was first described in 1957.[2] Later on, it was determined that serum from patients with certain autoimmune diseases may contain antibodies to nuclear antigens that are soluble in normal saline. Some of the nuclear constituents such as double-stranded DNA (dsDNA), deoxyribonucleoprotein (DNP), and histones are insoluble in saline, whereas others, such as the DNA and RNA binding proteins and proteins of the spliceosome complex, are soluble or are "extracted" in saline and have thus been called extractable nuclear antigens (ENAs).

LABORATORY TESTING
Indirect Immunofluorescence Assay

The IIF assay is still considered the gold standard for ANA testing.[3] In this assay, a cell substrate, usually permeabilized HEp-2 or HEp-2000 cells, is incubated with patient serum. Autoantibodies within patient serum bind to a target antigen, which are in turn recognized by a fluorochrome-linked secondary antibody specific for the Fc portion of human immunoglobulin (Ig)G.[4] Target antigens may be located in the nuclear or cytosolic compartments. Nuclear antigens include DNA, RNA, and their binding proteins, as well as antigens in the spliceosome complex. Cytosolic proteins include Golgi, mitochondrial, and lysosomal proteins.

HEp-2 cells are often favored for their large, distinct nuclei, which facilitate enhanced visualization of nuclear patterns.[5] HEp-2000 cells are a specialized cell line transfected to overexpress the 60 kDa Ro/SS-A antigen, allowing for streamlined detection of anti-Ro autoantibodies.[6] ANA by IIF testing is reported as a titer, which is the highest dilution of patient serum at which fluorescence can still be detected.[7]

Although IIF is considered the gold standard for ANA testing, there are a few drawbacks. First, the technique is labor-intensive and requires a skilled reader. Second, interobserver variability may lead to slight differences in reported titers, but these should ordinarily only vary within one dilution among trained readers. The availability of standardized control samples with distinct patterns and the routine use of positive and negative controls helps minimize any discrepancy. Third, interassay variability may exist, which may complicate interpretation of titers across different institutions. Due to interobserver variability and interassay variability, a change in titer of one dilution may not represent a major change in the disease state of the patient. Although HEp-2000 cells with overexpressed 60 kDa Ro/SS-A antigen may promote the detection of anti-Ro/SS-A antibodies, these cells may still fail to detect anti-La/SS-B and anti-Jo1 antibodies.[8]

Enzyme-Linked Immunosorbent Assay

Enzyme-linked immunosorbent assay (ELISA) testing is performed by incubating patient serum in autoantigen-coated wells to detect the presence of autoantibodies. Autoantigens may either be purified from nuclear extracts or generated as recombinant proteins. After initial steps of incubation and washing, an enzyme-linked secondary antibody to the Fc portion of the autoantibody is added to allow for quantitation. The linked enzyme cleaves a substrate resulting in a color change that can be detected and quantitated using an optical reader.[4] The advantage of this approach is that it is less labor-intensive and time-intensive due to increased automation and higher throughput. Results may be comparable between IIF and ELISA.[9] However, there are a few drawbacks. The lack of antigen standardization may lead to greater variability in reported values. Furthermore, although a quantitative numerical value can be reported, information about the nuclear staining pattern (eg, homogeneous, speckled, nucleolar, or centromeric) is lost. Finally, as the focus of this ELISA is on ANA, it does not provide information about autoantibodies to cytoplasmic antigens or cytoplasmic staining patterns and separate assays may need to be performed. For these reasons, ELISA has still not supplanted IIF as the gold standard.

Multiplex Bead Technology

Multiplex bead technology (MULTIPLEX-ANA) expands the advantages of solid-phase ANA assays by using specific autoantigen-coated and distinctly identifiable microspheres in an indirect immunofluorescence-based assay, allowing for an automated readout of many analytes.[10] Analysis may occur using an immunoassay analyzer or flow cytometer. Although multiplex technology has its advantages, including automation and high throughput, it may have a lower sensitivity for ANA in some contexts.[11] In addition, the lack of certain standardized and purified antigenic determinants, such as RNA polymerase III and nucleolar antigens, can lead to false-negative results compared with IIF testing, and there can be difficulty quantitating autoantibodies relevant in autoimmune liver diseases and scleroderma.[12,13]

INTERPRETATION OF LABORATORY TESTING

Although the availability of various assays for the detection of autoantibodies in patient serum facilitates the effective diagnosis of autoimmune diseases, interpretation of these test results needs to be performed with detailed knowledge of the patient's clinical situation. A positive ANA can be seen in healthy adults; importantly, detection of ANA has a high sensitivity but a low specificity and is prone to low-titer positive results that may not be clinically relevant. For example, a low 1:40 ANA titer may be seen in as many as 25% to 45% of healthy blood donors, with perhaps 10% to 15% exhibiting a 1:80 titer, and up to 5% with a 1:160 titer.[14,15] Furthermore, the prevalence of these antibodies increases with aging. The sensitivity of ANA averages for SLE is 90% to 95%,[15] which makes repeat testing low-yield.

ANA titers may persist over time in 91% of patients and in some patients may precede the development of any clinical signs or symptoms of autoimmune disease.[16,17] On repeat testing, a previously negative result only changes to a positive one (greater than 1:160) approximately 1% of the time, so repeat testing without a clear clinical change is not usually warranted.[18] Dilutions of 1:160 and higher have been proposed as being helpful to differentiate potentially true-positive ANA results from incidentally positive ANA results seen in healthy patients, and may serve as a threshold for deciding whether to order additional tests.[19–21] ANA may be elevated in rheumatoid arthritis (RA) as well, but it is not specific in this disease and may not be useful in diagnosis unless there is another comorbid illness.[15] If there is an elevated anti-cyclic citrullinated peptide (anti-CCP) or rheumatoid factor in addition to the positive ANA, these patients are more likely to develop RA compared with another rheumatologic disease.[22] A positive ANA pattern can also be seen in organ-specific autoimmune disease, such as thyroid disorders, liver diseases, inflammatory bowel disease, and rarely with malignancy.

Another method for differentiating between healthy patients with a positive ANA and those with connective tissue disease is identification of the ANA pattern. With IIF, ANA can be reported with a titer and a pattern. Among ANA patterns, the speckled pattern is the most common in healthy individuals. Healthy adults with a positive ANA usually have patterns of nuclear fine speckled or nuclear dense-fine speckled.[23] Nuclear dense-fine speckled pattern was found in 33% of healthy patients with a positive ANA, but only 0.01% of patients with a positive ANA with rheumatic disease.[24,25]

Detection of this pattern has been minimized with standardized commercial ANA kits and diluents. Despite this, the speckled ANA pattern remains the most common pattern, but it is also the least specific. If there is a high ANA titer or strong clinical suspicion of Sjögren syndrome, mixed connective tissue disease (MCTD), or SLE, additional testing for ENA antibodies may be warranted (for example, anti-Ro/SS-A, anti-La/SS-B, anti-RNP, or anti-Sm antibodies, respectively).[26,27] It is important to note that Ro/SS-A autoantibody detection is most relevant in Sjögren syndrome, but this is minimally expressed in the HEp-2 cell line, hence the utilization of the HEp-2000 cell line at some institutions. If one has a high clinical suspicion for Sjögren syndrome, direct quantitation of anti-Ro/SS-A by ELISA may be needed even if the ANA is negative.

A homogeneous ANA pattern is more specific for autoimmune disease than a speckled pattern. This pattern may be associated with SLE or drug-induced lupus. If there is detection of any homogeneous pattern with a high index of clinical suspicion for SLE or drug-induced lupus, or if a homogenous ANA pattern is seen at a high titer, more specific tests, such as those for anti-dsDNA and anti-histone autoantibodies, should be ordered.[28]

Nucleolar patterns may be seen in scleroderma, whereas the anti-centromere pattern is associated with CREST syndrome.[29,30] Sometimes, multiple patterns can be seen within the same sample. **Table 1** illustrates the different ANA patterns that are typically seen in various systemic and organ-specific autoimmune diseases. Other conditions associated with a positive ANA include use of certain medications,[31] thyroiditis,[32] hepatitis,[33] infection,[34] and malignancies such as leukemia and lymphoma,[35] hepatocellular carcinoma,[36] and malignant melanoma.[37] Thus, even a high-titer ANA may not be specific for a rheumatologic condition if there is no clinical history consistent with a rheumatologic condition or if there is the presence of one of the aforementioned confounding conditions.[38] Without a high pre-test probability, a

Table 1
Systemic and organ-specific autoimmune diseases with positive ANA test results

Disease	%ANA+, %	Titer	Common Patterns
SLE – active	95%–98%	High	Homogeneous > Speckled > Rim
SLE – in remission	90	Moderate-high	Homogeneous > Speckled
MCTD	93	High	Speckled > Nucleolar
Systemic sclerosis or CREST	85	High	Speckled > Centromere > Nucleolar
Sjögren syndrome	48	Moderate-high	Speckled > Homogeneous
DM/PM	61	Low-moderate	Speckled > Nucleolar
RA	41	Low-moderate	Speckled
Drug-induced lupus	95	Low-moderate	Homogeneous > Speckled
Pauciarticular JIA	71	Low-moderate	Speckled
Graves disease	50	Low-moderate	Speckled
Hashimoto thyroiditis	46	Low-moderate	Speckled
Autoimmune hepatitis	63–91	Low-moderate	Speckled
Primary biliary cirrhosis	10–40	Low-moderate	Speckled

Abbreviations: DM/PM, dermatomyositis/polymyositis; JIA, juvenile idiopathic arthritis; MCTD, mixed connective tissue disease; RA, rheumatoid arthritis; SLE, systemic lupus erythematosus.

Adapted from Murali MR. Autoimmune disorders involving the connective tissue and immunodeficiency diseases. In: Laposata M, editor. Laposata's laboratory medicine: the diagnosis of disease in clinical laboratory. 3rd ed. New York: McGraw-Hill; 2018; with permission.

positive ANA test may lead to unnecessary additional testing, which may result in delayed "normal" assessments and confusion for clinicians and patients.

EXTRACTABLE NUCLEAR ANTIGENS

Antigens that are extracted from saline extracts of nuclei are known as ENAs. Characterization of ENAs and their respective antibodies led first to the description of anti-Sm and anti-RNP antibodies,[39,40] which may be relevant in lupus and MCTD. Antibodies found to be relevant in Sjögren syndrome, anti-Ro/SS-A and anti-La/SS-B antibodies, were later discovered.[41] Scl-70 is an antibody to topoisomerase-I that is important in scleroderma.[42] Jo-1 is an autoantibody found to be important in dermatomyositis (DM).[43] Testing for ENA autoantibodies may be considered if the ANA titer is >1:160 or if there are clinical features suggestive of one of the aforementioned autoimmune diseases.

SS-A/SS-B

Ro/SS-A is a 60 kDa RNA binding protein and La/SS-B is a 52 kDa RNA binding protein. Autoantibodies to SS-A and/or SS-B are more specific than ANA alone for Sjögren syndrome. Positive ANA may be seen in up to 70% of cases of Sjögren syndrome, but has also been shown to disappear at follow-up in many cases.[44] As mentioned earlier, the cell substrate used for IIF (eg, HEp-2 vs HEp-2000) may affect the sensitivity for detecting anti-SS-A antibodies, with a lower sensitivity of HEp-2 cells and a higher reported sensitivity using HEp2000.[6] In a study of 445 patients with Sjögren syndrome, 48% were found to have anti-SS-A antibodies, with 39% being present at diagnosis.[44] SS-A and SS-B are highly specific, as these are found in only 0.44% of healthy individuals.[45] However, ANA and antibodies to SS-A and SS-B may not be detected in up to 23% of patients; if this is the case and clinical suspicion remains high, other diagnostic tests may be helpful.[15,46] Immunologic testing may also correlate with different phenotypes of the disease. For example, in patients who are ANA positive but have negative SS-A and SS-B antibodies, there is a lower incidence of peripheral neuropathy.[46] Some may also have secondary Sjögren syndrome rather than primary disease. Patients with subacute cutaneous lupus erythematosus often have positive antibodies to SS-A with or without a positive ANA on IIF. It is to be noted that anti-SS-A IgG antibodies from a pregnant mother can be transferred transplacentally to the neonate.[47] Due to the predilection of this antibody for affecting the conduction tissue of the heart, the neonate may manifest features of heart block. Therefore, the recommendation is to screen for this antibody in pregnant women with SLE and Sjögren syndrome.

Smith (Sm)

Smith (Sm) autoantibodies recognize an RNase-sensitive, but trypsin-resistant ENA composed of U1, 2, 4, 5, and 6 spliceosomal small nuclear ribonucleoproteins (snRNPs) complexed to Sm core proteins (SmB, SmB', SmN, SmD1, SmD2, SmD3, SmE, SmF, and SmG). Anti-Sm is considered a specific biomarker of SLE, but it is not as sensitive as ANA for initial screening and is found less frequently than positive dsDNA in SLE; it is found only in approximately one-third of patients with SLE.[48,49] However, due to its high specificity (96%–98%), Sm remains useful if positive in that it helps confirm the diagnosis.[50,51] At diagnosis, there may be a male predominance in Sm positivity compared with female, as well as a higher positivity in younger patients (<50 years of age).[52,53]

Ribonucleoprotein (RNP)

RNP is an RNase- and trypsin-sensitive ENA composed of U1 spliceosomal RNA complexed to 3 polypeptides (ie, 70 kD, A, and C proteins). A high-titer RNP antibody is specific for MCTD and is required for diagnosis, though it is also seen in patients whose clinical features overlap with SLE, DM, polymyositis (PM), and/or systemic sclerosis. Criteria for diagnosis of MCTD includes positive serology, Raynaud phenomenon, swollen hands, myositis, synovitis, and in some cases, acrosclerosis.[54]

Scl70

Scl70 is an autoantibody that was discovered[42] before its antigen, topoisomerase 1, was known.[55] Scl70 is observed to be positive in 40% to 70% of patients with progressive systemic sclerosis. It can be quantitated using ELISA as well as multiplex assays, and may be associated with a speckled ANA pattern on IIF. Clinical features of systemic sclerosis include skin thickening, sclerodactyly, telangiectasias, pulmonary arterial hypertension and/or interstitial lung disease (ILD), and Raynaud phenomenon.[56] Other systemic sclerosis-related antibodies include anti-centromere (seen in CREST syndrome)[30] and anti-RNA polymerase III (seen in more severe or rapidly progressive disease, with a greater risk of diffuse cutaneous disease and scleroderma renal crisis).[57]

Jo-1

Jo-1 is an autoantibody that recognizes a cytoplasmic protein, histidyl-tRNA synthetase, an enzyme important for incorporating histidine into proteins.[58] Jo-1 is a marker of immune-mediated ILD and may be helpful in its early evaluation.[59,60] ANA may be negative in patients positive for Jo-1, although granular histidyl-tRNA synthetase-specific cytoplasmic staining and nonspecific nuclear staining may be observed on IIF.[61] Jo-1 was first described as being present in the sera of patients with myositis; however, a positive Jo-1 is only seen in approximately 20% to 30% of patients with DM/PM, although it is fairly specific for myositis when found.[62,63] If positive, anti-Jo-1 antibody levels may correlate with disease activity in idiopathic inflammatory myopathy.[63,64]

Myositis-Specific Autoantibodies

Recently, the expanded identification of myositis-specific autoantibodies (MSAs) and a greater understanding of their clinical correlates has facilitated improvement in the diagnosis and management of patients with various forms of inflammatory myositis.[65–68] In addition to Jo-1, detection of antibodies to other aminoacyl tRNA synthetases (ARS) including to EJ, Ha, KS, OJ, PL-7, PL-12, or Zo antigens may be seen in the anti-synthetase syndrome, which is characterized by myositis, Raynaud phenomenon, ILD, and arthritis.[69] Anti-signal recognition particle (SRP) may be associated with severe, often treatment-refractory necrotizing myopathy.[70] On the other hand, anti-Mi-2, often associated with classic DM features including heliotrope rash, Gottron papules, and the "shawl sign," may portend a more treatment-responsive course.[71] Autoantibodies to transcription intermediary factor 1γ/α (TIF1γ/α, p155/140) are associated with malignancy-associated DM.[72] Anti-melanoma differentiation-associated gene 5 (MDA5, CADM140) is associated with clinically amyopathic DM (CADM), which may be complicated by rapidly progressive ILD.[73] Other important MSAs include anti-MJ/nuclear matrix protein 2 (NXP-2), which also may be associated with malignancy-associated DM,[74] and anti-small ubiquitin-like modifier-1 activating enzyme (SAE).[75] **Fig. 1** highlights the potential utility of Hep-2 IIF patterns in determining which

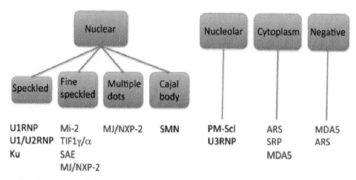

Fig. 1. Hep-2 patterns and MSAs or ENAs in PM/DM (*red*) and overlap syndrome (*black*).

MSAs may be present in patients with PM/DM or overlap syndromes, which may help guide decisions regarding confirmatory testing.

Double-Stranded DNA

If ANA is positive (especially if it is homogeneous), and there is high clinical suspicion for SLE, further testing for anti-dsDNA is warranted. dsDNA is composed of a double helix of DNA wrapped around an octameric histone core (pairs of H2A, H2B, H3, and H4 proteins). The gold standard for the detection of dsDNA is the detection of immunofluorescence in a certain protozoa, *Crithidia luciliae*, after incubation with human sera and a fluorescence-linked secondary antibody. Fortuitously, each of these flagellates possesses a giant mitochondrion containing coiled circular dsDNA with no other confounding antigens and no contamination with single-stranded DNA (ssDNA). Although some laboratories use ELISA and multiplex assays instead, immunofluorescence may have a leg up on these assays because the antigens used in ELISA and multiplex assays may be less stable and may contain ssDNA as contaminants. Immunofluorescence results are expressed as the highest dilution of sera at which signal is clearly detected. Anti-dsDNA is found in more than 70% of patients with SLE.[76,77] It is more commonly positive in childhood and early-onset SLE.[53] The specificity of the test, like the sensitivity, is dependent on the assay used and the population tested, and is quoted as being 90% to 98%.[77,78] Anti-dsDNA may be detected before clinical signs and symptoms of SLE.[79] Furthermore, anti-dsDNA may have utility in longitudinal follow-up as a marked increase in the anti-dsDNA may predict a severe flare of symptoms in the ensuing 6 months.[80] An assay for ssDNA may be more sensitive than dsDNA, and has been suggested as a tool for monitoring patients once a diagnosis of SLE has been established,[81] although there is incomplete validation and adoption of this approach.

SUMMARY

In summary, patients with clinical signs and symptoms suggestive of a connective tissue disease benefit from more definitive diagnosis aided by the detection and quantitation of ANA, with further confirmation achieved through the detection and quantitation of ENAs.

REFERENCES

1. Hargraves MM. Discovery of the LE cell and its morphology. Mayo Clin Proc 1969;44(9):579–99.

2. Holborow EJ, Weir DM, Johnson GD. A serum factor in lupus erythematosus with affinity for tissue nuclei. Br Med J 1957;2(5047):732–4.

3. Agmon-Levin N, Damoiseaux J, Kallenberg C, et al. International recommendations for the assessment of autoantibodies to cellular antigens referred to as anti-nuclear antibodies. Ann Rheum Dis 2014;73(1):17–23.

4. Mahler M, Meroni PL, Bossuyt X, et al. Current concepts and future directions for the assessment of autoantibodies to cellular antigens referred to as anti-nuclear antibodies. J Immunol Res 2014;2014:315179.

5. Vermeersch P, Bossuyt X. Prevalence and clinical significance of rare antinuclear antibody patterns. Autoimmun Rev 2013;12(10):998–1003.

6. Hoffman IE, Peene I, Veys EM, et al. Detection of specific antinuclear reactivities in patients with negative anti-nuclear antibody immunofluorescence screening tests. Clin Chem 2002;48(12):2171–6.

7. Volkmann ER, Taylor M, Ben-Artzi A. Using the antinuclear antibody test to diagnose rheumatic diseases: when does a positive test warrant further investigation? South Med J 2012;105(2):100–4.

8. Bossuyt X, Luyckx A. Antibodies to extractable nuclear antigens in antinuclear antibody-negative samples. Clin Chem 2005;51(12):2426–7.

9. Bizzaro N, Villalta D, Giavarina D, et al. Are anti-nucleosome antibodies a better diagnostic marker than anti-dsDNA antibodies for systemic lupus erythematosus? A systematic review and a study of metanalysis. Autoimmun Rev 2012; 12(2):97–106.

10. Sowa M, Hiemann R, Schierack P, et al. Next-generation autoantibody testing by combination of screening and confirmation-the CytoBead(R) technology. Clin Rev Allergy Immunol 2017;53(1):87–104.

11. Nifli AP, Notas G, Mamoulaki M, et al. Comparison of a multiplex, bead-based fluorescent assay and immunofluorescence methods for the detection of ANA and ANCA autoantibodies in human serum. J Immunol Methods 2006;311(1–2): 189–97.

12. Pisetsky DS. Antinuclear antibody testing - misunderstood or misbegotten? Nat Rev Rheumatol 2017;13(8):495–502.

13. Shanmugam VK, Swistowski DR, Saddic N, et al. Comparison of indirect immunofluorescence and multiplex antinuclear antibody screening in systemic sclerosis. Clin Rheumatol 2011;30(10):1363–8.

14. Dahle C, Skogh T, Aberg AK, et al. Methods of choice for diagnostic antinuclear antibody (ANA) screening: benefit of adding antigen-specific assays to immunofluorescence microscopy. J Autoimmun 2004;22(3):241–8.

15. Solomon DH, Kavanaugh AJ, Schur PH, American College of Rheumatology Ad Hoc Committee on Immunologic Testing Guidelines. Evidence-based guidelines for the use of immunologic tests: antinuclear antibody testing. Arthritis Rheum 2002;47(4):434–44.

16. Myckatyn SO, Russell AS. Outcome of positive antinuclear antibodies in individuals without connective tissue disease. J Rheumatol 2003;30(4):736–9.

17. Arbuckle MR, McClain MT, Rubertone MV, et al. Development of autoantibodies before the clinical onset of systemic lupus erythematosus. N Engl J Med 2003; 349(16):1526–33.

18. Man A, Shojania K, Phoon C, et al. An evaluation of autoimmune antibody testing patterns in a Canadian health region and an evaluation of a laboratory algorithm aimed at reducing unnecessary testing. Clin Rheumatol 2013;32(5):601–8.

19. Bonaguri C, Melegari A, Ballabio A, et al. Italian multicentre study for application of a diagnostic algorithm in autoantibody testing for autoimmune rheumatic disease: conclusive results. Autoimmun Rev 2011;11(1):1–5.

20. Tan EM, Feltkamp TE, Smolen JS, et al. Range of antinuclear antibodies in "healthy" individuals. Arthritis Rheum 1997;40(9):1601–11.

21. Selmi C, Ceribelli A, Generali E, et al. Serum antinuclear and extractable nuclear antigen antibody prevalence and associated morbidity and mortality in the general population over 15 years. Autoimmun Rev 2016;15(2):162–6.

22. Lee AN, Beck CE, Hall M. Rheumatoid factor and anti-CCP autoantibodies in rheumatoid arthritis: a review. Clin Lab Sci 2008;21(1):15–8.

23. Mariz HA, Sato EI, Barbosa SH, et al. Pattern on the antinuclear antibody-HEp-2 test is a critical parameter for discriminating antinuclear antibody-positive healthy individuals and patients with autoimmune rheumatic diseases. Arthritis Rheum 2011;63(1):191–200.

24. Mahler M, Fritzler MJ. The clinical significance of the dense fine speckled immunofluorescence pattern on HEp-2 cells for the diagnosis of systemic autoimmune diseases. Clin Dev Immunol 2012;2012:494356.

25. Mahler M, Hanly JG, Fritzler MJ. Importance of the dense fine speckled pattern on HEp-2 cells and anti-DFS70 antibodies for the diagnosis of systemic autoimmune diseases. Autoimmun Rev 2012;11(9):642–5.

26. Damoiseaux JG, Tervaert JW. From ANA to ENA: how to proceed? Autoimmun Rev 2006;5(1):10–7.

27. Craig WY, Ledue TB. The relationship between antinuclear antibody data and antibodies against extractable nuclear antigens in a large laboratory cohort. Clin Chem Lab Med 2011;50(3):497–502.

28. Craig WY, Ledue TB. The antinuclear antibody assay: developing criteria for reflexive anti-dsDNA antibody testing in a laboratory setting. Clin Chem Lab Med 2011;49(7):1205–11.

29. Bernstein RM, Steigerwald JC, Tan EM. Association of antinuclear and antinucleolar antibodies in progressive systemic sclerosis. Clin Exp Immunol 1982; 48(1):43–51.

30. Tan EM, Rodnan GP, Garcia I, et al. Diversity of antinuclear antibodies in progressive systemic sclerosis. Anti-centromere antibody and its relationship to CREST syndrome. Arthritis Rheum 1980;23(6):617–25.

31. He Y, Sawalha AH. Drug-induced lupus erythematosus: an update on drugs and mechanisms. Curr Opin Rheumatol 2018;30(5):490–7.

32. Nisihara R, Pigosso YG, Prado N, et al. Rheumatic disease autoantibodies in patients with autoimmune thyroid diseases. Med Princ Pract 2018;27(4):332–6.

33. Muratori L, Deleonardi G, Lalanne C, et al. Autoantibodies in autoimmune hepatitis. Dig Dis 2015;33(Suppl 2):65–9.

34. Berlin T, Zandman-Goddard G, Blank M, et al. Autoantibodies in nonautoimmune individuals during infections. Ann N Y Acad Sci 2007;1108:584–93.

35. Timuragaoglu A, Duman A, Ongut G, et al. The significance of autoantibodies in non-Hodgkin's lymphoma. Leuk Lymphoma 2000;40(1–2):119–22.

36. Covini G, von Muhlen CA, Pacchetti S, et al. Diversity of antinuclear antibody responses in hepatocellular carcinoma. J Hepatol 1997;26(6):1255–65.

37. Thomas PJ, Kaur JS, Aitcheson CT, et al. Antinuclear, antinucleolar, and anticytoplasmic antibodies in patients with malignant melanoma. Cancer Res 1983;43(3): 1372–80.

38. Abeles AM, Abeles M. The clinical utility of a positive antinuclear antibody test result. Am J Med 2013;126(4):342–8.

39. Tan EM, Kunkel HG. Characteristics of a soluble nuclear antigen precipitating with sera of patients with systemic lupus erythematosus. J Immunol 1966;96(3): 464–71.

40. Mattioli M, Reichlin M. Characterization of a soluble nuclear ribonucleoprotein antigen reactive with SLE sera. J Immunol 1971;107(5):1281–90.

41. Alspaugh MA, Tan EM. Antibodies to cellular antigens in Sjogren's syndrome. J Clin Invest 1975;55(5):1067–73.

42. Douvas AS, Achten M, Tan EM. Identification of a nuclear protein (Scl-70) as a unique target of human antinuclear antibodies in scleroderma. J Biol Chem 1979;254(20):10514–22.

43. Nishikai M, Reichlin M. Heterogeneity of precipitating antibodies in polymyositis and dermatomyositis. Characterization of the Jo-1 antibody system. Arthritis Rheum 1980;23(8):881–8.

44. Fauchais AL, Martel C, Gondran G, et al. Immunological profile in primary Sjogren syndrome: clinical significance, prognosis and long-term evolution to other autoimmune disease. Autoimmun Rev 2010;9(9):595–9.

45. Fritzler MJ, Pauls JD, Kinsella TD, et al. Antinuclear, anticytoplasmic, and anti-Sjogren's syndrome antigen A (SS-A/Ro) antibodies in female blood donors. Clin Immunol Immunopathol 1985;36(1):120–8.

46. Garcia-Carrasco M, Ramos-Casals M, Rosas J, et al. Primary Sjogren syndrome: clinical and immunologic disease patterns in a cohort of 400 patients. Medicine (Baltimore) 2002;81(4):270–80.

47. Zuppa AA, Riccardi R, Frezza S, et al. Neonatal lupus: follow-up in infants with anti-SSA/Ro antibodies and review of the literature. Autoimmun Rev 2017;16(4): 427–32.

48. Migliorini P, Baldini C, Rocchi V, et al. Anti-Sm and anti-RNP antibodies. Autoimmunity 2005;38(1):47–54.

49. Jearn LH, Kim TY. Anti-Sm faces a threat to its reigning position as the marker antibody. Rheumatol Int 2011;31(8):1119–20.

50. Benito-Garcia E, Schur PH, Lahita R, American College of Rheumatology Ad Hoc Committee on Immunologic Testing Guidelines. Guidelines for immunologic laboratory testing in the rheumatic diseases: anti-Sm and anti-RNP antibody tests. Arthritis Rheum 2004;51(6):1030–44.

51. Mahler M. Sm peptides in differentiation of autoimmune diseases. Adv Clin Chem 2011;54:109–28.

52. Ding Y, He J, Guo JP, et al. Gender differences are associated with the clinical features of systemic lupus erythematosus. Chin Med J (Engl) 2012;125(14): 2477–81.

53. Webb R, Kelly JA, Somers EC, et al. Early disease onset is predicted by a higher genetic risk for lupus and is associated with a more severe phenotype in lupus patients. Ann Rheum Dis 2011;70(1):151–6.

54. Amigues JM, Cantagrel A, Abbal M, et al. Comparative study of 4 diagnosis criteria sets for mixed connective tissue disease in patients with anti-RNP antibodies. Autoimmunity Group of the Hospitals of Toulouse. J Rheumatol 1996; 23(12):2055–62.

55. Maul GG, French BT, van Venrooij WJ, et al. Topoisomerase I identified by scleroderma 70 antisera: enrichment of topoisomerase I at the centromere in mouse mitotic cells before anaphase. Proc Natl Acad Sci U S A 1986;83(14):5145–9.

56. van den Hoogen F, Khanna D, Fransen J, et al. 2013 classification criteria for systemic sclerosis: an American College of Rheumatology/European League

Against Rheumatism collaborative initiative. Ann Rheum Dis 2013;72(11): 1747–55.

57. Harvey GR, Butts S, Rands AL, et al. Clinical and serological associations with anti-RNA polymerase antibodies in systemic sclerosis. Clin Exp Immunol 1999; 117(2):395–402.

58. Mathews MB, Bernstein RM. Myositis autoantibody inhibits histidyl-tRNA synthetase: a model for autoimmunity. Nature 1983;304(5922):177–9.

59. Yoshida S, Akizuki M, Mimori T, et al. The precipitating antibody to an acidic nuclear protein antigen, the Jo-1, in connective tissue diseases. A marker for a subset of polymyositis with interstitial pulmonary fibrosis. Arthritis Rheum 1983;26(5): 604–11.

60. Douglas WW, Tazelaar HD, Hartman TE, et al. Polymyositis-dermatomyositis-associated interstitial lung disease. Am J Respir Crit Care Med 2001;164(7): 1182–5.

61. Shi MH, Tsui FW, Rubin LA. Cellular localization of the target structures recognized by the anti-Jo-1 antibody: immunofluorescence studies on cultured human myoblasts. J Rheumatol 1991;18(2):252–8.

62. Vazquez-Abad D, Rothfield NF. Sensitivity and specificity of anti-Jo-1 antibodies in autoimmune diseases with myositis. Arthritis Rheum 1996;39(2):292–6.

63. Zampieri S, Ghirardello A, Iaccarino L, et al. Anti-Jo-1 antibodies. Autoimmunity 2005;38(1):73–8.

64. Stone KB, Oddis CV, Fertig N, et al. Anti-Jo-1 antibody levels correlate with disease activity in idiopathic inflammatory myopathy. Arthritis Rheum 2007;56(9): 3125–31.

65. Targoff IN. Autoantibodies and their significance in myositis. Curr Rheumatol Rep 2008;10(4):333–40.

66. Mammen AL. Dermatomyositis and polymyositis: clinical presentation, autoantibodies, and pathogenesis. Ann N Y Acad Sci 2010;1184:134–53.

67. Lazarou IN, Guerne PA. Classification, diagnosis, and management of idiopathic inflammatory myopathies. J Rheumatol 2013;40(5):550–64.

68. Satoh M, Tanaka S, Ceribelli A, et al. A comprehensive overview on myositis-specific antibodies: new and old biomarkers in idiopathic inflammatory myopathy. Clin Rev Allergy Immunol 2017;52(1):1–19.

69. Mahler M, Miller FW, Fritzler MJ. Idiopathic inflammatory myopathies and the anti-synthetase syndrome: a comprehensive review. Autoimmun Rev 2014;13(4–5): 367–71.

70. Picard C, Vincent T, Lega JC, et al. Heterogeneous clinical spectrum of anti-SRP myositis and importance of the methods of detection of anti-SRP autoantibodies: a multicentric study. Immunol Res 2016;64(3):677–86.

71. Muro Y, Sugiura K, Akiyama M. Cutaneous manifestations in dermatomyositis: key clinical and serological features-a comprehensive review. Clin Rev Allergy Immunol 2016;51(3):293–302.

72. Fiorentino D, Casciola-Rosen L. Autoantibodies to transcription intermediary factor 1 in dermatomyositis shed insight into the cancer-myositis connection. Arthritis Rheum 2012;64(2):346–9.

73. Gono T, Kawaguchi Y, Satoh T, et al. Clinical manifestation and prognostic factor in anti-melanoma differentiation-associated gene 5 antibody-associated interstitial lung disease as a complication of dermatomyositis. Rheumatology (Oxford) 2010;49(9):1713–9.

74. Fiorentino DF, Chung LS, Christopher-Stine L, et al. Most patients with cancer-associated dermatomyositis have antibodies to nuclear matrix protein NXP-2 or transcription intermediary factor 1gamma. Arthritis Rheum 2013;65(11):2954–62.
75. Betteridge Z, Gunawardena H, North J, et al. Identification of a novel autoantibody directed against small ubiquitin-like modifier activating enzyme in dermatomyositis. Arthritis Rheum 2007;56(9):3132–7.
76. Swaak T, Smeenk R. Detection of anti-dsDNA as a diagnostic tool: a prospective study in 441 non-systemic lupus erythematosus patients with anti-dsDNA antibody (anti-dsDNA). Ann Rheum Dis 1985;44(4):245–51.
77. Ghirardello A, Villalta D, Morozzi G, et al. Diagnostic accuracy of currently available anti-double-stranded DNA antibody assays. An Italian multicentre study. Clin Exp Rheumatol 2011;29(1):50–6.
78. Kavanaugh AF, Solomon DH, American College of Rheumatology Ad Hoc Committee on Immunologic Testing Guidelines. Guidelines for immunologic laboratory testing in the rheumatic diseases: anti-DNA antibody tests. Arthritis Rheum 2002; 47(5):546–55.
79. Arbuckle MR, James JA, Kohlhase KF, et al. Development of anti-dsDNA autoantibodies prior to clinical diagnosis of systemic lupus erythematosus. Scand J Immunol 2001;54(1–2):211–9.
80. Pan N, Amigues I, Lyman S, et al. A surge in anti-dsDNA titer predicts a severe lupus flare within six months. Lupus 2014;23(3):293–8.
81. Egner W. The use of laboratory tests in the diagnosis of SLE. J Clin Pathol 2000; 53(6):424–32.

Serologic Diagnosis of Rheumatoid Arthritis

Hugues Allard-Chamard, MD, PhD, FRCPC[a,b,c,d,*], Gilles Boire, MD, MSc, FRCPC[b,c,d]

KEYWORDS

- Rheumatoid arthritis • Rheumatoid factor • Anti–cyclic citrullinated peptide
- Biomarkers • Serology

KEY POINTS

- A stage of clinically silent immune dysfunction frequently precedes rheumatoid arthritis (RA) and offers a unique window into disease pathogenesis as well as opportunities for prevention and treatment.
- Despite good sensitivity and specificity, a positive rheumatoid factor (RF) should be interpreted in the clinical context, because many infectious and autoimmune diseases can present with arthritis and a positive RF.
- RF and anti–cyclic citrullinated peptide assays should be calibrated using reference sera to ensure harmonization across laboratories.
- Approximately 30% of patients with RA remain seronegative using current immunoassays, and evidence suggest that many may have a genetically and pathologically distinct disease.

INTRODUCTION

Rheumatoid arthritis (RA) is a chronic inflammatory disorder affecting the synovial lining of joints, tendon sheaths, and bursae. With a prevalence close to 1%, RA is the most widespread immune-mediated inflammatory arthropathy around the world.[1] The incidence of RA is highest in middle-aged women. Joint damage is characterized

The authors contributed equally to this work.

Disclosure Statement: Dr Hugues Allard-Chamard funding: Fellowship grant from the Faculté de médecine et des sciences de la santé de Sherbrooke; Dr Gilles Boire funding: Canadian Institutes for Health Research, Canadian Initiative for Outcomes in Rheumatology Care, and Centre de Recherche Clinique du Centre Hospitalier Universitaire de Sherbrooke.

[a] Ragon Institute of MGH, MIT and Harvard, Cambridge, MA, USA; [b] Division of Rheumatology, Faculty of Medicine and Health Sciences, Université de Sherbrooke, Sherbrooke, Québec, Canada; [c] Centre de Recherche Clinique du Centre Hospitalier Universitaire de Sherbrooke, Sherbrooke, Québec, Canada; [d] Division of Rheumatology, Centre intégré universitaire de santé et de service sociaux de l'Estrie – Centre hospitalier universitaire de Sherbrooke (CIUSSS de l'Estrie-CHUS), 3001, 12th Avenue North, Room 3853, Sherbrooke, Québec J1H 5N4, Canada
* Corresponding author. Division of Rheumatology, Centre intégré universitaire de santé et de service sociaux de l'Estrie – Centre hospitalier universitaire de Sherbrooke (CIUSSS de l'Estrie-CHUS), 3001, 12th Avenue North, Room 3857, Sherbrooke, Québec J1H 5N4, Canada.
E-mail address: hugues.allard-chamard@USherbrooke.ca

by bony erosions, thinning of articular cartilage, weakening of periarticular structures, joint deformities, and periarticular osteopenia, all contributing to increasing disability and loss of function. Before the advent of modern medicine, RA was severely disabling. Structural damage may be observed within the first few months after disease onset.[2] Early treatment of RA with the implementation of treat-to-target strategies, a judicious use of disease-modifying antirheumatic drugs (DMARDs) and the emergence of biologic drugs, starting in 1998 with the approval of etanercept by the US Food and Drug Administration, has profoundly modified the patient outcomes.

Although a plethora of autoantibodies and proteins are associated with RA and its various manifestations, only immunoglobulin (Ig) M rheumatoid factor (RF) and anti–citrullinated protein antibodies (ACPA), with a large predominance of IgG anti–cyclic citrullinated peptides (anti-CCPs), are widely used in clinical practice across the world.[3] Both antibodies are relatively sensitive and specific for the diagnosis of RA, and both predict a more severe course compared with seronegative RA[4]; however, this distinction according to seropositivity seems to be shrinking in the current treat-to-target era.[5] Although RF and ACPA are frequently found together in patient sera, they identify several single-positive patients in whom they represent an independent predictor of poorer outcomes.[6–8] It is important to keep in mind that a significant subset of patients with clinically defined RA are currently seronegative.[5] Moreover, both RF and anti-CCP antibodies can be present in non-RA rheumatic and nonrheumatic diseases, highlighting the need for novel RA biomarkers that are not correlated with these two antibodies.[9]

Rheumatoid Factor

RFs comprise autoreactive immunoglobulins that are directed toward the Fc portion of IgG. IgM RF is the clinically detected isotype and constitutes the major RF species in patients with RA. Although IgG and IgA RF are also produced, their role in disorder is less clear.[10] RF prevalence increases with age, being present in up to 10% of the elderly population.[11–13] RF production is also frequent in nonspecific chronic activation of the immune system; for example, in autoimmune diseases such as cryoglobulinemia and primary Sjögren syndrome, in which it is associated with an increased risk of lymphomatous transformation, and in subacute bacterial endocarditis and chronic infectious hepatitis, particularly hepatitis C.[9] The pathologic high-affinity IgG RF antibodies seen in RA are produced by B cells in the synovial membranes of RA-affected joints that show a high degree of somatic mutation, indicating cluster of differentiation (CD) 4+ T-cell help through CD40L, germinal center reaction, and affinity maturation.[14] Natural IgM antibodies with RF activity are commonly observed in various infectious and inflammatory conditions but, in contrast, they typically lack somatic hypermutation in their complementarity-determining regions.

Anti–citrullinated Protein Antibodies

ACPA autoantibodies in RA serum target several proteins that bear citrulline-containing epitopes, resulting from the deamination of arginine (**Fig. 1**). The first protein autoantigen other than IgG recognized by an RA-specific autoantibody was identified in 1964, as an antiperinuclear factor by indirect immunofluorescence on buccal epithelial cells.[15] In the following years, several additional autoantibodies were identified, such as antikeratin antibody (by indirect immunofluorescence on fixed sections of rat esophagus),[16] antivimentin (anti-Sa; by immunoblotting of soluble human spleen extracts),[17] and antifilaggrin.[18] It was later realized that these target specificities were critically dependent on a posttranslational modification, arginine deamination or citrullination.[19] In recent years, RA-specific autoantibodies have

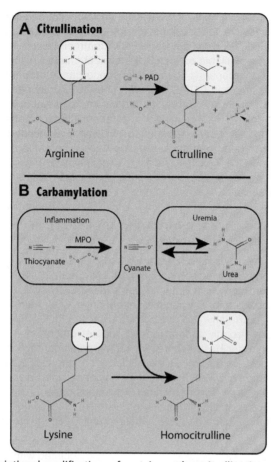

Fig. 1. Posttranscriptional modifications of proteins, such as citrullination and carbamylation, increase their immunogenicity and make them targets of autoantibodies in rheumatoid arthritis. (*A*) Citrullination, or arginine deamination, results from the catalytic removal by peptidylarginine deiminase (PAD) of a terminal amine group (leading to the formation of a ketone group) from the R chain of arginine, converting it to citrulline. (*B*) Carbamylation consists of the nonenzymatic binding of cyanate to an amine group. Carbamylation may occur at the amino terminus of any peptide, as well as at the side chains of lysine (yielding homocitrulline; shown) and arginine. In inflamed tissue, cyanate can arise from the catalytic activity of myeloperoxidase (MPO) on thiocyanate; cyanate (and ammonium ion) may also result from the spontaneous reversible dissociation of urea in water.

been found to target several citrullinated antigens, such as citrullinated mutated vimentin,[20] citrullinated fibrinogen,[21] alpha-enolase,[22] and many others.[23,24]

When it became apparent that citrulline was essential for recognition by ACPA, a synthetic library of CCP antigens was developed for designing enzyme-linked immunosorbent assay (ELISA) assays with optimal diagnostic sensitivity and specificity for RA.[25] The antibodies detected by these assays are called anti-CCP. The reactivity to particular CCP epitopes is shared to varying degrees among ACPA-positive persons.[26] The cyclic conformation of the antigenic peptides used in the assay reduces conformational flexibility and enhances the recognition of the citrullinated epitopes.[25] Pools of CCPs used in anti-CCP ELISAs have evolved over the years, resulting in improvements in sensitivity and specificity. Successive generations of anti-CCP assays are designated anti-CCP, anti-CCP2, and anti-CCP3. Anti-CCP2 and anti-CCP3 were developed and commercialized independently using public information available on anti-CCP, and both have similar sensitivities and specificities. Assay comparisons have shown concordance rates greater than 95% between anti-CCP2 and anti-CCP3; however, anti-CCP3 may perform slightly better in RF-negative patients.[27] Efforts to further improve anti-CCP assay performance are still ongoing.[28,29] For instance, a recent study explored the potential benefits of detecting individual responses to 16 distinct citrullinated peptides using an addressable laser bead immunoassay approach. The assay performed better than a standard anti-CCP2 ELISA, yielding a sensitivity of 57% and a specificity of 96%, allowing the reclassification of 10% of the anti-CCP2–negative patients with RA as seropositive.[30]

OTHER CLINICALLY SIGNIFICANT RHEUMATOID ARTHRITIS BIOMARKERS
Anti-Sa (Citrullinated Vimentin) Antibodies

Anti-Sa antibodies were identified and their target shown to be vimentin by mass spectrometry,[17] long before recognition of the citrulline specificity of ACPA. Targeting of citrullinated rather than native vimentin was subsequently confirmed.[31] The specificity of anti-Sa antibodies for RA parallels that of anti-CCP2. Although less sensitive than anti-CCP2 for both early and established disease (20%–30% vs 50%–70%),[32] anti-Sa seems more strongly associated with poorer outcomes (refractory disease and higher Sharp/van der Heijde scores for radiographic damage in particular) than anti-CCP2.[33] The behavior of anti-Sa also differs from anti-CCP2 both before onset of RA and after initiation of DMARD therapy. For instance, anti-Sa antibodies were absent in healthy relatives of North American indigenous patients with RA, in contrast with 15% anti-CCP2 positivity.[34] Following treatment with DMARDs, anti-Sa titers decreased and often became negative, whereas anti-CCP2 levels usually remained stable.[35]

Anti–carbamylated Proteins Antibodies

Anti–carbamylated protein (CarP) antibodies target proteins and peptides containing homocitrulline residue rather than citrulline. Homocitrulline formation involves nonenzymatic chemical carbamylation by cyanate of the primary amine group of lysine (see **Fig. 1**).[36] Dietary or smoking-derived cyanides are detoxified to thiocyanate, which in turn can be oxidized to cyanate under the action of myeloperoxidase at inflammatory sites,[37,38] where citrullination also occurs under the action of peptidylarginine deiminase.[39] Cyanate is also produced as a result of the spontaneous reversible dissociation of urea.[40,41] Antibodies to homocitrullinated peptides and to citrullinated peptides may be cross reactive, or may discriminate between peptides identical otherwise.[42] Anti-CarP antibodies are present in 40% to 55% of patients with established RA and in 38% to 73% of patients with early disease.[43] Anti-CarP antibodies are correlated with anti-CCP antibodies, being found in less than 10% of seronegative patients.[43] Our study found a strong correlation of anti-CarP with anti-Sa and with more extensive radiographic damage.[43] The role of anti-CarP beyond or in addition to anti-CCP for RA diagnosis and prognosis remains undetermined.

Anti–immunoglobulin Binding Protein

The human stress protein immunoglobulin binding protein (BiP) was found to stimulate synovial T-cell proliferation and levels are increased in RA. Anti-BiP antibodies were reported in patients with RA, in whom they have moderate (67%) sensitivity and good specificity (90%).[44,45] However, a significant proportion of the antibodies seem to target citrullinated BiP.[46] Therefore, the independent contribution of anti-BiP antibodies to RA diagnosis remains unclear.

Anti-RA33

Antibodies to RA33 are uncommon and moderately specific RA-associated antibodies. RA33, also called heterogeneous nuclear ribonucleoprotein A2/B1, associates with nascent pre–messenger RNAs and various other single-stranded RNA and DNA. Antibodies to both native and citrullinated RA33 are present in distinct subsets of patients with RA,[47] antibodies to native RA33 being present only in early RA, and antibodies to citrullinated RA33 being markers of longer disease duration and poorer prognosis.[48]

Antibodies to Type II Collagen

Anti–type II collagen antibodies are rare (<10%) in patients with RA but may represent patients with high disease activity at disease onset but not over time. They are not helpful for diagnosis, and their prognostic significance remains controversial.[49,50]

14-3-3η

The functions of 14-3-3η are not well known. It is a member of a family of proteins regulating intracellular processes and signaling. The serum levels of 14-3-3η are associated with increased risk of developing RA in healthy individuals with arthralgia and positive for RF or ACPA.[51] In early RA, the baseline levels of 14-3-3η were higher in patients later developing erosive arthritis and did not correlate with CRP.[52,53]

PATHOGENICITY OF RHEUMATOID ARTHRITIS ANTIBODIES

RF-containing immune complexes are thought to contribute to vasculitic manifestations in RA, such as the rheumatoid nodules[54] and rheumatoid vasculitis.[55,56] However, there is little evidence that RF, on its own, is involved in triggering the initial events in RA and thus may be secondary to the chronic inflammation. However, RF synergizes with ACPA by promoting the formation of ACPA-containing immune complexes.[57] The combined effect of RF and ACPA is in keeping with the clinical observation that double-positive patients present more severe arthritis.[4] ACPA have been observed in early RA, and there is growing evidence to suggest that they may be more tightly linked to the pathogenesis of RA.[24]

MEASUREMENT OF RHEUMATOID ARTHRITIS–ASSOCIATED ANTIBODIES
Antigens Used in Conventional Commercially Available Tests

Most RF assays use gamma globulins or the isolated Fc fraction from rabbit, human, or cattle sera.[9,58] Rabbits only have 1 IgG isotype (Cγ gene),[59] cattle have 2 (IgG1, IgG2),[60] and humans 4 (IgG1, IgG2, IgG3, and IgG4). Some studies suggest that using single-isotype rabbit IgG increases the specificity of RF detection but leads to significantly lower sensitivity.[61] The antibody titers reported in these assays are the reciprocal of the last serial serum dilution that yields a positive signal. The antigen used for detecting anti-CCP is a proprietary pool of CCPs that have been optimized for their sensitivity and specificity in large cohorts. Although RF is detected by using either particle aggregation or ELISA approaches, the detection of anti-CCP relies solely on ELISA assays.

Agglutination and Nephelometry

Historically, RF was detected using the agglutination of rabbit IgG–coated sheep erythrocytes.[62,63] Nonetheless, the agglutination methods were hard to standardize and have now been largely phased out. They have been replaced by more sensitive nephelometric techniques that are highly reproducible, easily automated, and cheap. Fixed amounts of immunoglobulins in the form of heat-aggregated,[64] chemically cross-linked IgG,[65] or IgG immobilized on latex beads,[66] are used to trigger the formation of light-scattering immune complexes at a controlled temperature. The degree of light scattering is highly correlated with RF concentration. This technique is particularly vulnerable to the prozone effect, also called the hook effect, in which the presence of extremely high concentrations of the analyte leads to a decrease in signal as the antibodies saturate and are not able to form a network anymore.[67]

Enzyme-Linked Immunosorbent Assay

Indirect ELISAs are widely used bioassays because of their precision and are available in a variety of automated formats. For RF determination by ELISA, whole IgGs or their Fc portion are adsorbed to the bottom of microwells and sequential dilutions of a patient serum are added. The immunoglobulins that reacted to the solid phase immobilized antigen are revealed using an antihuman immunoglobulin coupled to a quantifiable detection modality. The antihuman immunoglobulin used can be specific for IgM, IgG, or IgA, hence allowing the quantification of IgM RF, IgG RF, or IgA RF. Anti-CCP antibodies are also determined by indirect ELISA using proprietary mixtures of citrullinated peptide antigens. ELISAs are not suitable for determining antibody titers; these results are expressed as international units (IU) per milliliter, based on normalized sera.[68,69]

FACTORS THAT INTERFERE WITH SEROLOGIC TESTING

Aggregation assays are prone to a variety of interferences. For instance, C1q is an acute phase reactant triggered by systemic inflammation, which can cross-link and precipitate IgG on its own.[70] High levels of C1q could thus result in false-positive RF results. However, C1q is heat labile and denatured by heating at 56°C for 15 to 30 minutes.[71] Similarly, depending on the residual concentration of clotting factors remaining in an incompletely clotted serum, both fibrin and fibrinogen can interfere with the ability of RF to cross-link Fc, or they may simply continue to coagulate and entrap analytes, leading to false-positives.[72]

Temperature is a well-known determinant of the kinetics of immune complex formation. Furthermore, cryoglobulins can present with a strong RF activity, but they may precipitate if the serum is prepared or stored at colder temperatures, leading to falsely negative or low RF titers.[73] In some nephelometric assays, the reaction buffer is enriched in polyethylene glycol or other macromolecular crowding agents that promote protein interaction. This interaction may cause false-positive results by favoring the aggregation of fibrin, cryoglobulins, or other immune complexes.[74] Moreover, chylomicrons and lipoproteins have the capacity to induce light scattering on their own and can give false-positive results when their levels are increased or when their solubility is decreased, as after a freeze-thaw cycle.[75] Clinicians should thus avoid using nephelometry when the serum is lipemic, and, in mild cases, subtract the light-scattering capacity of a sample prepared without the addition of the IgG-based cross-linking agent.

High levels of histidine-rich glycoprotein (HRG), an abundant plasma protein, can interfere with RF testing and result in false-negatives. HRG levels inversely correlate with the capacity to detect RF activity by standard nephelometric assays.[76] HRG interferes with RF detection in 3 ways: (1) it inhibits the generation of IgG-containing immune complexes by RF, (2) it inhibits the insolubilization by RF of IgG-containing immune complexes, and (3) it can solubilize already formed immune complexes.[77] A correction factor for RF titers, based on the concentration of serum HRG, has been proposed.[76]

Naturally occurring polyreactive antibodies can also interfere with RF detection. They are sometimes called heterophilic antibodies because of their ability to bind immunoglobulins of nonself-species. Although a small percentage of these antibodies target the Fc portion of IgG and are therefore bona fide RF, most of the polyreactive antibodies are of poorly defined specificity and react with the variable Ig domain, leading to false-positive RF activity in immunoassays using intact IgG rather than its purified Fc fragment as an antigen. In principle, such an interference can be neutralized by the addition of rabbit F(ab) fragments.[78]

HARMONIZATION AND CALIBRATION OF RHEUMATOID ARTHRITIS–ASSOCIATED ANTIBODIES

Accuracy and reproducibility of laboratory testing are essential to ensure consistency in clinical diagnosis. Both the World Health Organization (WHO) and the Centers for Disease Control and Prevention (CDC) provide standardized sera for RF assay calibration. The reference sera provided are devoid of IgG RF or IgA RF, and only contain a purely IgM RF activity.[79]

Based on their recommendations, and like any serologic diagnostic tests, all ELISA and nephelometric RF assays should be performed with both positive and negative controls. Preferably 2 positive controls should be included, 1 with a strong positive signal and 1 slightly greater than the cutoff for positivity. The high positive control is used to monitor for the prozone effect (false-negative or inaccurately low results resulting from very high concentrations of antibodies) and the low positive control helps ensure consistency in the measurement of weakly positive samples, which represent the most vulnerable part of the assay.[80,81] Based on standards provided by the WHO, 1 IU of RF is the activity contained in 0.171 mg of the reference lyophilisate (half-life estimate to be longer than 2000 years). Storage of the reconstituted standard serum at $-10°C$ leads to a loss of half of its activity after about 8 years (95% confidence interval, 1–250).[79]

Given the widespread clinical adoption of anti-CCP testing and the concurrent use of different versions of the assays (anti-CCP, anti-CCP2, and anti-CCP3) that have different cutoffs and sensitivities, there is a critical need for assay harmonization. This endeavor is led by 3 institutions: (1) the CDC, (2) The International Union of Immunological Societies (IUIS), and (3) The European AutoCure consortium.[26,82,83] The CDC provides reference serum for calibrating solid-phase anti-CCP assays. This calibration standard was developed using the plasma from a single donor positive for anti-CCP. This international standard is set to contain 100 IU/mL (catalog IS2723). The IUIS Autoantibody Standardization Committee proposed the first reference serum for anti-CCP testing in 2006. The serum of an index patient with RA was diluted with normal serum to create lyophilized reference standards with various levels of reactivities. Using these standards, they tested 12 commercially available ELISAs using the serum of 20 patients with RA. This method allowed a reduction in the mean coefficient of variation from 76.4% to 27.9% for low positive sera, and from 85.9% to 33.5% for negative samples.[84] The European AutoCure consortium is a serum repository from patients with RA and other rheumatic diseases. This biobank has been designed to allow the validation of new anti-CCP tests, allowing the use of the same core bank of sera to increase consistency between the old and newly developed assays.[85]

PRECLINICAL ARTHRITIS

As irreversible harm may occur early in the disease, intensive attempts have been made to identify specific biomarkers, both at the preclinical stage and in very early RA.[86] At present, no test efficiently screens for preclinical RA, but positive RF or ACPA assays increase the likelihood of developing RA in predisposed individuals. Before the onset of RA, ACPA specificities were shown to gradually spread to encompass a broader range of citrullinated antigens supporting a form of antigen spreading targeted by B cells.[86,87] The onset of clinical RA is linked to a switch to more inflammatory isotypes and Fc glycosylation patterns.[88,89] Similarly, RF and anti-CCP frequently appear before the onset of clinical RA, with increasing titers and prevalence close to onset.[90] In early undifferentiated arthritis, the presence of either RF or anti-CCP antibodies was independently associated with an increased likelihood of developing RA.[91]

A crucial piece of information came from a Dutch arthralgia cohort, in which patients with inflammatorylike arthralgia without synovitis were screened and followed for the development of RA over 2 years. In this setting, 40% of patients doubly positive for RF and anti-CCP2 at baseline developed RA. This risk increased to 50% when anti-CCP2 titers were greater than the 75th percentile.[92] Development of anti-CCP antibodies is strongly influenced by the human leukocyte antigen background.[93] IgM and IgA anti-CCP isotypes may predominate in first-degree relatives without arthritis, whereas the IgG isotype predominated in established inflammatory arthritis.[94]

Although progressive loss of tolerance and development of autoantibodies preceding RA onset are strongly supported observations, the rate of conversion of arthralgia to RA remains only 50% at 2 years, even with high anti-CCP and RF titers. Furthermore, close to 50% of patients with early RA, and about 30% with established RA, remain seronegative using current immunoassays. Therefore, exclusive reliance on serologic diagnosis may delay essential therapeutic interventions in patients with early seronegative RA. Furthermore, it is presently not recommended to screen patients without active arthritis for the presence of antibodies, because well-supported and safe preventive treatments are still lacking.

SUMMARY

The rapid growth in the number and types of RA biomarkers in recent years has led to an improved understanding of the disease pathogenesis. The development of robust anti-CCP assays has helped translate this knowledge to the clinic. However, a significant proportion of patients are still seronegative by current assays for RA-specific antibodies. There are still unmet needs for better biomarkers of disease activity and treatment response, and for preclinical and early detection of RA. Thus, this field is likely to continue to evolve rapidly.

REFERENCES

1. Silman AJ, Pearson JE. Epidemiology and genetics of rheumatoid arthritis. Arthritis Res 2002;4(Suppl 3):S265–72.
2. Van der Heijde DM. Joint erosions and patients with early rheumatoid arthritis. Br J Rheumatol 1995;34(Suppl 2):74–8.

3. Mc Ardle A, Flatley B, Pennington SR, et al. Early biomarkers of joint damage in rheumatoid and psoriatic arthritis. Arthritis Res Ther 2015;17:141.
4. Lingampalli N, Sokolove J, Lahey LJ, et al. Combination of anti-citrullinated protein antibodies and rheumatoid factor is associated with increased systemic inflammatory mediators and more rapid progression from preclinical to clinical rheumatoid arthritis. Clin Immunol 2018;195:119–26.
5. Barra L, Pope JE, Orav JE, et al. Prognosis of seronegative patients in a large prospective cohort of patients with early inflammatory arthritis. J Rheumatol 2014;41:2361–9.
6. De Rycke L, Peene I, Hoffman IEA, et al. Rheumatoid factor and anticitrullinated protein antibodies in rheumatoid arthritis: diagnostic value, associations with radiological progression rate, and extra-articular manifestations. Ann Rheum Dis 2004;63:1587–93.
7. Berglin E, Johansson T, Sundin U, et al. Radiological outcome in rheumatoid arthritis is predicted by presence of antibodies against cyclic citrullinated peptide before and at disease onset, and by IgA-RF at disease onset. Ann Rheum Dis 2006;65:453–8.
8. Humphreys JH, van Nies JAB, Chipping J, et al. Rheumatoid factor and anti-citrullinated protein antibody positivity, but not level, are associated with increased mortality in patients with rheumatoid arthritis: results from two large independent cohorts. Arthritis Res Ther 2014;16:483.
9. Ingegnoli F, Castelli R, Gualtierotti R. Rheumatoid factors: clinical applications. Dis Markers 2013;35:727–34.
10. Houssien DA, Jónsson T, Davi E. Rheumatoid factor isotypes, disease activity and the outcome of rheumatoid arthritis: comparative effects of different antigens. Scand J Rheumatol 2009;27:46–53.
11. Dequeker J, Van Noyen R, Vandepitte J. Age-related rheumatoid factors. Incidence and characteristics. Ann Rheum Dis 1969;28:431–6.
12. Nielsen SF, Bojesen SE, Schnohr P, et al. Elevated rheumatoid factor and long term risk of rheumatoid arthritis: a prospective cohort study. BMJ 2012;345: e5244.
13. Waller M, Toone EC, Vaughan E. Study of rheumatoid factor in a normal population. Arthritis Rheum 1964;7:513–20.
14. Williams DG, Moyes SP, Mageed RA. Rheumatoid factor isotype switch and somatic mutation variants within rheumatoid arthritis synovium. Immunology 1999; 98:123–36.
15. Nienhuis RLF, Mandema E, Smids C. New serum factor in patients with rheumatoid arthritis: the antiperinuclear factor. Ann Rheum Dis 1964;23:302–5.
16. Aho K, Essen von R, Kurki P, et al. Antikeratin antibody and antiperinuclear factor as markers for subclinical rheumatoid disease process. J Rheumatol 1993;20: 1278–81.
17. Despres N, Boire G, Lopez-Longo FJ, et al. The Sa system: a novel antigen-antibody system specific for rheumatoid arthritis. J Rheumatol 1994;21:1027–33.
18. Aho K, Palosuo T, Heliövaara M, et al. Antifilaggrin antibodies within "normal" range predict rheumatoid arthritis in a linear fashion. J Rheumatol 2000;27:2743–6.
19. Schellekens GA, de Jong BA, van den Hoogen FH, et al. Citrulline is an essential constituent of antigenic determinants recognized by rheumatoid arthritis-specific autoantibodies. J Clin Invest 1998;101:273–81.
20. Poulsom H, Charles PJ. Antibodies to citrullinated vimentin are a specific and sensitive marker for the diagnosis of rheumatoid arthritis. Clin Rev Allergy Immunol 2008;34:4–10.

21. Joshua V, Schobers L, Titcombe PJ, et al. Antibody responses to de novo identified citrullinated fibrinogen peptides in rheumatoid arthritis and visualization of the corresponding B cells. Arthritis Res Ther 2016;18:284.

22. Lundberg K, Wegner N, Yucel-Lindberg T, et al. Periodontitis in RA—the citrullinated enolase connection. Nat Rev Rheumatol 2010;6:727–30.

23. Steiner G. Auto-antibodies and autoreactive T-cells in rheumatoid arthritis. Clin Rev Allergy Immunol 2007;32:23–35.

24. Wegner N, Lundberg K, Kinloch A, et al. Autoimmunity to specific citrullinated proteins gives the first clues to the etiology of rheumatoid arthritis. Immunol Rev 2010;233:34–54.

25. Schellekens GA, Visser H, de Jong BA, et al. The diagnostic properties of rheumatoid arthritis antibodies recognizing a cyclic citrullinated peptide. Arthritis Rheum 2000;43:155–63.

26. Aggarwal R, Liao K, Nair R, et al. Anti-citrullinated peptide antibody assays and their role in the diagnosis of rheumatoid arthritis. Arthritis Rheum 2009;61: 1472–83.

27. Swart A, Burlingame RW, Gürtler I, et al. Third generation anti-citrullinated peptide antibody assay is a sensitive marker in rheumatoid factor negative rheumatoid arthritis. Clin Chim Acta 2012;414:266–72.

28. van Venrooij WJ, van Beers JJBC, Pruijn GJM. Anti-CCP antibodies: the past, the present and the future. Nat Rev Rheumatol 2011;7:391–8.

29. van Venrooij WJ, Pruijn GJM. How citrullination invaded rheumatoid arthritis research. Arthritis Res Ther 2014;16:103.

30. Wagner CA, Sokolove J, Lahey LJ, et al. Identification of anticitrullinated protein antibody reactivities in a subset of anti-CCP-negative rheumatoid arthritis: association with cigarette smoking and HLA-DRB1 "shared epitope" alleles. Ann Rheum Dis 2015;74:579–86.

31. Vossenaar ER, Després N, Lapointe E, et al. Rheumatoid arthritis specific anti-Sa antibodies target citrullinated vimentin. Arthritis Res Ther 2004;6:R142–50.

32. Guzian M-C, Carrier N, Cossette P, et al. Outcomes in recent-onset inflammatory polyarthritis differ according to initial titers, persistence over time, and specificity of the autoantibodies. Arthritis Care Res 2010;62:1624–32.

33. Boire G, Cossette P, de Brum-Fernandes AJ, et al. Anti-Sa antibodies and antibodies against cyclic citrullinated peptide are not equivalent as predictors of severe outcomes in patients with recent-onset polyarthritis. Arthritis Res Ther 2005; 7:R592–603.

34. El-Gabalawy HS, Wilkins JA. Anti-Sa antibodies: prognostic and pathogenetic significance to rheumatoid arthritis. Arthritis Res Ther 2004;6:86–9.

35. Goldbach-Mansky R, Lee J, McCoy A, et al. Rheumatoid arthritis associated autoantibodies in patients with synovitis of recent onset. Arthritis Res 2000;2: 236–43.

36. Stark GR, Stein WH, Moore S. Reactions of the cyanate present in aqueous urea with amino acids and proteins. J Biol Chem 1960;235:3177–81.

37. Ospelt C, Bang H, Feist E, et al. Carbamylation of vimentin is inducible by smoking and represents an independent autoantigen in rheumatoid arthritis. Ann Rheum Dis 2017;76:1176–83.

38. Sirpal S. Myeloperoxidase-mediated lipoprotein carbamylation as a mechanistic pathway for atherosclerotic vascular disease. Clin Sci 2009;116:681–95.

39. Kinloch A, Lundberg K, Wait R, et al. Synovial fluid is a site of citrullination of autoantigens in inflammatory arthritis. Arthritis Rheum 2008;58:2287–95.

40. Flückiger R, Harmon W, Meier W, et al. Hemoglobin carbamylation in uremia. N Engl J Med 1981;304:823–7.
41. Erill S, Calvo R, Carlos R. Plasma protein carbamylation and decreased acidic drug protein binding in uremia. Clin Pharmacol Ther 1980;27:612–8.
42. Shi J, Willemze A, Janssen GMC, et al. Recognition of citrullinated and carbamylated proteins by human antibodies: specificity, cross-reactivity and the "AMC-Senshu" method. Ann Rheum Dis 2013;72:148–50.
43. Challener GJ, Jones JD, Pelzek AJ, et al. Anti-carbamylated protein antibody levels correlate with anti-Sa (citrullinated vimentin) antibody levels in rheumatoid arthritis. J Rheumatol 2016;43:273–81.
44. Liu Y, Wu J, Shen G, et al. Diagnostic value of BiP or anti-BiP antibodies for rheumatoid arthritis: a meta-analysis. Clin Exp Rheumatol 2018;36:405–11.
45. Bodman-Smith MD, Corrigall VM, Berglin E, et al. Antibody response to the human stress protein BiP in rheumatoid arthritis. Rheumatology (Oxford) 2004;43: 1283–7.
46. Shoda H, Fujio K, Shibuya M, et al. Detection of autoantibodies to citrullinated BiP in rheumatoid arthritis patients and pro-inflammatory role of citrullinated BiP in collagen-induced arthritis. Arthritis Res Ther 2011;13:R191.
47. Mediwake R. Use of anti-citrullinated peptide and anti-RA33 antibodies in distinguishing erosive arthritis in patients with systemic lupus erythematosus and rheumatoid arthritis. Ann Rheum Dis 2001;60:67–8.
48. Nell VPK, Machold KP, Stamm TA, et al. Autoantibody profiling as early diagnostic and prognostic tool for rheumatoid arthritis. Ann Rheum Dis 2005;64:1731–6.
49. Manivel VA, Mullazehi M, Padyukov L, et al. Anticollagen type II antibodies are associated with an acute onset rheumatoid arthritis phenotype and prognosticate lower degree of inflammation during 5 years follow-up. Ann Rheum Dis 2017;76: 1529–36.
50. Mullazehi M, Wick MC, Klareskog L, et al. Anti-type II collagen antibodies are associated with early radiographic destruction in rheumatoid arthritis. Arthritis Res Ther 2012;14:R100.
51. van Beers-Tas MH, Marotta A, Boers M, et al. A prospective cohort study of 14-3-3η in ACPA and/or RF-positive patients with arthralgia. Arthritis Res Ther 2016; 18:76.
52. Maksymowych WP, van der Heijde D, Allaart CF, et al. 14-3-3η is a novel mediator associated with the pathogenesis of rheumatoid arthritis and joint damage. Arthritis Res Ther 2014;16:R99.
53. Carrier N, Marotta A, de Brum-Fernandes AJ, et al. Serum levels of 14-3-3η protein supplement C-reactive protein and rheumatoid arthritis-associated antibodies to predict clinical and radiographic outcomes in a prospective cohort of patients with recent-onset inflammatory polyarthritis. Arthritis Res Ther 2016; 18:37.
54. Ziff M. The rheumatoid nodule. Arthritis Rheum 1990;33:761–7.
55. Makol A, Matteson EL, Warrington KJ. Rheumatoid vasculitis: an update. Curr Opin Rheumatol 2015;27:63–70.
56. Vollertsen RS, Conn DL. Vasculitis associated with rheumatoid arthritis. Rheum Dis Clin North Am 1990;16:445–61.
57. Sokolove J, Johnson DS, Lahey LJ, et al. Rheumatoid factor as a potentiator of anti-citrullinated protein antibody-mediated inflammation in rheumatoid arthritis. Arthritis Rheum 2014;66:813–21.
58. Dresser DW, Popham AM. Induction of an IgM anti-(bovine)-IgG response in mice by bacterial lipopolysaccharide. Nature 1976;264:552–4.

59. Weber J, Peng H, Rader C. From rabbit antibody repertoires to rabbit monoclonal antibodies. Exp Mol Med 2017;49:e305.

60. Butler JE. Bovine immunoglobulins: an augmented review. Vet Immunol Immuno-pathol 1983;4:143–52.

61. Tuomi T. Which antigen to use in the detection of rheumatoid factors? Comparison of patients with rheumatoid arthritis and subjects with "false positive" rheumatoid factor reactions. Clin Exp Immunol 1989;77:349–55.

62. Rose HM, Ragan C. Differential agglutination of normal and sensitized sheep erythrocytes by sera of patients with rheumatoid arthritis. Proc Soc Exp Biol Med 1948;68:1–6.

63. Waaler E. On the occurrence of a factor in human serum activating the specific agglutination of sheep blood corpuscles. 1939. Reprinted from Acta Path Micro-biol Scand 1940;17:172-188. APMIS 2007;115:422–38.

64. Roberts-Thomson PJ, Wernick RM, Ziff M. Quantitation of rheumatoid factor by laser nephelometry. Rheumatol Int 1982;2:17–20.

65. Wedgwood JF, Hatam L, Bonagura VR. Expression of large quantities of rheuma-toid factor major cross-reactive idiotype in the serum of adults with seropositive rheumatoid arthritis. Arthritis Rheum 1991;34:840–5.

66. Wolfe F. A comparison of IgM rheumatoid factor by nephelometry and latex methods: clinical and laboratory significance. Arthritis Care Res 1998;11:89–93.

67. Borque L, Yago M, Mar C, et al. Turbidimetry of rheumatoid factor in serum with a centrifugal analyzer. Clin Chem 1986;32:124–9.

68. Bampton JL, Cawston TE, Kyle MV, et al. Measurement of rheumatoid factors by an enzyme-linked immunosorbent assay (ELISA) and comparison with other methods. Ann Rheum Dis 1985;44:13–9.

69. Ulvestad E, Wilfred LL, Kristoffersen EK. Measurement of IgM rheumatoid factor by ELISA. Scand J Rheumatol 2001;30:366.

70. Levinson SS, Goldman J. Absorbance nephelometry of C1q-precipitable immune complexes: method comparisons and clinical correlations. Clin Chem 1983;29: 2082–6.

71. Borque L, Rus A, Ruiz R. Automated turbidimetry of rheumatoid factor without heat inactivation of serum. Eur J Clin Chem Clin Biochem 1991;29:521–7.

72. Virella G, Hipp WA, John JF Jr, et al. Nephelometric detection of soluble immune complexes: methodology and clinical applications. Int Arch Allergy Appl Immunol 1979;58:402–10.

73. Motyckova G, Murali M. Laboratory testing for cryoglobulins. Am J Hematol 2011; 86:500–2.

74. Whitsed H, McCarthy WH, Hersey P. Nephelometric detection of circulating im-mune complexes using monoclonal rheumatoid factor. J Immunol Methods 1979;29:311–21.

75. Hirst CF, Poller L. The cause of turbidity in lyophilised plasmas and its effects on coagulation tests. J Clin Pathol 1992;45:701–3.

76. Kim D, Mun S, Lee J, et al. Proteomics analysis reveals differential pattern of widespread protein expression and novel role of histidine-rich glycoprotein and lipopolysaccharide-binding protein in rheumatoid arthritis. Int J Biol Macromol 2018;109:704–10.

77. Gorgani NN, Altin JG, Parish CR. Histidine-rich glycoprotein prevents the forma-tion of insoluble immune complexes by rheumatoid factor. Immunology 1999;98: 456–63.

78. Hassan J, Feighery C, Bresnihan B, et al. Prevalence of anti-Fab antibodies in patients with autoimmune and infectious diseases. Clin Exp Immunol 1992;89: 423–6.
79. Anderson SG, Bentzon MW, Houba V, et al. International reference preparation of rheumatoid arthritis serum. Bull World Health Organ 1970;42:311–8.
80. Taylor RN, Fulford KM, Jones WL. Reduction of variation in results of rheumatoid factor tests by use of a serum reference preparation. J Clin Microbiol 1977; 5:42–5.
81. Goddard DH, Moore ME. Common tests for rheumatoid factors: poorly standardized but ubiquitous. Arthritis Rheum 1988;31:432–5.
82. Bossuyt X, Louche C, Wiik A. Standardisation in clinical laboratory medicine: an ethical reflection. Ann Rheum Dis 2008;67:1061–3.
83. Pruijn GJ, Wiik A, van Venrooij WJ. The use of citrullinated peptides and proteins for the diagnosis of rheumatoid arthritis. Arthritis Res Ther 2010;12:203.
84. Bizzaro N, Pregnolato F, van Boekel MAM, et al. Preliminary evaluation of the first international reference preparation for anticitrullinated peptide antibodies. Ann Rheum Dis 2012;71:1388–92.
85. Taylor P, Gartemann J, Hsieh J, et al. A systematic review of serum biomarkers anti-cyclic citrullinated Peptide and rheumatoid factor as tests for rheumatoid arthritis. Autoimmune Dis 2011;2011:815038.
86. Deane KD. Preclinical rheumatoid arthritis (autoantibodies): an updated review. Curr Rheumatol Rep 2014;16:419.
87. van der Woude D, Rantapää-Dahlqvist S, Ioan-Facsinay A, et al. Epitope spreading of the anti-citrullinated protein antibody response occurs before disease onset and is associated with the disease course of early arthritis. Ann Rheum Dis 2010;69:1554–61.
88. Ercan A, Cui J, Chatterton DEW, et al. Aberrant IgG galactosylation precedes disease onset, correlates with disease activity, and is prevalent in autoantibodies in rheumatoid arthritis. Arthritis Rheum 2010;62:2239–48.
89. Rombouts Y, Ewing E, van de Stadt LA, et al. Anti-citrullinated protein antibodies acquire a pro-inflammatory Fc glycosylation phenotype prior to the onset of rheumatoid arthritis. Ann Rheum Dis 2015;74:234–41.
90. del Puente A, Knowler WC, Pettitt DJ, et al. The incidence of rheumatoid arthritis is predicted by rheumatoid factor titer in a longitudinal population study. Arthritis Rheum 1988;31:1239–44.
91. van der Helm-van Mil AHM, Detert J, le Cessie S, et al. Validation of a prediction rule for disease outcome in patients with recent-onset undifferentiated arthritis: moving toward individualized treatment decision-making. Arthritis Rheum 2008; 58:2241–7.
92. Bos WH, Wolbink GJ, Boers M, et al. Arthritis development in patients with arthralgia is strongly associated with anti-citrullinated protein antibody status: a prospective cohort study. Ann Rheum Dis 2010;69:490–4.
93. Nordang GBN, Flåm ST, Maehlen MT, et al. HLA-C alleles confer risk for anti-citrullinated peptide antibody-positive rheumatoid arthritis independent of HLA-DRB1 alleles. Rheumatology (Oxford) 2013;52:1973–82.
94. Ioan-Facsinay A, Willemze A, Robinson DB, et al. Marked differences in fine specificity and isotype usage of the anti-citrullinated protein antibody in health and disease. Arthritis Rheum 2008;58:3000–8.

Antineutrophil Cytoplasmic Antibodies Testing and Interpretation

Hugues Allard-Chamard, MD, PhD, FRCPC[a,b,c,d,*],
Patrick Liang, MD, FRCPC[b,c,d]

KEYWORDS

- ANCA • pANCA • cANCA • Proteinase-3 • Myeloperoxidase • Immunoassay
- ELISA • Immunofluorescence

KEY POINTS

- Used in the clinical setting of patients with a high suspicion of vasculitis, ANCAs testing is highly specific for AAV.
- ANCA positivity is a frequent manifestation of non-AAV diseases, such as infective endocarditis, Crohn's disease, ulcerative colitis, anti-glomerular basement membrane (GBM) syndrome, and autoimmune hepatitis.
- Indirect immunofluorescence (IIF) for ANCA is performed on ethanol-fixed formalin-fixed neutrophils (PMNs); a cANCA pattern on ethanol maintains the same staining pattern on formalin, whereas pANCAs adopt a cANCA pattern on formalin.
- ANCA patterns are most reliable at a high titer; low cANCA titer frequently mimics pANCA pattern or other cytoplasmic fluorescence patterns, such as anti-Jo-1 or antiribosomal nucleoprotein, despite not being associated with AAV.
- ANCA testing is not yet standardized across clinical laboratories; however, new techniques are emerging to streamline and increase the robustness of ANCAs testing.

BRIEF HISTORY OF ANTINEUTROPHIL CYTOPLASMIC ANTIBODY TESTING

Since their initial discovery as an antileukocyte factor in the blood of patients with various autoimmune disorders in 1959,[1] antineutrophil cytoplasmic antibodies (ANCAs) have become integral to the clinical investigation and diagnosis of small

The authors contributed equally to this work.
[a] Ragon Institute of MGH, MIT and Harvard, Cambridge, MA, USA; [b] Division of Rheumatology, Faculty of Medicine and Health Sciences, Université de Sherbrooke; [c] Centre de Recherche Clinique du Centre Hospitalier Universitaire de Sherbrooke, Sherbrooke, Québec, Canada; [d] Division of Rheumatology, Centre intégré universitaire de santé et de service sociaux de l'Estrie – Centre hospitalier universitaire de Sherbrooke (CIUSSS de l'Estrie-CHUS), 3001, 12th Avenue North, Room 3853, Sherbrooke, Québec J1H 5N4, Canada
* Corresponding author. Division of Rheumatology, Centre intégré universitaire de santé et de service sociaux de l'Estrie – Centre hospitalier universitaire de Sherbrooke (CIUSSS de l'Estrie-CHUS), 3001, 12th Avenue North, Room 3857, Sherbrooke, Qc J1H 5N4, Canada.
E-mail address: hugues.allard-chamard@USherbrooke.ca

Clin Lab Med 39 (2019) 539–552
https://doi.org/10.1016/j.cll.2019.07.003
0272-2712/19/© 2019 Elsevier Inc. All rights reserved.

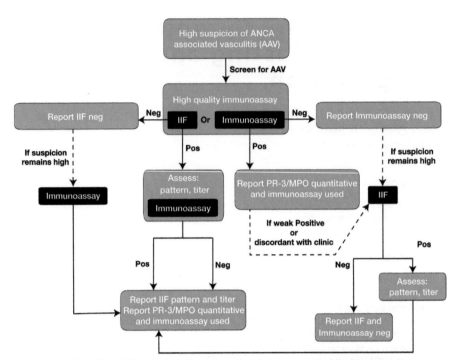

Fig. 1. Algorithm for ANCA testing. Based on the development of high-quality immunoassays to assess for the presence of antimyeloperoxidase and anti- proteinase-3 antibodies, it has now become acceptable to directly screen for ANCA using an antigen-specific test. In the presence of a high clinical suspicion of AAV, despite a negative screening test, a second immunoassay could be performed to reveal possible false negatives. In the presence of a weak positive signal in a screening immunoassay, confirmatory testing using indirect immunofluorescent might help to distinguish false-positive from true-positive signal. IIF, indirect immunofluorescence; MPO, myeloperoxidase; PR-3, proteinase-3.

vessel vasculitis (**Fig. 1**). The significance of the cytoplasmic (cANCA) or perinuclear (pANCA) varieties of ANCA was apparent about 20 years after their original description. Indeed, the importance of ANCA became more evident from 1982 to 1985 when cANCA were identified in patients with glomerulonephritis[2] and subsequently linked to granulomatosis with polyangiitis (formerly called Wegener granulomatosis) using indirect immunofluorescence (IIF).[3] This interest in the staining pattern of ANCA in autoimmunity led to the identification of a new pattern of ANCA in 1988, with a specificity for myeloperoxidase (MPO). Thus, the pANCAs were born.[4] Within a year of identification of MPO as the target of pANCA, intensive research culminated in the identification of proteinase-3 (PR3) as the major target of cANCA.[5]

WHY WERE THE CURRENT GUIDELINES ADOPTED?

Wide clinical availability of ANCA testing led to the identification of additional patterns, besides the well-characterized pANCA and cANCA (**Fig. 2**). These "new ANCA" included nuclear ANCA,[6] atypical ANCA (or flat ANCA without interlobular accentuation),[7] and double-positive pANCA and cANCA.[8] Thus, ANCA reporting has become more complex and the sensitivity and specificity of readings have been impacted as a result.[7] The somewhat subjective reading of IIF patterns

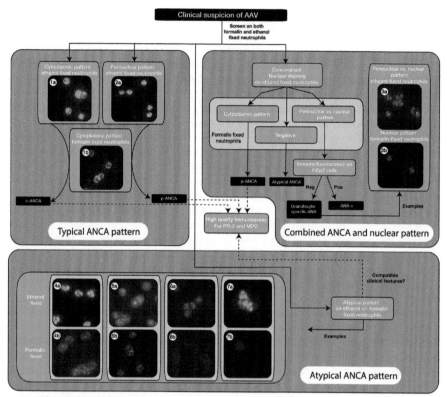

Fig. 2. Indirect immunofluorescence for ANCA. (1a) Typical cytoplasmic pattern on ethanol-fixed neutrophils. (1b) Typical cytoplasmic pattern on formalin-fixed neutrophils. (2a) Typical perinuclear pattern on ethanol-fixed neutrophils. (3a) Perinuclear pattern on ethanol-fixed neutrophils that remains (3b) perinuclear with some nuclear extension in formalin-fixed neutrophils. Antinuclear antibody (ANA) assay must be performed to distinguish between granulocyte-specific ANA and classic ANA. (4a) Atypical perinuclear ANCA with a mixture of homogenous and punctate nuclear staining with (4b) a perinuclear pattern on formalin-fixed neutrophils. (5a) Atypical cytoplasmic ANCA on ethanol-fixed neutrophils that look like a classic cytoplasmic ANCA on formalin-fixed neutrophils; enzyme-linked immunosorbent assay for PR3 was positive. (6a) Atypical intranuclear punctate staining combined with (6b) weak cytoplasmic fluorescence on formalin-fixed cells. (7a) Atypical ANCA, showing combined strong nuclear and cytoplasmic staining on ethanol-fixed neutrophils with (7b) a negative fluorescence on formalin-fixed neutrophils. cANCA, cytoplasmic ANCA; pANCA, perinuclear ANCA.

seeded the need for a more specific ANCA assay and called for guidelines framing ANCA usage and interpretation. In 1999, a group of experts came to the conclusion that ANCA immunofluorescence in a clinical setting of probable vasculitis had only a mild specificity and should probably be combined with antigen-specific enzyme-linked immunosorbent assay (ELISA) for MPO in case of pANCA or PR3 in the case of cANCA.[9] Relying exclusively only on IIF failed to capture an unacceptably high, 10% to 15%, of patients with ANCA-associated vasculitis (AAV). The combined use of IIF and first-generation ANCA ELISAs resulted in an increase in the diagnostic performance from a sensitivity of 81% to 85% and a specificity of 76% to a favorable specificity approaching 98% and a sensitivity of 67% to 82%.[9]

WHEN SHOULD ANTINEUTROPHIL CYTOPLASMIC ANTIBODY ENZYME-LINKED IMMUNOSORBENT ASSAY BE ORDERED?

ANCA should only be ordered in patients with a reasonable clinical suspicion of vasculitis (**Box 1**). These clinical testing guidelines are aimed at focusing ANCA testing on a population with a high likelihood of AAV. Adherence to these guidelines reduces unnecessary testing and also improves the predictive values of the test. ANCA measured by IIF or ELISA are frequently positive in several clinical settings that are unrelated to AAV; it is therefore imperative to be careful in interpreting positive ANCA results, especially if the test was ordered outside the recommended clinical scenario. As a result of this promiscuity, ANCAs exhibit a positive predictive value of 54% and negative predictive value of 99% in conventional clinical settings.[10] It is important to keep in mind that these metrics are highly dependent on the prevalence of AAV in the population examined; hence the variability across studies using this test. In theory, if ANCA tests are restricted to a subset of patients with a high pretest probability, better predictive values would be obtained. Carefully selecting the patients that will be screened is therefore crucial for the test interpretation.[11] Furthermore, ANCA titers generally correlate with disease activity. They have higher titer at presentation and decline with treatment-induced stabilization of the disease. Disease relapse is seen in approximately half of the patients whose titers bounce back.[12,13]

Hitherto, the chronologic relationship between disease relapse and the rise in ANCA is not yet fully understood. Moreover, the threshold to call an ANCA increase clinically significant, the speed of the increase, and the delay between the change in titer and relapse are not known. It is also still not known which test should be used to monitor ANCA titer (IIF, ELISA, or newer tests). Recent meta-analysis suggests that a rise in ANCA titers or persistence of ANCA during remission only mildly predicts the risk of relapse.[14] Therefore, rheumatology societies currently do not support serial testing of ANCAs.[9,15] The current practice guidelines suggest that ANCA testing should be restricted to establishing AAV diagnosis because ANCA are present in virtually all

---

Box 1
Indications for ANCA testing[a]

- Glomerulonephritis, especially rapidly progressive glomerulonephritis
- Pulmonary hemorrhage, especially pulmonary renal syndrome
- Cutaneous vasculitis with systemic features
- Multiple lung nodules
- Chronic destructive disease of the upper airways
- Long-standing sinusitis or otitis
- Subglottic tracheal stenosis
- Mononeuritis multiplex or other peripheral neuropathy
- Retro-orbital mass
- Scleritis

[a] Unless there are other obvious explanation for the clinical presentation (eg, retro-orbital mass with biopsy-proven lymphoma).
Modified from Savige J, Gillis D, Benson E, et al. International consensus statement on testing and reporting of antineutrophil cytoplasmic antibodies (ANCA). Am J Clin Pathol. 1999;111(4):508; with permission.

patients with severe AAV and 80% of limited disease.[16] It could also be useful in assessing the likelihood that new manifestations (eg, new undiagnosed respiratory features) are linked to AAV, because vasculitic relapses are usually associated with positive ANCAs once relapses occur. ANCA could also be of use for disease prognostication, because some evidence suggests that PR3-positive AAV are more likely to relapse than MPO-positive AAV.[17,18]

The 1999 consensus had suggested that in an ideal world, IIF and ELISA should be performed on patients with a suspicion of AAV.[9] However, testing all patients with suspected AAV using both methods was not considered suitable in a clinical setting because it could delay diagnosis and increase costs; the authors had proposed that the initial screening for ANCAs be done using IIF. To optimize specificity, positive results were to be confirmed by an immunoassay, usually ELISA, for identification of antigenic specificity to either MPO or PR3. These recommendations reflected that 10% of the ANCAs were detectable by IIF while remaining negative by first-generation ELISAs in use in 1999. The consensus also stipulated that clinicians could consider ordering ELISA, despite negative IIF, because in 5% of the cases of AAV, only the ELISA is positive. The reason for this discrepancy was not well understood.[9]

The most recent consensus published in 2017 by Bossuyt and colleagues[15] proposes to tackle the sensitivity/specificity issue of ANCA testing with a new point of view, in light of improved technologies for ANCA testing. Indeed, the newly available second- and third-generation ELISAs for PR3 and MPO outperform classic IIF for sensitivity and specificity in most clinical contexts. They are also arguably cheaper and faster to perform. Therefore, the 2017 consensus proposed a strategy where MPO or PR3 ELISA are performed as a first-line screening in patients with reasonable suspicion of AAV, based on a list of compatible clinical scenarios (see **Box 1**). Because no biomarker is 100% reliable, if the ELISA is negative and the clinical suspicion is high, a second assay, potentially IIF, is ordered to increase sensitivity. The role of a second assay could be extended to weak positive signals that are suspected of being false positive, in which case a second immunoassay can increase marginally the specificity. The 2017 consensus also opens the door to new confirmatory immunoassays that are not necessarily IIF as long as they are internally validated by a positive control using known ANCA-positive serum and appropriate negative controls. Clinicians must not forget that the most robust means of making a diagnosis of AAV remains a biopsy of affected organs, especially if the suspicion remains elevated after negative testing with both ELISA and IIF. Therefore, despite being counterintuitive, ANCAs are not *sine qua non* for AAV diagnosis.

HOW SHOULD CLASSIC ANTINEUTROPHIL CYTOPLASMIC ANTIBODY STAINING BE APPROACHED?

ANCA were first detected by IIF, using polymorphonuclear neutrophils (PMNs) and monocytes as the substrate. When ethanol is used for fixation, two principal patterns of fluorescence can readily be identified. cANCA, or classic pattern (because it was the first to be identified), designates a cytoplasmic, granular pattern often with central, perinuclear, interlobar accentuation. It is most often caused by antibodies directed against PR3, a neutral serine proteinase found in PMN primary granules. Other antigenic targets with a cANCA pattern include bactericidal permeability-increasing peptide and, more rarely, MPO.[19]

The perinuclear pattern, or pANCA, is the second pattern that is seen on ethanol-fixed neutrophils. It is caused by an artifact that allows migration of positively charged granule components toward the nuclear membrane, which is negatively charged. A pANCA pattern may be associated with many target antigens. MPO is the most clinically relevant because it is associated with AAV. Other targets include lysozyme, lactoferrin, cathepsin G, azurocidin, elastase, and bactericidal permeability-increasing peptide; however, they do not have clinical use in AAV except for elastase, which may be found in drug-induced AAV.[20] PR3 may rarely give a pANCA pattern. Other yet to be identified targets can also produce a pANCA pattern.[21]

Formalin is a cross-linking fixative, and when used instead of ethanol, prevents the perinuclear migration of positively charged antigens. Thus, a pANCA pattern as seen on an ethanol-fixed preparation has a cANCA appearance when formalin is used as the fixative. This distinction is used when trying to distinguish true pANCA from antinuclear antibodies (ANA). On formalin, ANAs are either negative or retain their nuclear distribution, whereas a true pANCA adopts a cytoplasmic granular pattern. The cANCA pattern is similar on formalin- and ethanol-fixed preparations.[19]

Double positivity for cANCA and pANCA is fairly rare in clinic and is only consistently associated with levamisole-induced vasculopathy. In this mimicker of AAV, 50% of patients exhibit a dual positivity for cANCA and pANCA, whereas the remaining fraction are largely pANCA single positive.[22]

A third ANCA pattern termed atypical ANCA refers to staining that may have features of pANCA and cANCA and/or nuclear autoantibodies. It is associated with multiple antigenic specificities and may be observed in conditions other than primary AAV, including rheumatoid arthritis, connective tissue diseases, autoimmune hepatitis, inflammatory bowel diseases, infections, and various drugs.[7,23]

Recent studies propose that ANCA are more than surrogate markers of AAV, and could be actively involved in the pathogenesis of AAV by triggering PMN activation, reactive oxygen species production, and degranulation.[24] It is also notable that neonatal transmission of ANCA through placental transfer has been linked to AAV in the newborn.[25] The exact mechanisms are still not fully understood; however, tentative models based on current knowledge have been developed. Briefly, epigenetically dysregulated neutrophils start expressing abnormally elevated level of PR3 and MPO. Molecular mimicry, epitope spreading, or dysregulated regulatory T cells leads to the escape and maturation of B cells producing IgG able to engage the highly expressed ANCA antigens. Neutrophils primed by environmental factors, such as inflammatory cytokines, expose their PR3/MPO. Freshly exposed antigens are hence made available to react with the ANCAs. Cross-linking of ANCA antigens or Fc receptor binding results in constitutive activation of neutrophils, triggering a cascade of inflammatory events. Activated neutrophils release properdin that binds to their membrane creating a platform for C3 convertase activity. The alternative complement pathway is consequently activated culminating in greater neutrophil recruitment and in neutrophil extracellular trap (NET) generation. The NETs expose an increasing quantity of neutrophil antigens leading to more activation, endothelial damage, thus creating a spiral of activation. The accumulation of activated neutrophils and their cellular contents disrupts the endothelial barrier and leads to the small vessel vasculitis (**Table 1**).[26]

Despite widespread effort to standardize ANCA testing, many hurdles can still easily arise when trying to get valuable clinical information from IIF-derived ANCAs. Beyond just experience with interpretation of ANCA IIF patterns, several technical factors can hinder ANCA interpretation and testing. Extensive manuals exist on how to test and troubleshoot ANCA testing.[21] Here, we focus on the most common pitfalls. Nonspecific fluorescence background is always a concern in any clinical IIF. Most of the time, it is decreased by adding 1% of bovine serum albumin in the wash solution and the serum diluent. The use of Evans blue counterstain can also help reduce

Table 1
ANCA visualization and classification using IIF[27]

Pattern	Immunohistochemistry Definition	Antigen Associated with the Pattern
Classic ANCAs (associated with AAV)		
cANCA	Cytoplasmic staining with marked interlobular accentuation	PR3, bactericidal permeability-increasing peptide, lysozyme
pANCA	Perinuclear staining with nuclear extension	MPO, azurocidin, bacterial permeability increasing protein, cathepsin G, lactoferrin, lysozyme, human leukocyte elastase, β-glucuronidase
Atypical ANCA		
Atypical cANCA	Cytoplasmic staining without a clear interlobular accentuation	
Atypical pANCA	Perinuclear staining without any extension inside the nuclear membrane rim	Lactoferrin
Nuclear ANCA	Analogous to an ANA-like pattern with homogenous staining of the nuclear constituents	
Double positive	Feature both homogenous cytoplasm staining concomitantly with some nuclear protrusion	Elastase
Undefined	Any staining pattern not herein defined	

background but it should be used judiciously, because it can obliviate weak true-positive signals and create discordance between IIF and ELISA.[28] Heat-inactivated serum should not be used because it creates aggregates that artificially increase staining and lead to some false positives. "ANCAs" of IgM and IgA isotype are fairly common in the serum of healthy young individuals,[29] but do not strongly bind complement and are not associated with AAV. Therefore, only IgG isotype should be detected for AAV prediction.[9] A nonspecific haze or film caused by various proteins, antibodies, or caused by hemolyzed serum may make proper interpretation a challenge and may be difficult to correct, despite using fresh and nonhemolyzed serum samples. Consequently, technical controls should accompany every ANCA test.

As mentioned in the in the 1999 consensus on ANCA testing, the training to read ANCA involves a steep learning curve. Titration of ANCA should also be considered, especially in the presence of another source of fluorescence in the cytoplasm. For example, anti-Jo-1 or antiribosomal nucleoprotein lead to fluorescence in the cytoplasm resembling cANCA. Titration could help to discern the source of the fluorescence observed, because the fluorescence produced by one of the two components should vanish before the other with progressive dilution allowing for the determination of the underlying ANCA positivity or lack of ANCA.[9] The approach toward serum samples with accompaning ANA should be dictated by the pattern of the ANA. If the pattern of ANA does not interfere with the reading of the ANCA (eg, anti-centromeric pattern) no further action is required. However, if it does interfere with interpretation (eg, homogenous pattern of antihistone) an ANCA ELISA should be ordered.[9] Local knowledge is also crucial for ANCA interpretation because the threshold for positivity slightly varies according to the light source used and the optical machinery of the microscope. The First International ANCA Workshop proposed a starting dilution of 1:20,[30] but despite this attempt at standardization, local factors should be taken into account and the starting dilution should be tailored to the local context. Indeed, in some centers, a starting dilution of 1:40 could lead to fewer false positives.[9] Thus, given the many potential pitfalls that can influence IIF specificity, a positive result should always be confirmed by a high-quality antigen-specific immunoassay.

THE EVOLUTION OF ANTINEUTROPHIL CYTOPLASMIC ANTIBODY TESTING FROM A LABORATORY PERSPECTIVE: WHERE DO WE STAND IN 2019, AND WHAT ARE THE CUTTING EDGE TECHNOLOGIES THAT WE SHOULD START USING TODAY

Propelled by the ever-growing clinical demand, the face of ANCA testing has rapidly shifted since the first commercial ELISA became available on the market in 1990. Not only were the ELISAs improved, but the IIF was also revisited. Indeed, this lengthy and expensive process is now being automated by borrowing technology developed in oncology, and relying on pattern recognition driven by machine learning and neural networks.[13] Other technologies are challenging the role of classic IIF and ELISA by trying to convert those classic assays into more streamlined methods using flow cytometry and microbeads coated with various antigen or neutrophil NETs and the use of the most recent biochip technology. In the following paragraphs we describe the incremental evolution of the ELISAs that are still used in most clinical laboratory and focus the rest of the discussion on newer techniques that increase precision and the possibility of automation.

Enzyme-Linked Immunosorbent Assay

The ELISAs to assess PR3 and MPO have undergone three main stages in their evolution. First-generation ELISA consisted of direct ELISA, called immobilization-based ELISA. The antigen was directly adsorbed with or without carrier to the well where the ELISA was performed. The process of adsorbing the antigen resulted in masking many potentially antigenic sites and therefore resulted in low sensitivity. To overcome this problem, a second-generation ELISA known as capture ELISA was developed. In this assay, each well is precoated with monoclonal antibody targeting the analyte to be captured (MPO and PR3). The masked epitopes of captured antigens are standardized because the monoclonal capture antibody always binds the same epitope. Despite outperforming the previous version of ELISA, the second-generation ELISA still, to some extent, suffered from epitope masking. Indeed, it is formally possible that the site of interface between the capture antibody is the main antigenic determinant of a targeted ANCA antibody. With this in mind, a third-generation of ELISA was developed. In this version of ELISA, the analyte is bound to the plate through a linker molecule. The limited steric hindrance of the linker molecule prevents occluding any potential antigen-binding site resulting in a slightly better performance than the second-generation ELISA.[31]

Although the fourth-generation of ELISA is not yet defined, many new approaches are percolating from the biotechnology world and promise to further improve the currently available ANCA immunoassays. For instance, approaches using liquid complexing of the antigen-antibody duet in liquid phase could completely resolve the steric hindrance encountered in the current assays.[32] These new technologies should also be calibrated against the International Union of Immunologic Societies-Centres for Disease Control (IUIS-CDC) reference sera to ensure reproducibility across techniques and studies.[15]

Fluorescent-Enzyme Immunoassay

Direct alternatives to ELISA, in the form of fluorescent-enzyme immunoassay (FEIA), are currently being tested in the research context and some clinical laboratories. These techniques, which can be fully automated, were moderately sensitive for PR3-ANCA in their first generation (60%–74%) when compared with direct ELISA (64%) and capture ELISA (74%).[12,13] However, because of the broad dynamic range of the test and improved analytical sensitivity and accuracy, investigators started to evaluate if the rise of ANCA titers evaluated by this new technique could better predict relapse of AAV. Among those studies, Damoiseaux and colleagues[12] in 2005 showed a promising positive predictive value of 69% for relapse in the context of rising ANCA and a negative predictive value of 75% for patients with stable titers of PR3-ANCAs. It was also shown in an Italian cohort of AAV that changes in ANCA titer, especially PR3 ANCA, were tightly correlated with the Birmingham Vasculitis Activity Score.[13] Moreover, as for ELISA, new generation of FEIA are emerging. A third-generation anchor-FEIA is now being commercialized by Thermo Fisher Scientific (Waltham, MA) and has been tested against the IUIS-CDC reference sera. It exhibits limited antigenic masking during the process of antigenic immobilization on the plate. As a result, it exhibits a sensitivity of 90% and a specificity of 95% that can now rival traditional ELISA.[33]

Chemiluminescent Immunoassays

Chemiluminescent immunoassays (CLIA) are also being developed. The performance of CLIA from Inova (San Diego, CA, USA) CLIA is comparable with ELISA and FEIA with a sensibility of 90% and a specificity of 94.5%. It is also validated against the IUIS-CDC reference sera.[15,34] Compared with other ANCA testing, this assay is linear at very low and very high titer and is more rapid to perform; only 30 minutes are required from the beginning to the end of the assay. This CLIA is highly concordant with ELISA except at low titer, where there seems to be some discrepancies.[35]

Addressable-Laser-Bead Immunoassays

Despite being fast and accurate, plate-based assays, such has ELISA, FEIA, and CLIA, are not easily amenable to multiplexing. This hurdle is elegantly resolved by a technology called addressable-laser-bead immunoassays (ALBIA). This technique is a hybrid between classic ELISA and flow cytometry, where wells are transposed into beads, with the added bonus of being easily multiplexed and automated. The concept relies on the immobilization of antigens, in this case PR3 and MPO, on polystyrene microspheres instead of in classic wells. Then the beads are mixed with the patient serum containing the putative autoantibodies. The beads that react with the serum are then revealed by a fluorescent secondary antibody and analyzed on a flow cytometer. If beads of different color or shape are used, then multiple analytes can be tested simultaneously. ALBIA performs similar to IIF and ELISA[36] and multiplexed versions are already in use based on the Luminex platform (Austin, TX), that is, the FIDIS Vasculitis immunoassay. This assay includes the concomitant detection of anti-GBM with PR3 and MPO.[37] Recently, Biorad (Hercules, CA) has also commercialized an ALBIA integrating anti-GBM detection with MPO and PR3, the Bio-Plex 2200 Vasculitis assay.[38] To ameliorate possible antigen-masking effects that occur with antigen immobilization, ALBIAs are currently being developed using neutrophils NETs to coat microbeads instead of purified antigen.[39]

Dot Blot and Lateral Flow Blot

Dot blot technology represents a simplified version of Western blot, where proteins are fixed on a membrane and the analyte applied to the membrane. Euroimmun (Luebeck, Germany) released a dot blot for ANCA as a stand-alone or coupled with an immuno-chip. Dot blot is not quantitative but is extremely fast and cheap. It is not as reliable as classical ELISA and therefore should be reserved for situations where IIF and ELISA are not available in a timely fashion.[40] A dot blot may be more suited for an emergency setting or for remote areas because it comes in formats that accommodate testing individual samples. The same company also commercialized a lateral flow strip based on the same principle. Lateral flow assays are a modified version of dot blot where the analyte diffuses laterally along a membrane up to the point where the protein of interest has been immobilized. The Euroimmun lateral flow assay can detect MPO, PR3, and anti-GBM in parallel. The main shortcoming of lateral flow assays is their lack of sensitivity secondary to epitope masking.[41] Although still not quantitative or prospectively tested, this assay presents a potentially interesting alternative for remote communities where the need for such testing is rare. Moreover, some new lateral flow assays propose the use of antigens in solution or in an emulsion. These improvements could raise the detection performance of lateral flow assays closer to the efficacy of classic ELISA.[42]

Biochips

The BioCHIP designed by Euroimmun combines immunoblotting with IIF.[43] BioCHIP technology can help when ANCA IIF interpretation is puzzling. On one chip, it is possible to assess the ANCA on ethanol- and formalin-fixed neutrophils, a composite substrate of HEp-2 cells + granulocytes, and a dot blot for PR3, MPO, and anti-GBM. The composite substrate of HEP-2 cells combined with granulocytes allows the easy distinction of ANA versus ANCA. In the presence of ANCA, only the neutrophils light up by immunofluorescence; in the case of ANA all nuclei capture the antibody and fluoresce. This clever combination of several assays and biomarkers on one chip captures the clinical trajectory of sequential tests that are sometimes necessary to correctly interpret ANCA titer. Biochips in their current format are also suitable for bedside medicine and could provide rapid diagnosis in rural communities.

Future Technological Developments

Advances in the biotechnological industry have led to more sophisticated laboratory techniques. Development of procedures, such as FRET, FRET-PINCER, and nanowire-based ELISAs, could provide an unprecedented increase in sensitivity while requiring less analytical material. Such techniques as ImmunoPCR show great promise because they are easily amenable to multiplexing without compromising on the sensitivity lent by their ELISA backbone. Aiming at providing fast and reliable IIF, artificial intelligence algorithms and computer-assisted pattern recognition devices are being developed and compared head to head with current state-of-the-art assays.[44,45]

SUMMARY

ANCA testing has witnessed a profound transformation technically and conceptually since its early implementation and is now a cornerstone laboratory test for vasculitis investigation, especially when AAV is suspected. In an appropriate clinical context, a positive ANCA test with proven specificity to either PR3 or MPO is strongly suggestive of AAV. In practice, ANCA should be used to support AAV diagnosis and suspected relapses. However, despite the association between the risk of AAV relapse in the context of a rising ANCA titer, current recommendation does not support serial ANCA testing to monitor AAV activity; more evidence is needed in this area.

Alongside its success as a useful biomarker universally adopted in clinic, the ANCA testing algorithm and ANCA assays have greatly evolved. Currently, the two main approaches to ANCA testing (IIF and ELISA) remain complementary and should, in an ideal world, be jointly ordered to support AAV diagnosis because both tests detect some cases that the other would have missed. Nonetheless, because of the limited availability of resources in clinical settings, the most recent guideline proposes to use high-quality immunoassay as a screening test followed by a confirmatory test in ambiguous cases. Because of the burgeoning of high-performance ANCA assays, more specifically third-generation ELISAs, a change in ANCA testing paradigm was proposed in 2017.[34] Indeed, with the faster results using ELISA over IIF for screening and its good negative predictive value, ELISA could inform clinical decision making in a timely fashion. If, however, IIF is used for screening, a positive result should be followed by an antigen-specific immunoassay to assess whether the ANCA visualized by IIF is of a PR3 or MPO nature because the other antigenic ANCA targets are not associated with AAV. There is no doubt that the availability of newer technologies to detect ANCAs will lead to further evolution of the clinical testing scheme with a more tailored algorithm for ANCA testing reflecting the clinical setting and economicogeographic constraints.

ACKNOWLEDGMENTS

This work was supported by a fellowship grant from the Faculté de médecine et des sciences de la santé de Sherbrooke (H. A.-C.); No source of funding that might influence views expressed in this paper (P. L.).

REFERENCES

1. Calabresi P, Edwards EA, Schilling RF. Fluorescent antiglobulin studies in leukopenic and related disorders. J Clin Invest 1959;38(11):2091–100.
2. Davies DJ, Moran JE, Niall JF, et al. Segmental necrotising glomerulonephritis with antineutrophil antibody: possible arbovirus aetiology? Br Med J (Clin Res Ed) 1982;285(6342):606.
3. van der Woude FJ, Rasmussen N, Lobatto S, et al. Autoantibodies against neutrophils and monocytes: tool for diagnosis and marker of disease activity in Wegener's granulomatosis. Lancet 1985;1(8426):425–9.
4. Falk RJ, Jennette JC. Anti-neutrophil cytoplasmic autoantibodies with specificity for myeloperoxidase in patients with systemic vasculitis and idiopathic necrotizing and crescentic glomerulonephritis. N Engl J Med 1988;318(25):1651–7.
5. Niles JL, McCluskey RT, Ahmad MF, et al. Wegener's granulomatosis autoantigen is a novel neutrophil serine proteinase [see comments]. Blood 1989;74(6):1888–93.
6. Lee SS, Lawton JW, Chak W. Distinction between antinuclear antibody and P-ANCA. J Clin Pathol 1991;44(11):962–3.
7. Wong RC, Silvestrini RA, Savige JA, et al. Diagnostic value of classical and atypical antineutrophil cytoplasmic antibody (ANCA) immunofluorescence patterns. J Clin Pathol 1999;52(2):124–8.

8. Kumar D, Batal I, Jim B, et al. Unusual case of levamisole-induced dual-positive ANCA vasculitis and crescentic glomerulonephritis. BMJ Case Rep 2018;2018 [pii:bcr-2018-225913].

9. Savige J, Gillis D, Benson E, of DDAJ, 1999. International consensus statement on testing and reporting of antineutrophil cytoplasmic antibodies (ANCA). Academicoupcom 2003;120(3):312–8.

10. Mandl LA, Solomon DH, Smith EL, et al. Using antineutrophil cytoplasmic antibody testing to diagnose vasculitis: can test-ordering guidelines improve diagnostic accuracy? Arch Intern Med 2002;162(13):1509–14.

11. Baldessarini RJ, Finklestein S, Arana GW. The predictive power of diagnostic tests and the effect of prevalence of illness. Arch Gen Psychiatry 1983;40(5): 569–73.

12. Damoiseaux JGMC, Slot MC, Vaessen M, et al. Evaluation of a new fluorescent-enzyme immuno-assay for diagnosis and follow-up of ANCA-associated vasculitis. J Clin Immunol 2005;25(3):202–8.

13. Sinico RA, Radice A, Corace C, et al. Value of a new automated fluorescence immunoassay (EliA) for PR3 and MPO-ANCA in monitoring disease activity in ANCA-associated systemic vasculitis. Ann N Y Acad Sci 2005;1050:185–92.

14. Tomasson G, Grayson PC, Mahr AD, et al. Value of ANCA measurements during remission to predict a relapse of ANCA-associated vasculitis: a meta-analysis. Rheumatology (Oxford) 2012;51(1):100–9.

15. Bossuyt X, Cohen Tervaert J-W, Arimura Y, et al. Position paper: revised 2017 international consensus on testing of ANCAs in granulomatosis with polyangiitis and microscopic polyangiitis. Nat Rev Rheumatol 2017;13(11):683–92.

16. Finkielman JD, Lee AS, Hummel AM, et al. ANCA are detectable in nearly all patients with active severe Wegener's granulomatosis. Am J Med 2007;120(7): 643.e9-14.

17. Fussner LA, Hummel AM, Schroeder DR, et al. Factors determining the clinical utility of serial measurements of antineutrophil cytoplasmic antibodies targeting proteinase 3. Arthritis Rheumatol 2016;68(7):1700–10.

18. Terrier B, Pagnoux C, Perrodeau É, et al. Long-term efficacy of remission-maintenance regimens for ANCA-associated vasculitides. Ann Rheum Dis 2018;77(8):1150–6.

19. Beauvillain C, Delneste Y, Renier G, et al. Antineutrophil cytoplasmic autoantibodies: how should the biologist manage them? Clin Rev Allergy Immunol 2008;35(1–2):47–58.

20. Nässberger L, Johansson AC, Björck S, et al. Antibodies to neutrophil granulocyte myeloperoxidase and elastase: autoimmune responses in glomerulonephritis due to hydralazine treatment. J Intern Med 1991;229(3):261–5.

21. Wiik A, Rasmussen N, of JWMOBM, 1993. Methods to detect autoantibodies to neutrophilic granulocytes, ii(6). Dordrecht (Netherlands): Springer; 1996. p. 135–48.

22. Jin Q, Kant S, Alhariri J, et al. Levamisole adulterated cocaine associated ANCA vasculitis: review of literature and update on pathogenesis. J Community Hosp Intern Med Perspect 2018;8(6):339–44.

23. Hagen EC, Ballieux BE, van Es LA, et al. Antineutrophil cytoplasmic autoantibodies: a review of the antigens involved, the assays, and the clinical and possible pathogenetic consequences. Blood 1993;81(8):1996–2002.

24. Kettritz R. How anti-neutrophil cytoplasmic autoantibodies activate neutrophils. Clin Exp Immunol 2012;169(3):220–8.

25. Schlieben DJ, Korbet SM, Kimura RE, et al. Pulmonary-renal syndrome in a newborn with placental transmission of ANCAs. Am J Kidney Dis 2005;45(4): 758–61.
26. Jennette JC, Falk RJ, Gasim AH. Pathogenesis of antineutrophil cytoplasmic autoantibody vasculitis 2011;20(3):263–70.
27. Hagen C. Standardization of solid phase assays for ANCA determination. Nephrology 1997;3(s2):s764–5.
28. Closs O, Aarli JA. Evans blue as counterstain in the demonstration of muscle antibodies by immunofluorescence in myasthenia gravis. J Clin Pathol 1974;27(2): 162–7.
29. Wiik A. Antinuclear factors in sera from healthy blood donors. Acta Pathol Microbiol Scand C 1976;84(3):215–20.
30. Wiik A. Delineation of a standard procedure for indirect immunofluorescence detection of ANCA. APMIS Suppl 1989;6:12–3.
31. Cohen Tervaert J-W, Damoiseaux J. Antineutrophil cytoplasmic autoantibodies: how are they detected and what is their use for diagnosis, classification and follow-up? Clin Rev Allergy Immunol 2012;43(3):211–9.
32. Hamblin C, Barnett IT, Hedger RS. A new enzyme-linked immunosorbent assay (ELISA) for the detection of antibodies against foot-and-mouth disease virus. I. Development and method of ELISA. J Immunol Methods 1986;93(1):115–21.
33. Bossuyt X, Rasmussen N, van Paassen P, et al. A multicentre study to improve clinical interpretation of proteinase-3 and myeloperoxidase anti-neutrophil cytoplasmic antibodies. Rheumatology (Oxford) 2017;56(9):1533–41.
34. Bossuyt X, Cohen Tervaert J-W, Arimura Y, et al. Position paper: revised 2017 international consensus on testing of ANCAs in granulomatosis with polyangiitis and microscopic polyangiitis. Nat Rev Rheumatol 2017;30:i8.
35. Pucar PA, Hawkins CA, Randall KL, et al. Comparison of enzyme-linked immunosorbent assay and rapid chemiluminescent analyser in the detection of myeloperoxidase and proteinase 3 autoantibodies. Pathology 2017;49(4):413–8.
36. Trevisin M, Pollock W, Dimech W, et al. Evaluation of a multiplex flow cytometric immunoassay to detect PR3- and MPO-ANCA in active and treated vasculitis, and in inflammatory bowel disease (IBD). J Immunol Methods 2008;336(2): 104–12.
37. Damoiseaux J, Vaessen M, Knapen Y, et al. Evaluation of the FIDIS vasculitis multiplex immunoassay for diagnosis and follow-up of ANCA-associated vasculitis and Goodpasture's disease. Ann N Y Acad Sci 2007;1109:454–63.
38. Kaul R, Johnson K, Scholz H, et al. Performance of the BioPlex 2200 autoimmune vasculitis kit. Autoimmun Rev 2009;8(3):224–7.
39. Roitsch S, Gößwein S, Neurath MF, et al. Detection by flow cytometry of antineutrophil cytoplasmic antibodies in a novel approach based on neutrophil extracellular traps. Autoimmunity 2018;51(6):288–96.
40. Rutgers A, Damoiseaux J, Roozendaal C, et al. ANCA-GBM dot-blot: evaluation of an assay in the differential diagnosis of patients presenting with rapidly progressive glomerulonephritis. J Clin Immunol 2004;24(4):435–40.
41. Posthuma-Trumpie GA, Korf J, van Amerongen A. Lateral flow (immuno)assay: its strengths, weaknesses, opportunities and threats. A literature survey. Anal Bioanal Chem 2008;393(2):569–82.
42. Offermann N, Conrad K, Fritzler MJ, et al. Development and validation of a lateral flow assay (LFA) for the determination of IgG-antibodies to Pr3 (cANCA) and MPO (pANCA). J Immunol Methods 2014;403(1–2):1–6.

43. Damoiseaux J, Steller U, Buschtez M, et al. EUROPLUS ANCA BIOCHIP mosaic: PR3 and MPO antigen microdots improve the laboratory diagnostics of ANCA-associated vasculitis. J Immunol Methods 2009;348(1–2):67–73.

44. Knütter I, Hiemann R, Brumma T, et al. Automated interpretation of ANCA patterns: a new approach in the serology of ANCA-associated vasculitis. Arthritis Res Ther 2012;14(6):R271.

45. Csernok E, Moosig F. Current and emerging techniques for ANCA detection in vasculitis. Nat Rev Rheumatol 2014;10(8):494–501.

Laboratory Evaluation of Antiphospholipid Syndrome

An Update on Autoantibody Testing

Anne E. Tebo, PhD, D(ABMLI)

KEYWORDS

- Antiphospholipid syndrome • Antiphospholipid antibodies • Criteria • Noncriteria
- Diagnostic approach

KEY POINTS

- Criterial antiphospholipid antibodies are relevant for the diagnosis of antiphospholipid syndrome.
- Antiphosphatidylserine/prothrombin antibodies can contribute to the diagnosis of at-risk seronegative antiphospholipid syndrome patients.
- The presence of anti–domain I IgG antibodies is associated with triple antiphospholipid antibody positivity and risk for thrombosis.
- Correlation between anti–domain I IgG and triple antiphospholipid positivity depends on the characteristics of the immunoassays used.

INTRODUCTION
Laboratory Evaluation of Antiphospholipid Syndrome

Antiphospholipid (aPL) syndrome (APS) is an autoimmune disorder characterized by thrombosis and/or certain pregnancy-related complications in association with persistence of specific aPL antibodies as defined by the revised Sapporo Sydney Criteria.[1] The aPL autoantibodies are directed against phospholipid (PL), PL-binding proteins, or PL-binding protein complexes detected by solid phase immunoassays, and by coagulation assays named lupus anticoagulant (LAC) tests. The current laboratory criteria for APS include the LAC tests as well as the anticardiolipin (aCL) IgG/IgM, and anti-beta2 glycoprotein I (anti-β_2GPI) IgG/IgM that are routinely determined by diverse types of solid phase immunoassays.

Why more laboratory tests for evaluating antiphospholipid syndrome?
The detection and interpretation of aPL antibodies is challenging partly due to heterogeneity of autoantibodies that target PLs, PL-binding plasma proteins, and PL–protein

Disclosure Statement: The author has nothing to disclose.
Department of Pathology, ARUP Laboratories, University of Utah School of Medicine, 500 Chipeta Way, MS 115, Salt Lake City, UT 84108-1221, USA
E-mail address: anne.tebo@hsc.utah.edu

Clin Lab Med 39 (2019) 553–565
https://doi.org/10.1016/j.cll.2019.07.004
0272-2712/19/© 2019 Elsevier Inc. All rights reserved.

labmed.theclinics.com

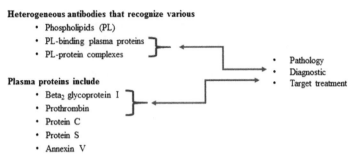

Heterogeneous antibodies that recognize various
- Phospholipids (PL)
- PL-binding plasma proteins
- PL-protein complexes

Plasma proteins include
- Beta$_2$ glycoprotein I
- Prothrombin
- Protein C
- Protein S
- Annexin V

- Pathology
- Diagnostic
- Target treatment

Fig. 1. The aPL antibodies are heterogeneous.

complexes (**Fig. 1**). In addition, available immunoassays for detecting aPL antibodies demonstrate variable performance characteristics likely owing to the absence of reference materials necessary for harmonization.[2,3] Significant problems with harmonizing aPL antibody assays and reports of APS seronegativity in patients with a strong suspicion of APS indicate the need for improvement of existing tests and/or the development of additional assays for diagnosis and management. These factors have led to a persistent search for alternative and more robust biomarkers to effectively diagnose and predict specific clinical manifestations, as well as to guide therapeutic management in APS.

Several autoantibodies directed against plasma proteins (β_2GPI, prothrombin [PT], protein C, protein S, and annexin V) or certain PLs (antiphosphatidic acid [aPA], antiphosphatidylinositol [aPI], antiphosphatidylserine [aPS]) and/or their complexes APhL [a proprietary mixture of PL antigens], and anti-PT/phosphatidylserine [aPS/PT]) have been recognized and suggested to have diagnostic and/or prognostic relevance for APS.[4–8] **Table 1** shows a list of these antibodies by categories. In addition to aCL and anti-β_2GPI antibodies of IgG and IgM isotypes, aCL IgA, and anti-β_2GPI IgA specificities have also been reported to be of diagnostic usefulness in some patients at risk for APS.[5,6] Studies on the

Table 1
Main noncriteria aPL antibodies associated with APS

Antibody Type or Category	Specificity or Isotype
aCL	aCL IgA
Anti-β_2GPI	Anti-β_2GPI IgA Anti–domain I IgG
Annexin A5	Anti–annexin A5 IgG and IgM
APhL	Proprietary mixture of PLs and PL-binding proteins (IgG and IgM)
Negatively charged PL antibodies	Antiphosphatidyl serine (aPS) IgG and IgM; antiphosphatidic acid (aPA) IgG and IgM; antiphosphatidyl inositol (aPI); antiphosptatidyl glycerol (aPG) IgG and IgM
PT	Antiprothrombin (aPT) IgG and IgM Antiprothrombin/phosphatidylserine complex (aPT/PS) IgG and IgM
Others	Antiphosphatidyl ethanolamine (aPE) IgG and IgM; antiphosphatidyl choline (aPC) IgG and IgM

use on negatively charges PLs assays such as aPS, antiphosphatidylinositol and antiphosphatidic do not demonstrate significant improvement in the diagnosis APS, except for possibly aPS in patients with pregnancy-related morbidities associated with disease (reviewed in[4,6]). A better understanding of specific immune targets such PS/PT and domain I of β_2GPI protein in APS and their potential role(s) in the pathophysiology of disease suggests that these molecules may provide diagnostic, prognostic, and/or therapeutic clues.[7] A number of recent studies focused on the performance characteristics of the aPS/PT IgG/IgM[9–17] and anti–domain I IgG[12–14,18–22] tests in the diagnosis and stratification of patients with APS have recently been published with some interesting outcomes.

This review discusses the criteria and noncriteria (aPS/PT IgG and IgM and anti–domain I IgG) aPL antibodies detected by solid phase immunoassays and the different types of immunoassays for detecting these antibodies, as well as challenges for reporting and interpreting these tests in clinical diagnostic laboratories. In addition, possible diagnostic approaches for using these noncriteria aPL autoantibody tests in combination or after evaluation with current criteria aPL tests for the diagnosis and management of APS are highlighted.

Criteria Antiphospholipid Antibody Immunoassays for Antiphospholipid Syndrome

The aCL (IgG and IgM) and the anti-β_2GPI (IgG and IgM) assays are included in the revised classification criteria for definite APS, which were published in 2006.[1] These criteria presented a significant step in improving the diagnosis and management of patients with APS. The major changes compared with the original Sapporo classification criteria published in 1999[23] were the inclusion of medium- or high-titer IgG and IgM anti-β_2GPI antibodies among the laboratory classification criteria, the addition of pregnancy morbidity symptoms, and a change in the definition of the interval for persistent aPL positivity from other significant improvements included 2 suggestions to categorize patients with APS according to the presence or absence of other acquired or inherited risk factors that may contribute to thrombosis and to subclassify patients with APS into 4 different categories according to the extent or type of aPL positivity. The latter is based on evidence suggesting that multiple aPL positivity is associated with a more severe course of the disease.[24] The expert committee also attempted to clarify the definition of medium and high antibody titers and introduced a statement that the threshold for medium antibody titers should be greater than 40 IgG PL units or IgM PL units (for aCL assays), which can be traced to the Harris standard (reviewed in[1]) or greater than the 99th percentile of the reference population (for both aCL and anti-β_2GPI assays).

Rationale for revised classification criteria for antiphospholipid syndrome

It is important to recognize that the main purpose of the original and revised classification criteria was to create common ground for conducting clinical research, exchanging and comparing results, and analyzing data originating from different cohorts, and not for routine clinical diagnosis. Therefore, in reality, the diagnosis of APS may still be made by the physician in patients who do not fulfill the requirement of 1 laboratory or 1 clinical classification criterion. A main challenge of the laboratory criteria is the definition of the cutoff for medium-positive antibody titers or levels. The suggested threshold of 40 IgG PL or IgM P units for aCL assays is frequently significantly different from the 99th percentile value derived from the reference population.[25,26] In fact, the definition of medium-positive antibody titers depends on the performance characteristics of the particular assay, the calculation method used to determine the cutoff values, and the reference population that is being tested. The revised classification criteria guidance mentioned the lack of suitable evidence and specifically commented that these values are to be used "until an international consensus is reached." The publication also mentioned that the measurement of aCL and anti-β_2GPI antibodies should be performed by "standardized ELISA [enzyme-linked immunosorbent assay]" methods. In reality, the standardization of these assays is still far from complete.[2] Moreover, a number of aPL immunoassays had been approved before the publication of these guidance and other newly developed immunoassays may have superior analytical performance compared with the traditional ELISA methodology. Overall, the 2006 revised Sapporo classification criteria was a major milestone in the diagnosis and management of APS, as new evidence emerges, the classification criteria will require further revision and validation.

Clinical attributes of criteria antiphospholipid antibody tests

Testing for aCL antibodies can be traced to the development of radioimmunoassay by Harris and colleagues[27] in 1983, which was subsequently replaced with a semiquantitative ELISA method.[28] The aCL ELISA is sensitive but not specific for APS particularly at low positive levels and certain infections. Despite these limitations, testing for aCL antibodies continues to play a significant role in the diagnosis and management of APS owing to its high sensitivity, absence of interference with anticoagulants, and ability to test in serum and plasma, as well as ease of testing. With respect to anti-β_2GPI IgG and IgM testing, 3 groups in 1990 independently reported the identification of β_2GPI (also termed apolipoprotein H), as a critical plasma protein required for the binding of aCL antibodies to cardiolipin.[29–31] These studies demonstrated that purified aCL antibodies from patients with APS could bind to cardiolipin only in the presence of β_2GPI (β_2GPI-dependent aCL). In contrast, aCL found in patients with syphilis bound to cardiolipin in the absence of β_2GPI (β_2GPI-independent aCL). Therefore, aCL associated with autoimmune disease (and an increased thrombotic risk) could be distinguished from aCL found in syphilis and other infectious diseases that generally were not associated with an increased thrombotic risk. An early study on anti-β_2GPI IgG and IgM tests in patients with APS, systemic lupus erythematosus, and other connective tissue diseases demonstrated that these antibodies were generally not as sensitive (ie, some aCL-positive patients with definite APS were negative by these assays) as aCL or LAC but are more specific for APS.[32]

A number of epidemiologic studies as well as a systematic review of the literature show that anti-β_2GPI antibodies are heterogeneous and the IgG isotype is more strongly associated with thrombosis than IgM and tends to coexist with aCL autoantibodies and/or LAC activity.[32–35] A systemic review (literature search from 1988 to 2000) by Galli and colleagues[34] reported that aCL antibodies did not have such strong risk factors for thrombosis as LAC and were associated with cerebral stroke and myocardial infarction and not deep vein thrombosis. In a more recent review of the literature from 2001 to 2014, Kelchtermans and colleagues[35] found more significant correlations with thrombosis for aCL IgG and anti-b2GPI IgG than for their IgM isotype counterparts. Based on this review, the unavailability of paired IgG and IgM results for aCL and anti-b2GPI hampers evaluating the added value of IgM positivity. Thus, the role of IgM isotype testing in the evaluation of APS remains controversial.

A systemic review (literature search from 1988 to 2000) by Galli and colleagues[34] reported that aCL antibodies did not have such strong risk factors for thrombosis as LAC and were associated with cerebral stroke and myocardial infarction and not deep vein thrombosis. In a more recent review of the literature from 2001 to 2014, Kelchtermans and colleagues[35] found more significant correlations with thrombosis for aCL IgG and anti-β_2GPI IgG than for their IgM isotype counterparts. Based on this review, the unavailability of paired IgG and IgM results for aCL and anti-β_2GPI hampers evaluating the added value of IgM positivity. Thus, the role of IgM isotype testing in the evaluation of APS remains controversial.

Noncriteria Antiphospholipid Antibody Tests for Antiphospholipid Syndrome

Recent efforts for better diagnose, categorize or stratify patients with APS or at-risk for specific clinical manifestations have focused on understanding the performance characteristics of aPS/PT IgG/IgM and anti–domain I IgG antibodies. To address these needs, both markers have been evaluated with respect to current criteria aPL in various areas; alternative to current diagnostic paradigms, additional benefits to current tests ("seronegative" gaps), markers of disease stratification as well as risk assessment in case of aPL carriers.

Antiprothrombin/phosphatidylserine antibodies

Antibodies targeting human PT alone (aPT) by ELISA was first reported in 1995.[36] Subsequent studies demonstrated that aPT antibodies bind not only to PT coated on gamma-irradiated or activated polyvinyl chloride ELISA plates, but also to PT exposed to immobilized phosphatidylserine (phospatidylserine-dependent antiprothrombin antibodies: aPS/PT).[37,38] Galli and colleagues[37] showed that aPS/PT antibodies occurred in 95% of their patients with thrombosis, but no difference in prevalence was found between those with thrombosis and those without. Funke and colleagues[38] reported that aPS–PT conferred an odds ratio of 2.8 for venous thrombosis and of 4.1 for arterial thrombosis in patients with systemic lupus erythematosus and Atsumi and colleagues[39] reported that the presence of aPS/PT antibodies conferred an odds ratio of 3.6 for APS in Japanese patients with systemic autoimmune diseases. In a subsequent study, Bertolaccini and colleagues[40] confirmed the association between aPS/PT IgG and/or IgM isotype with arterial and/or venous thrombosis. In this study, both the sensitivity and specificity of aPS/PT for the diagnosis of APS have been shown to be higher than that of aCL and their presence was not attributable to cross-reactivity with aCL or anti-β_2GPI. In addition, aPS/antibodies strongly correlated with the presence of LAC suggesting that aPS/PT marker may be used as a screening or confirming assay for APS-associated LAC.[39,40] Early recognition of the relative increased sensitivies and correlations with LAC of aPS/PT compared with aPT antibodies has prompted a number of recent studies that have examined the relationships between APS-related clinical features, current criterial aPL tests and the presence of aPS/PT.[9–17] Some of these studies have confirmed the diagnostic role for aPS/PT antibodies for APS,[10,12–14] the positive correlation between aPS/PT IgG and LAC,[10,12,13] as well as the relevance of aPS/PT IgG in stratification of patients with thrombosis[11–15,17] and intrauterine growth retardation[16] in APS. In a recent study, types I and II novel subpopulations of aPS/PT IgG antibodies had different mechanisms of PT recognition and function,[41] indicating the possibility of further stratifying patients with thrombosis if independently confirmed. Based on these studies, some of the gaps on the role of aPS/PT antibodies in the diagnosis APS such antibody persistence[42] are beginning to emerge aPL carriers positive for this marker.[14,17]

Anti–domain I IgG antibodies

β_2GPI is recognized as one of the most important antigens implicated in the pathophysiology of APS.[43] The protein consists of 326 amino acids organized in 5 complement control protein domains with the first 4 composed of 60 amino acids, except for domain 5, which has 82 amino acids.[44] Autoantibodies targeting β_2GPI are recognized to be diverse and may target different epitopes in the different domains. De Laat and colleagues were amongst the first to show that the presence of anti–domain I antibodies associated more strongly with venous thrombosis when compared with reactivities against the whole protein or other domains.[45] This observation was confirmed in a double-blinded multicenter study including 442 patients all positive for anti-β_2GPI antibodies.[46] Anti–domain I antibodies were shown to be present in the plasma of 243 of 442 patients (55%). Of these patients, 83% had a history of thrombosis resulting in an odds ratio of 3.5 (95% confidence interval, 2.3–5.4) for thrombosis. Interestingly, it was also found that anti–domain I antibodies were associated with pregnancy morbidity. An early study by Banzato and colleagues[47] showed that APS patients with triple positivity have the highest risk for thrombosis and that this population of patients had a significantly higher prevalence of anti–domain I antibodies when compared with those with single or double aPL positivity. There is considerable evidence for a central role for domain I of β_2GPI in APS disease stratification based on several recent in patients with APS[18–21] as well as aPL antibody carriers.[22]

Immunoassays for Antiphospholipid Antibodies (Criteria and Noncriteria)

Immunoassays to detect aPL antibodies provide clinicians with additional information that is not obtainable with the LAC tests. This information includes detection of specific aPL analytes, their isotype class (IgG or IgM), and their relative concentrations (levels). More important, the solid phase immunoassays are not significantly affected by analytical variables like the functional-based LAC assays. For example, the use of anticoagulation (oral or subcutaneous) or antiplatelet therapy may interfere with LAC testing.

Since the development of the initial ELISA to detect aCL antibodies, a number of immunoassays of similar principles as those of the ELISA have been developed and implemented in clinical laboratories (**Table 2**). These non-ELISA methods include test to detect single or multiple antibody specificities such as the line immunoassays, multiplex bead assay, the chemiluminescent immunoassays, or the fluorescence enzyme immunoassay for single aPL measurements.[2,3,5,6,48–53] Except for line immunoassays which is not widely used, criteria aPL are routinely tested by ELISA, multiplex bead assay, chemiluminescent immunoassays, and fluorescence enzyme immunoassay in clinical diagnostic laboratories. Testing for aPS/PT antibodies are limited to the ELISA method (reviewed in[42]) and the anti–domain I to the CIA and ELISA methodologies.[53] The immunoassays for the detection of all aPL tests have been developed in the absence of internationally acceptable standards[2–5,42,53]; as such, their performance characteristics are largely dependent on conditions established by the respective manufacturers. These conditions include the assay plates and other types of solid support, buffers (blocking, sample diluents, and washing), standards, and reference preparations for quality control and assurance as well as units of measurements. Recent studies comparing the detection of aCL and anti-β_2GPII antibodies across platforms indicate that there seems to be differences between methods without significant influence on the diagnostic outcome for APS.[51,52]

With respect to aPS/PT and anti–domain I antibodies, very few groups have examined the relative performance of available aPS/PT tests[54–56] and anti–domain I antibodies.[57] However, investigations from independent studies have demonstrated similar diagnostic performance characteristics in APS for the most part. For aPS/PT assays, these investigations report acceptable agreements (Cohen's kappa) and/or positive correlations as well as predictions for clinical manifestations for APS with the aPS/PT IgG assays.[54–56] However, the correlation between the aPS/PT IgM kits range from weak to moderate, and do not consistently associate with the APS

Table 2
Characteristics of ELISAs and other immunologic methods for detecting aPL antibodies

Characteristics	ELISAs	Other Solid Phase Immunoassays (Except Multiplex)	Multiplexed Bead Immunoassays
Type of solid phase	Usually 96-well microtiter plate	Uniformly sized paramagnetic microparticles or individual wells	Uniformly sized paramagenetic microparticles
aCL/β_2GPI attachment/wash buffer	Adsorption/detergent in aCL wash buffer may not be allowed	Passive absorption or covalent coupling/detergent in aCL wash buffer may not be allowed	Covalent coupling/detergent in aCL wash buffer allowed
Antihuman immunoglobulin reagent	Enzyme-conjugated antihuman immunoglobulin	Enzyme-, isoluminol-, or acridinium-conjugated antihuman immunoglobulin	Fluorochrome-conjugated antihuman immunoglobulin
Detection method/ readout	Colorimetric/absorbance	Light detection/chemiluminescence, fluorescence	Fluorescence
Automated vs manual	Manual or semiautomated	Fully automated	Fully automated
Internal (equipment) controls	Internal controls not included	Internal controls included	Internal controls included
Equipment type	Basic laboratory equipment and microplate reader with special filters, or semiautomated ELISA processing instruments	Specialized equipment, closed system	Specialized equipment, closed system
Economic use	Sample batching required, but large number of specimens can be run at the same time	Generally continuous random access, with no batching required	Continuous random access, no batching required, multiplexed results

(continued on next page)

Table 2
(continued)

Characteristics	ELISAs	Other Solid Phase Immunoassays (Except Multiplex)	Multiplexed Bead Immunoassays
Sensitivity to environmental factors	Sensitive	Not sensitive; controlled reaction conditions	Not sensitive; controlled reaction conditions
Time to first result	1.5–2.0 h	<1 h	<1 h
Random access	No	Yes	Yes
Calibration	Calibrators have to be assayed with every run	Stored calibration curves	Stored calibration curves
Analytical sensitivity	Medium to high	High to very high	Very high
AMR	Narrow	Potentially wide	Potentially wide
Precision	Medium to high (10% to 15%)	Very high (<10%)	Very high (<10%)
Calculation of results	Manual (plotting) or with special software	Automatic (stored curve)	Automated (stored curve)

Abbreviations: AMR, analytical measurement range; ELISA, enzyme-linked immunosorbent.

manifestations. With respect to anti–domain I IgG antibodies, a recent report by Yin and colleagues[57] suggested that optimal exposure of the highly cryptic epitope containing glycine40–arginine43 is critical and may responsible for inconsistent results in the correlations between assays and for clinical symptoms.

With respect to the units and cutoff values for reporting aPL antibody test results, aPS/PT and anti–domain I assays have been developed without strict adherence to the revised Sapporo guidance. For the aPS/PT assays, Bardin and colleagues[58] reported using a cutoff based on 97th percentile of 120 sera from normal controls, Sciascia and colleagues[59] based on 99th percentile using about 100 healthy controls, and Vlagea and colleagues[60] established ranges based on mean + 10 standard deviations using samples from 150 blood donors. While most studies on anti–domain I antibodies have been performed using the in-house ELISA and commercial CIA methods, no formal direct comparisons have been published. Thus, the same challenges experienced with other aPL tests are likely to apply.

Diagnostic Approaches for Antiphospholipid Antibody Testing

Testing for LAC as well as aCL and anti-β_2GPI antibodies (IgG and IgM) is currently recommended for the evaluation of APS. A number studies have examined the use of aPS/PT antibodies and/or anti–domain IgG in various combinations with current criteria aPL tests to determine the optimal diagnostic approach for evaluating patients at-risk for disease.[9–16,18–21,49,56,58,59] Given the heterogeneity of the APS disease cohorts, the variability of the analytes (aPL), diversity of platforms as well as the way patients are diagnose with APS, no consensus has emerged. In a very elegant study, De Craemer and colleagues[19] 2016 investigated the role of anti–domain I antibodies in the diagnosis and risk stratification of APS and showed its relevance in predicting thrombosis and triple aPL positivity. A subsequent study by Chayoua and colleagues[53] showed that identification of APS patients with a high risk for thrombosis associated with triple aPL positivity depends on the assays used to detect aCL and anti-β_2GPI antibodies. This observation implies careful examination between existing tests for APS and their correlations with anti–domain I antibodies by clinical laboratories before their adoption. Compared with anti–domain I antibodies, the evaluation of aPS/PT as a diagnostic marker has focused on its correlations with LAC as well as alternative to aCL testing given its high sensitivity.[10,12,13,39,40] In a recent investigation, the use of aPS/PT antibodies and anti–domain I antibodies were proposed as first-line noncriteria aPL tests. Given the consistent characterizations and availability of commercial tests with comparable analytical performance characteristics to current criteria aPL antibody assays, it seems to be logical to integrate aPS/PT antibodies and anti–domain I testing in patients at-risk for APS who are seronegative in criteria tests. In addition, both markers may be useful when current tests are equivocal for APS or in the case of aPL carriers.

SUMMARY

Although APS is well-described, it is difficult to diagnose definitively because there are numerous nonautoimmune causes of thrombosis and pregnancy-related morbidity. Misdiagnosis of APS can have significant adverse consequences, but a missed diagnosis can result in devastating consequences. Thus, the goal is to develop and standardize the most comprehensive, sensitive, specific, reliable, robust, and cost-effective panel of aPL tests that ideally will only detect clinically relevant antibodies. Data from multiple studies demonstrate that testing for aPS/PT antibodies offers comparable sensitivity to aCL antibodies with significant overlap with LAC, whereas anti–

domain I antibodies are significantly associated with the risk for thrombosis and triple aPL positivity.

REFERENCES

1. Miyakis S, Lockshin MD, Atsumi T, et al. International consensus statement on an update of the classification criteria for definite antiphospholipid syndrome (APS). J Thromb Haemost 2006;4:295–306.
2. Lakos G, Favaloro EJ, Harris EN, et al. International consensus guidelines on anti-cardiolipin and anti-β2-glycoprotein I testing: report from the 13th International Congress on antiphospholipid antibodies. Arthritis Rheum 2012;64:1–10.
3. Favaloro EJ. Variability and diagnostic utility of antiphospholipid antibodies including lupus anticoagulants. Int J Lab Hematol 2013;35:269–74.
4. Tebo AE. Antiphospholipid syndrome and the relevance of antibodies to negatively charged phospholipids in diagnostic evaluation. Lupus 2014;23:1313–6.
5. Bertolaccini ML, Amengual O, Atsumi T, et al. Non-criteria' aPL tests: report of a task force and preconference workshop at the 13th International Congress on Antiphospholipid Antibodies, Galveston, TX, USA, April 2010. Lupus 2011;20:91–205.
6. Bertolaccini ML, Amengual O, Andreoli L, et al. 14th international congress on antiphospholipid antibodies task force. Report on antiphospholipid syndrome laboratory diagnostics and trends. Autoimmun Rev 2014;13:917–30.
7. Alessandri C, Conti F, Pendolino M, et al. New autoantigens in the antiphospholipid syndrome. Autoimmun Rev 2011;10:609–16.
8. Atsumi T, Koike K. Antiprothrombin antibody: why do we need more assays? Lupus 2010;19:436–9.
9. Pregnolato F, Chighizola CB, Encabo S, et al. Anti-phosphatidylserine/prothrombin antibodies: an additional diagnostic marker for APS? Immunol Res 2013;56:432–8.
10. Heikal N, Jaskowski TD, Malmberg E, et al. Laboratory evaluation of antiphospholipid syndrome: a preliminary prospective study of phosphatidylserine/prothrombin antibodies in an at –risk patient cohort. Clin Exp Immunol 2015;180:218–26.
11. Lee JS, Gu J, Park HS, et al. Coexistence of anti-β2-glycoprotein I domain I and anti-phosphatidylserine/prothrombin antibodies suggests strong thrombotic risk. Clin Chem Lab Med 2017;55:882–9.
12. Litvinova E, Darnige L, Kirilovsky A, et al. Prevalence and significance of non-conventional antiphospholipid antibodies in patients with clinical APS criteria. Front Immunol 2018;9:2971.
13. Nakamura H, Oku K, Amengual O, et al. First-line, non-criterial antiphospholipid antibody testing for the diagnosis of antiphospholipid syndrome in clinical practice: a combination of anti-β2 glycoprotein I domain I and phosphatidylserine-dependent antiprothrombin antibodies. Arthritis Care Res 2018;4:627–34.
14. Žigon P, Podovšovnik A, Ambrožič A, et al. Added value of non-criteria antiphospholipid antibodies for antiphospholipid syndrome: lessons learned from year-long routine measurements. Clin Rheumatol 2019;38:371–8.
15. Núñez-Álvarez CA, Hernández-Molina G, Bermúdez-Bermejo P, et al. Prevalence and associations of anti-phosphatidylserine/prothrombin antibodies with clinical phenotypes in patients with primary antiphospholipid syndrome: aPS/PT antibodies in primary antiphospholipid syndrome. Thromb Res 2019;174:141–7.

16. Canti V, Del Rosso S, Tonello M, et al. Antiphosphatidylserine/prothrombin antibodies in antiphospholipid syndrome with intrauterine growth restriction and pre-eclampsia. J Rheumatol 2018;45:1263–72.

17. Tonello M, Mattia E, Favaro M, et al. IgG phosphatidylserine/prothrombin antibodies as a risk factor of thrombosis in antiphospholipid antibody carriers. Thromb Res 2019;177:157–60.

18. Meneghel L, Ruffatti A, Gavasso S, et al. Detection of IgG anti-Domain I beta2 Glycoprotein I antibodies by chemiluminescence immunoassay in primary antiphospholipid syndrome. Clin Chim Acta 2015;446:201–5.

19. De Craemer AS, Musial J, Devreese KM. Role of anti-domain 1-β2 glycoprotein I antibodies in the diagnosis and risk stratification of antiphospholipid syndrome. J Thromb Haemost 2016;14:1779–87.

20. Zhang S, Wu Z, Zhang F, et al. Role of anti-domain 1- β_2 glycoprotein I antibodies in the diagnosis and risk stratification of antiphospholipid syndrome: comment. J Thromb Haemost 2016;14:2076–8.

21. Iwaniec T, Kaczor MP, Celińska-Löwenhoff M, et al. Clinical significance of anti-domain 1 β2-glycoprotein I antibodies in antiphospholipid syndrome. Thromb Res 2017;153:90–4.

22. Tonello M, Mattia E, Del Ross T, et al. Clinical value of anti-domain I-β2Glycoprotein 1 antibodies in antiphospholipid antibody carriers. A single centre, prospective observational follow-up study. Clin Chim Acta 2018;485:74–8.

23. Wilson WA, Gharavi AE, Koike T, et al. International consensus statement on preliminary classification criteria for definite antiphospholipid syndrome: report of an international workshop. Arthritis Rheum 1999;42:1309–11.

24. Pengo V, Biasiolo A, Pegoraro C, et al. Antibody profiles for the diagnosis of antiphospholipid syndrome. Thromb Haemost 2005;93:1147–52.

25. Budd R, Harley E, Quarshie A, et al. A re-appraisal of the normal cut-off assignment for anticardiolipin IgM tests. J Thromb Haemost 2006;4:2210–4.

26. Ruffatti A, Olivieri S, Tonello M, et al. Influence of different IgG anticardiolipin antibody cut-off values on antiphospholipid syndrome classification. J Thromb Haemost 2008;6:1693–6.

27. Harris EN, Gharavi AE, Boey ML, et al. Anticardiolipin antibodies: detection by radioimmunoassay and association with thrombosis in systemic lupus erythematosus. Lancet 1983;2:1211–4.

28. Loizou S, McCrea JD, Rudge AC, et al. Measurement of anti-cardiolipin antibodies by an enzyme-linked immunosorbent assay (ELISA): standardization and quantitation of results. Clin Exp Immunol 1985;62:738–45.

29. McNeil HP, Simpson RJ, Chesterman CN, et al. Anti-phospholipid antibodies are directed against a complex antigen that includes lipid-binding inhibitor of coagulation: beta 2-glycoprotein I (apolipoprotein H). Proc Natl Acad Sci U S A 1990;87:4120–4.

30. Matsuura E, Igarashi Y, Fujimoto M, et al. Anticardiolipin cofactor(s) and differential diagnosis of autoimmune disease. Lancet 1990;336:177–8.

31. Galli M, Comfurius P, Maassen C, et al. Anticardilipoin antibodies (ACA) directed not to cardiolipin but to a plasma protein cofactor. Lancet 1990;335:1544–7.

32. Day HM, Thiagarajan P, Ahn C, et al. Autoantibodies to beta2-glycoprotein I in systemic lupus erythematosus and primary antiphospholipid antibody syndrome: clinical correlations in comparison with other antiphospholipid antibody tests. J Rheumatol 1998;25:667–74.

33. Danowski A, Kickler TS, Petri M. Anti–beta2-glycoprotein I: prevalence, clinical correlations, and importance of persistent positivity in patients with antiphospholipid syndrome and systemic lupus erythematosus. J Rheumatol 2006;33:1775–9.
34. Galli M, Luciani D, Bertolini G, et al. Lupus anticoagulants are stronger risk factors for thrombosis than anticardiolipin antibodies in the antiphospholipid syndrome: a systematic review of the literature. Blood 2003;101:1827–32.
35. Kelchtermans H, Pelkmans L, de Laat B, et al. IgG/IgM antiphospholipid antibodies present in the classification criteria for the antiphospholipid syndrome: a critical review of their association with thrombosis. J Thromb Haemost 2016; 14:1530–48.
36. Arvieux J, Darnige L, Caron C, et al. Development of an ELISA for autoantibodies to prothrombin showing their prevalence in patients with lupus anticoagulants. Thromb Haemost 1995;74:1120–5.
37. Galli M, Beretta G, Daldossi M, et al. Different anticoagulant and immunological properties of anti-prothrombin antibodies in patients with antiphospholipid antibodies. Thromb Haemost 1997;77:486–91.
38. Funke A, Bertolaccini ML, Atsumi T, et al. Autoantibodies to prothrombin-phosphatidylserine complex: clinical significance in systemic lupus erythematosus. Arthritis Rheum 1998;41:S240.
39. Atsumi T, Ieko M, Bertolaccini ML, et al. Association of autoantibodies against the phosphatidylserine-prothrombin complex with manifestations of the antiphospholipid syndrome and with the presence of lupus anticoagulant. Arthritis Rheum 2000;43:1982–93.
40. Bertolaccini ML, Atsumi T, Koike T, et al. Antiprothrombin antibodies detected in two different assay systems. Prevalence and clinical significance in systemic lupus erythematosus. Thromb Haemost 2005;93:289–97.
41. Chinnaraj M, Planer W, Pengo V, et al. Discovery and characterization of 2 novel subpopulations of aPS/PT antibodies in patients at high risk of thrombosis. Blood Adv 2019;3:1738–49.
42. Peterson LK, Willis R, Harris EN, et al. Antibodies to phosphatidylserine/prothrombin complex in antiphospholipid syndrome: analytical and clinical perspectives. Adv Clin Chem 2016;73:1–28.
43. de Laat B, Mertens K, de Groot PG. Mechanisms of disease: antiphospholipid antibodies-from clinical association to pathologic mechanism. Nat Clin Pract Rheumatol 2008;4:192–9.
44. Steinkasser A, Barlow PN, Willis AC, et al. Activity, disulfide mapping and structural modeling of the fifth domain of human β2-glycoprotein I. FEBS Lett 1992; 313:193–7.
45. de Laat B, Derksen RH, Urbanus RT, et al. IgG antibodies that recognize epitope Gly40-Arg43 in domain I of beta 2-glycoprotein I cause LAC, and their presence correlates strongly with thrombosis. Blood 2005;105:1540–5.
46. de Laat B, Pengo V, Pabinger I, et al. The association between circulating antibodies against domain I of beta2-glycoprotein I and thrombosis: an international multicenter study. J Thromb Haemost 2009;7:1767–73.
47. Banzato A, Pozzi N, Frasson R, et al. Antibodies to Domain I of beta(2)Glycoprotein I are in close relation to patients risk categories in Antiphospholipid Syndrome (APS). Thromb Res 2011;128:583–6.
48. Persijn L, Decavele AS, Schouwers S, et al. Evaluation of a new set of automated chemiluminescence assays for anticardiolipin and anti-beta2-glycoprotein I antibodies in the laboratory diagnosis of the antiphospholipid syndrome. Thromb Res 2011;128:565–9.

49. Zhang S, Wu Z, Li P, et al. Evaluation of the clinical performance of a novel chemi-luminescent immunoassay for detection of anticardiolipin and anti-beta2-glycoprotein 1 antibodies in the diagnosis of antiphospholipid syndrome. Medicine (Baltimore) 2015;94:e2059.

50. Montaruli B, De Luna E, Erroi L, et al. Analytical and clinical comparison of different immunoassay systems for the detection of antiphospholipid antibodies. Int J Lab Hematol 2016;38:172–82.

51. Martins TB, Heikal N, Miller J, et al. Assessment of diagnostic methods for the detection of anticardiolipin and anti-βeta2 glycoprotein I antibodies in patients under routine evaluation for antiphospholipid syndrome. Clin Chim Acta 2018; 485:7–13.

52. Chayoua W, Kelchtermans H, Moore GW, et al. Detection of anti-cardiolipin and anti-β2glycoprotein I antibodies differs between platforms without influence on association with clinical symptoms. Thromb Haemost 2019;119:797–806.

53. Chayoua W, Kelchtermans H, Moore GW, et al. Identification of high thrombotic risk triple-positive antiphospholipid syndrome patients is dependent on anti-cardiolipin and anti-β2glycoprotein I antibody detection assays. J Thromb Haemost 2018;16:2016–23.

54. Jaskowski TD, Wilson AR, Hill HR, et al. Autoantibodies against phosphatidylserine, prothrombin and phosphatidylserine-prothrombin complex: identical or distinct diagnostic tools for antiphospholipid syndrome? Clin Chim Acta 2009; 410:19–24.

55. Amengual O, Horita T, Binder W, et al. Comparative analysis of different enzyme immunoassays for assessment of phosphatidylserine-dependent antiprothrombin antibodies. Rheumatol Int 2014;32:1225–30.

56. Amengual O, Forastiero R, Sugiura-Ogasawara M, et al. Evaluation of phosphatidylserine-dependent antiprothrombin antibody testing for the diagnosis of antiphospholipid syndrome: results of an international multicentre study. Lupus 2017;26:266–76.

57. Yin D, de Laat B, Devreese KMJ, et al. The clinical value of assays detecting antibodies against domain I of β2-glycoprotein I in the antiphospholipid syndrome. Autoimmun Rev 2018;17:1210–8.

58. Bardin N, Alessi MC, Dignat-George F, et al. Does the anti-prothrombin antibodies measurement provide additional information in patients with thrombosis? Immunobiology 2007;212:557–65.

59. Sciascia S, Murru V, Sanna G, et al. Clinical accuracy for diagnosis of antiphospholipid syndrome in systemic lupus erythematosus: evaluation of 23 possible combinations of antiphospholipid antibody specificities. J Thromb Haemost 2012;10:2512–8.

60. Vlagea A, Gil A, Cuesta MV, et al. Antiphosphatidylserine/prothrombin antibodies (aPS/PT) as potential markers of antiphospholipid syndrome. Clin Appl Thromb Hemost 2013;19:289–96.

Diagnostic Pitfalls in Immunology Testing

Lewena Maher, MD[a], Cory Perugino, DO[b,c,*]

KEYWORDS

- Autoantibody • Rheumatoid factor • ANA • ANCA • Antiphospholipid • IgG4

KEY POINTS

- Rheumatoid factor is linked to the pathogenesis of seropositive rheumatoid arthritis, but low-titer values are unlikely to be of clinical importance.
- Both rheumatoid factor and antinuclear antibodies may precede the onset of their associated clinical presentations by upwards of a decade.
- Low-titer antiphospholipid antibodies and isolated IgM antiphospholipid antibodies are not strongly associated with the clinical syndrome of antiphospholipid syndrome.
- Both drug-induced positives and false positives are important considerations in indirect immunofluorescence testing that require confirmatory enzyme-linked immunosorbent assay testing.
- Serum IgG4 elevation is not specific to IgG4-related disease and the prozone phenomenon can result in spuriously low IgG4 levels.

RHEUMATOID FACTOR AND THE PATHOGENESIS OF RHEUMATOID ARTHRITIS

Rheumatoid factor (RF) was originally discovered by Erik Waaler in 1940 with his observation that sera from patients with rheumatoid arthritis caused agglutination of sheep red blood cells sensitized with rabbit antisheep red cell serum.[1,2] Subsequent work demonstrated that this reaction was due to a specific antibody in the sera of rheumatoid arthritis patients directed against human gamma globulin.[3,4] These autoantibodies are most commonly of the IgM isotype, which is routinely tested for, but IgA- and IgG-RF are also described and may be of diagnostic value.[5] Testing for RF is relevant when the diagnoses of rheumatoid arthritis, Sjögren's syndrome, or cryoglobulinemic vasculitis are being considered.

Disclosure Statement: The authors have nothing to disclose.
[a] Internal Medicine, Beth Israel Lahey Health, Burlington, MA, USA; [b] Division of Rheumatology, Allergy and Immunology, Massachusetts General Hospital, Boston, MA, USA; [c] Ragon Institute of MGH, MIT and Harvard, Cambridge, MA, USA
* Corresponding author. Ragon Institute of MGH, MIT and Harvard, 400 Technology Square, Cambridge, MA 02139.
E-mail address: cperugino@mgh.harvard.edu

Clin Lab Med 39 (2019) 567–578
https://doi.org/10.1016/j.cll.2019.07.005
0272-2712/19/© 2019 Elsevier Inc. All rights reserved.

labmed.theclinics.com

The Pathogenic Role of Rheumatoid Factor in Rheumatoid Arthritis

Despite the considerable time since its discovery and in contrast with the significant understanding related to anticitrullinated protein antibodies in the pathogenesis of rheumatoid arthritis, many unknowns persist regarding the pathogenic role of RF.[6] A prevailing hypothesis with supportive experimental data posits that RF binds to anticitrullinated protein antibodies–immune complexes and potentiates the proinflammatory responses to anticitrullinated protein antibodies.[7,8] Additionally, it is very unusual for a patient with rheumatoid arthritis that is seronegative at the time of presentation to seroconvert to RF (or anticitrullinated protein antibodies) positivity after the onset of clinically evident joint inflammation.[9,10] This observation supports the notion that RF has a causal or permissive role in the disease pathogenesis rather than occurring as an immunologic epiphenomenon of chronic inflammation. Epidemiologic studies have also demonstrated a strong correlation between the RF titer observed preclinically and the risk of developing rheumatoid arthritis.[11] In the context of interpreting a positive RF test, it is important to realize that RF positivity can precede the clinical syndrome of rheumatoid arthritis by more than a decade.[11]

Diagnostic Value of Rheumatoid Factor in Seropositive Rheumatoid Arthritis

The diagnostic value of RF is largely dependent on the clinical setting from which it is tested. In the general internal medicine setting, RF testing is of limited value as a screening tool carrying a low positive predictive value of only approximately 30%.[12] In contrast, the diagnostic value of the test is enhanced in a setting that is enriched for rheumatoid arthritis patients, such as a rheumatology subspecialty clinic, when the sensitivity of the test approximates 70%.[13–15] Although IgM-RF is the isotype most commonly observed and the one routinely tested for in most clinical laboratories, IgA-RF has also been linked to disease pathogenesis and prognosis in rheumatoid arthritis.[8,16,17] Moreover, IgA-RF has been shown to have comparable sensitivity with greater specificity to IgM-RF in the setting of rheumatoid arthritis.[5]

Rheumatoid Factor Is Not Specific to Rheumatoid Arthritis

Although most commonly tested by clinicians in the evaluation of inflammatory arthritis, RF is not specific for this condition.[18] RF has been reported in association with many rheumatologic and nonrheumatologic conditions (**Box 1**). Numerically, RF positivity carries a specificity of approximately 80% for rheumatoid arthritis but increases to 98% when combined with dual positivity for both RF and anticitrullinated protein antibodies.[14] Depending on the clinical context in which the test was sent, high-titer positive results are diagnostically consistent with preclinical rheumatoid arthritis, seropositive rheumatoid arthritis, Sjögren's syndrome, and cryoglobulinemic vasculitis.[6,19–22] Although 4% of healthy individuals will test positive for RF without

---

Box 1
RF disease associations

Rheumatologic diseases
  Rheumatoid arthritis, primary Sjögren's syndrome, juvenile idiopathic arthritis, psoriatic arthritis, reactive arthritis, SLE, systemic sclerosis, mixed connective tissue disease, polymyositis/dermatomyositis, sarcoidosis, mixed cryoglobulinemia

Nonrheumatologic diseases
  Hepatitis C virus, subacute bacterial endocarditis, tuberculosis, parvovirus, human immunodeficiency virus, primary biliary cirrhosis, malignancy

clinically evident disease, approximately 30% will go on to develop rheumatoid arthritis and this risk is directly correlated with the titer of RF observed.[23] Additionally, the RF seen in healthy individuals has been found to have limited evidence of having undergone somatic hypermutation and binds to Fc-IgG with a low affinity.[24] These observations suggest that a continuum of transient to chronic antigen exposure culminates in high-affinity, high-titer RF and joint inflammation in a minority of seemingly healthy individuals with a positive RF test.

THE UBIQUITOUS NATURE OF ANTINUCLEAR ANTIBODIES

Antinuclear antibody (ANA) testing is an essential feature of the diagnostic evaluation of many autoimmune diseases including systemic lupus erythematosus (SLE), systemic sclerosis, mixed connective tissue disease, Sjögren's syndrome, autoimmune hepatitis, and primary biliary cirrhosis. The most widely used assay for testing the presence of ANAs is indirect immunofluorescence and understanding the mechanics of this assay and rationale behind reporting the test are important in the interpretation of the results.

Indirect Immunofluorescence and Stipulations of Antinuclear Antibody Interpretation

The presence of autoantibodies specific to a nuclear antigen are assessed by the steps of fixing human cells to a glass slide, permeabilizing the cells, incubating the cells with patient plasma, washing off any unbound antibody, detecting bound immunoglobulin using a fluorescently labeled antihuman IgG antibody, and observing nuclear reactivity by fluorescent microscopy. The gold standard assay uses the human epidermoid carcinoma (HEp-2) cell line as a substrate partially because HEp-2 cells express the vast majority of autoantigens relevant to clinical diagnosis. Serial plasma dilutions are tested for reactivity as a surrogate measure of antibody affinity and abundance, with greater dilutions indicating more mature and/or abundant ANAs. Because ANAs occur at a high frequency in the putatively healthy population, a titer of 1:40 as the cut-off for positivity and a titer of 1:160 as a more specific indicator of autoimmune disease has been proposed.[25] The low titer of 1:40, which is observed in approximately 30% of the putatively healthy population, was chosen as an appropriate lower limit of positivity so as to maximize the sensitivity of this test in detecting suspected autoimmune disease.[25] A positive ANA at a 1:40 titer provides sensitivities of 100% for systemic sclerosis, 97% for SLE, and 84% for Sjögren's syndrome whereas the specificities for these diagnoses at this low titer are substantially less, 68% for each.[25] In contrast, a positive result at a 1:160 titer offers specificity of 95% for all 3 of these diagnoses.[25] An international consensus statement has recommended that each laboratory define their own positive cut-off values based on a sampling of the healthy population at each institution.[26]

Like the preclinical development of autoantibodies reported in rheumatoid arthritis, positive ANA results are observed in the majority of patients with SLE up to approximately 10 years before the clinical diagnosis.[27] Moreover, a positive ANA is one of the strongest predictors of subsequent development of lupus among family members of patients with lupus.[28] Therefore, although of low specificity, a low-titer ANA does not in and of itself indicate inconsequentiality and needs to be interpreted in the appropriate clinical context. However, with an estimated prevalence of ANA-associated connective tissue disease of less than 1% and 30% of healthy individuals testing positive for an ANA at a titer of 1:40, the vast majority of such results will ultimately be of little importance. Titers of 1:160 or greater are generally used as indicators to pursue additional and more specific autoantibody testing.[29]

Negative Antinuclear Antibody Results with High Clinical Suspicion for a Rheumatologic Disease

One limitation of using HEp-2 cells as the substrate for detecting the presence of ANAs is that this cell line does not express or expresses only at low levels, certain clinically important autoantigens. These include the Ro60 protein, with anti-Ro60 antibodies being most relevant to subacute cutaneous lupus erythematosus, neonatal lupus and primary Sjögren's syndrome, and ribosomal P proteins, with antibodies being specific for a diagnosis of SLE.[30–32] Additionally, antibodies directed against the melanoma differentiation-associated protein, histidyl-tRNA synthetase, and 3-hydroxy-3-methylglutaryl-coenzyme A reductase, all associated with idiopathic inflammatory myositis are poorly detected by indirect immunofluorescence assays on HEp-2 cells.[26,33,34] When these diagnoses are strongly suspected based on clinical grounds, more sensitive solid phase assays such as enzyme-linked immunosorbent assays (ELISA) are needed to assess antibodies to these antigens. In contrast to other more specific autoantibodies such as anti-dsDNA antibodies, the ANA titer does not correlate with disease activity and serial testing in an individual patient has no clinical value.

THE CONUNDRUM OF ANTIPHOSPHOLIPID ANTIBODY TESTING

Antiphospholipid syndrome is a disease of recurrent vascular thrombosis and/or obstetric complications occurring in the context of persistently positive autoantibodies directed against phospholipids (antiphospholipid antibodies [aPL]).[35] This disease is most often diagnostically considered in the setting of a patient presenting with idiopathic deep venous thrombosis, pulmonary embolism, arterial thrombosis, or recurrent pregnancy complications without an otherwise more evident explanation. The cornerstone of confirming the diagnosis relies on the demonstration of specific autoantibodies, usually by a solid phase assay such as ELISA, directed against phospholipids (anticardiolipin and anti–beta-2-glycoprotein I antibodies) or the presence of a lupus anticoagulant by a liquid phase coagulation assay.[35] Here, we focus on solid phase assays to detect aPL antibodies, which are commonly performed by clinical immunology laboratories as opposed to liquid phase assays, which are generally performed by hematology laboratories.

Assays to Detect Antiphospholipid Antibodies Are Not Standardized and Overly Sensitive

The aPL are reported in arbitrary GPL or MPL units, reflecting IgG aPL or IgM aPL antibodies, respectively, in reference to a set of calibrator standards. However, the variable use of monoclonal or polyclonal aPL antibodies as standards and the lack of an agreed upon international standard to use results in striking interlaboratory variation in reported results.[36] Although the extreme interlaboratory variability confounds epidemiologic studies related to these autoantibodies, in clinical practice this topic is only of relevance if the standards used for the assay were to change, thereby making older results not comparable with subsequent confirmatory results, or in the interpretation of results from outside institutions.

In addition to these issues with lack of standardization, these solid phase assays are also hypersensitive resulting in the very common identification of low-titer positive results of equivocal diagnostic usefulness. Furthermore, although many aPL antibodies are pathogenic, particularly antibodies directed against domain I of beta-2-glycoprotein I, a protein expressed on the surface of cells involved in coagulation, not all anticardiolipin antibodies are pathogenic.[37–39] The high sensitivity of solid phase assays results in the detection of both pathogenic and nonpathogenic aPL antibodies, including transiently positive antibodies that often arise in the acute inflammatory setting of an infectious process.[36,40,41] Additionally, the pathogenicity and clinical relevance of isolated IgM-aPL antibodies without IgG-aPL antibodies remain unresolved matters of debate.[39] Knowledge of the possibility of detecting nonpathogenic and transient aPL antibodies is essential in clinical decision making, particularly in the hospital setting when many of these tests are ordered (**Box 2**). Although low-titer aPL antibody results (20–40 GPL or MPL units) are statistically abnormal compared with the controls used in the assay, they are generally considered nonspecific, unlikely to be of pathologic importance, and not associated with the clinical syndrome of antiphospholipid syndrome.[42] These results need to be interpreted in the clinical context of the patient. Owing to the myriad issues with aPL testing (see **Box 2**), the laboratory criteria to stratify patients at risk for antiphospholipid syndrome require a moderate to high-titer aPL antibody result (>40 GPL or MPL units) that is persistently positive on 2 or more occasions at least 12 weeks apart.[43]

ANTINEUTROPHIL CYTOPLASMIC ANTIBODIES IN CONSIDERATION OF VASCULITIS

Antineutrophil cytoplasmic antibody (ANCA)-associated vasculitides (AAV) constitute a collection of diseases marked by inflammation of small and medium-sized blood vessels in association with ANCA.[44] The specific disease labels within this group include granulomatosis with polyangiitis, microscopic polyangiitis, and eosinophilic granulomatosis with polyangiitis. Histologically defined by the presence of leukocytoclastic infiltration of the walls of small blood vessels paired with tissue necrosis, these conditions are potentially fatal but fortunately treatable when diagnosed early.[45,46] Specifically, B-cell–depleting therapy with rituximab has demonstrated great efficacy in treating these diseases, highlighting the important role of B cells as disease drivers.[46–48]

The Pathogenicity of Antineutrophil Cytoplasmic Antibodies and the Central Role of Neutrophils in Antineutrophil Cytoplasmic Antibody–Associated Vasculitides

ANCAs occur in 2 major forms: those directed against proteinase-3 (PR-3) and those directed against myeloperoxidase (MPO), 2 proteins expressed by neutrophils. Antibodies targeting MPO are observed on indirect immunofluorescence as peri-nuclear staining and termed p-ANCA, whereas those targeting PR-3 result in a more diffuse cytoplasmic staining pattern and are referred to as c-ANCA. Numerous animal models have demonstrated the pathogenic potential of ANCAs, with both passive transfer and active immunization resulting in a vasculitic syndrome consistent with human

---

Box 2
Considerations in aPL antibody testing

- Isolated IgM aPL antibodies of unclear pathogenic relevance
- Transiently positive aPL antibodies arise in the setting of infection
- Solid phase assays detect both pathogenic and nonpathogenic aPL antibodies
- Low-titer aPL antibodies not clearly associated with clinical syndrome

AAV.[49,50] The prevailing disease model of AAV entails primed neutrophils expressing target antigens (MPO, PR-3) on the cell surface, ANCAs binding to these antigens, bound ANCA-Fc activating neighboring neutrophils via Fc receptors resulting in the release of lytic enzymes, reactive oxygen species and neutrophil extracellular traps, thereby driving tissue inflammation and damage.[51,52]

Indirect Immunofluorescence Is Imperfect and Not All Antineutrophil Cytoplasmic Antibodies Are Pathogenic

A not infrequent clinical scenario is the identification of a positive ANCA by indirect immunofluorescence paired with a negative ELISA for PR-3 or MPO. How to interpret this discrepant result is a source of confusion for clinicians. Indirect immunofluorescence of fixed and permeabilized neutrophils to detect a perinuclear or cytoplasmic staining pattern is the gold standard test to screen for the presence of ANCAs. However, it is important to recognize the limitations of this test. A positive indirect immunofluorescence test is not specific for the diagnosis of AAV and carries a positive predictive value of less than 50%.[53] In contrast, the high sensitivity of this screening test is evinced by the very high negative predictive value, which approaches 100%.[53] A portion of false positive ANCAs by this approach is related to the subjectivity in interpreting an immunofluorescent pattern. An established confounding factor in this interpretation is nuclear staining in a patient with a positive ANA that can result in the mislabeling of a positive p-ANCA.[54]

Although PR-3 and MPO are considered to be important autoantigens in the pathogenesis of AAV, there are many other proteins expressed by neutrophils that can be the target of autoantibody responses. These minor ANCA targets include α-enolase, cathepsin G, elastase, and lysosome-associated membrane protein 2, among others.[55–57] However, the pathogenic role of these minor ANCAs is not clearly established.[44] If present, antibodies targeting any of these minor antigens will produce a positive indirect immunofluorescence result that is unlikely to be clinically relevant. When present, antibodies against minor ANCAs only will cause a positive indirect immunofluorescence result with negative ELISA testing for MPO or PR-3. Taken together, these technical issues highlight the necessity of confirming the screening assay with more specific solid phase assays, most often ELISA, to confirm the presence of antibodies targeting PR-3 or MPO.[53]

Culprit Medications Can Induce Antineutrophil Cytoplasmic Antibodies Seropositivity or Even Antineutrophil Cytoplasmic Antibody–Associated Vasculitides

Contributing to the issues related to false-positive ANCA testing as described is a collection of commonly used medications that can induce the development of ANCAs (**Box 3**). Of these, hydralazine, propylthiouracil, minocycline, and

---

Box 3
Medications associated with drug-induced ANCA

Thyroid related: Propylthiouracil, methimazole, thiamazole, carbimazole

Cardiovascular medications: hydralazine, procainamide

Gout related: allopurinol, indomethacin

Anti-infectives: minocycline, rifampicin, cefotaxime, isoniazid, levamisole

Neuroleptic medications: clozapine, phenytoin

levamisole-adulterated cocaine are considered to be the most common offending agents, resulting in the clinical syndrome of drug-induced AAV.[58] In particular, these 4 molecules can induce a positive p-ANCA with MPO antibodies, most often at very high titers, along with the clinical syndrome of AAV.[58–61] Levamisole, a contaminant in a majority of illicit cocaine consumed in the United States, classically induces double positivity of both MPO and PR-3 antibodies, which is considered nearly pathognomonic for levamisole-induced AAV and should prompt testing the urine for the presence of cocaine and levamisole.[58,62]

SERUM IgG4 LEVEL IN CONSIDERATION OF IgG4-RELATED DISEASE

IgG4-related disease (IgG4-RD) is a relatively recently described immune-mediated fibrotic disease clinically phenotyped by tumor-like masses, often with multiorgan involvement, resulting in organ dysfunction.[63] The disease is defined both by a typical organ distribution of involvement (lacrimal glands, salivary glands, pancreas, bile ducts, kidneys, retroperitoneum) and the histopathologic findings of a dense lymphoplasmacytic infiltrate, fibrosis in a swirling or storiform pattern, and obliterative phlebitis.[64] The relevance to the IgG4 molecule lies in the plasma cells infiltrating the tissues being largely skewed to expressing this isotype, typically with greater than 40% of IgG^+ plasma cells being $IgG4^+$.[64] Furthermore, the serum IgG4 level is elevated in a majority of patients and seems to correlate with the extent of organ involvement, as well as the likelihood for the disease to relapse after treatment-induced remission.[65,66] Finally, multiple autoantibodies have been described in the context of IgG4-RD, most of which are specifically of the IgG4 isotype and some data suggest a pathogenic role of IgG4 autoantibodies in this disease.[67–71]

Elevated Serum IgG4 is Not Specific to the Diagnosis of IgG4-Related Disease

IgG4 class switching is an immunologic phenomenon that is only observed in the setting of chronic antigen-driven B-cell activation.[72] A classic example of this process is the observation that bee keepers develop a progressively skewed IgG response that is eventually dominated by IgG4 specific to bee venom antigens over the course of their careers.[73] Mildly elevated serum IgG4 levels are also seen in the context of chronic allergen exposure, which has been documented in patients receiving immunotherapy in the treatment of chronic allergic disease.[74] More broadly, it is important to consider an increased serum IgG4 level as indicative of chronic antigen exposure rather than diagnostic of IgG4-RD. In one of the largest studies relevant to this topic, 34% of all comers with an elevated serum IgG4 level at a tertiary referral center specializing in IgG4-RD were due to definite or probable IgG4-RD with 24% accounted for by chronic sinusitis and 18% by recurrent pneumonia.[75] In this study, it was rare for a non-IgG4-RD diagnosis to drive an IgG4 serum level of greater than 500 mg/dL, except for 2 cases of leukemia, 1 of 11 cases of connective tissue disease, and 1 of 29 cases of recurrent pneumonia included in the 190 patients examined.[75] In this regard, elevated serum IgG4 carries very low specificity for diagnosing IgG4-RD, but the degree of expansion may be relevant. Similarly, an exuberant IgG4-skewed B-cell response can be observed in various chronically inflamed tissues, such as the synovium of rheumatoid arthritis and cancer tissues with associated immune responses, in addition to IgG4-RD.[76] Relevant to the differential diagnosis of IgG4-RD, it is essential to realize that the common disease mimickers of AAV and malignancy can mirror the tissue and blood IgG4 expansions.[64,75,77,78]

The Prozone Phenomenon Is an Important Cause of Falsely Normal IgG4 Results

IgG4 serum concentrations are most often quantified by nephelometry. This assay measures the amount of light scattered by immune complexes that have formed in solution and the measurement is translated into plasma concentration based on concurrently run standards of known concentration to generate a standard curve. In a scenario of excessive antigen (plasma IgG4 in this case), the abundant antigen itself can interfere with the normal formation of antigen–antibody complexes, thereby preventing the development of lattices large enough to scatter light, which is termed the prozone effect.[79] The solution to this problem is to perform serial dilutions on a plasma sample so as to dilute the antigen excess into a range that is detectable by the assay. The prozone effect was investigated in a small cohort of IgG4-RD patients and found to have caused erroneously normal IgG4 results in over 20% of the patients studied.[80] Upon appropriately diluting a sample to account for this possibility, the resulting and more accurate serum IgG4 concentration may increase up to 600-fold compared with the undiluted sample.[80] This is an important laboratory consideration that may have grave implications on clinical decision making, for example, whether or not pursuing a biopsy is necessary or act in delaying the institution of effective treatment. Recognizing and creating a system to prevent the prozone effect in the nephelometric quantification of serum IgG4 is important for the reliability of such results from any immunology laboratory.

REFERENCES

1. Waaler E. On the occurrence of a factor in human serum activating the specific agglutination of sheep blood corpuscles. APMIS 1940;17:172–88.
2. Fraser KJ. The Waaler-Rose Test: anatomy of the eponym. Semin Arthritis Rheum 1988;18(1):61–71.
3. Epstein W, Johnson A, Ragan C. Observations on a precipitin reaction between serum of patients with rheumatoid arthritis and a preparation (Cohn fraction II) of human gamma globulin. Proc Soc Exp Biol Med 1956;91(2):235–7.
4. Franklin EC, Holman HR, Muller-Eberhard HJ, et al. An unusual protein component of high molecular weight in the serum of certain patients with rheumatoid arthritis. J Exp Med 1957;105(5):425–38.
5. Greiner A, Plischke H, Kellner H, et al. Association of anti-cyclic citrullinated peptide antibodies, anti-citrulline antibodies, and IgM and IgA rheumatoid factors with serological parameters of disease activity in rheumatoid arthritis. Ann N Y Acad Sci 2005;1050:295–303.
6. Malmström V, Catrina AI, Klareskog L. The immunopathogenesis of seropositive rheumatoid arthritis: from triggering to targeting. Nat Rev Immunol 2017;17(1):60–75.
7. Sokolove J, Johnson DS, Lahey LJ, et al. Rheumatoid factor as a potentiator of anti-citrullinated protein antibody-mediated inflammation in rheumatoid arthritis. Arthritis Rheumatol 2014;66(4):813–21.
8. Anquetil F, Clavel C, Offer G, et al. IgM and IgA rheumatoid factors purified from rheumatoid arthritis sera boost the Fc receptor- and complement-dependent effector functions of the disease-specific anti-citrullinated protein autoantibodies. J Immunol 2015;194(8):3664–74.
9. Rönnelid J, Wick MC, Lampa J, et al. Longitudinal analysis of citrullinated protein/peptide antibodies (anti-CP) during 5 year follow up in early rheumatoid arthritis: anti-CP status predicts worse disease activity and greater radiological progression. Ann Rheum Dis 2005;64(12):1744–9.

10. Nordberg LB, Lillegraven S, Aga A-B, et al. Comparing the disease course of patients with seronegative and seropositive rheumatoid arthritis fulfilling the 2010 ACR/EULAR classification criteria in a treat-to-target setting: 2-year data from the ARCTIC trial. RMD Open 2018;4(2):e000752.

11. Nielen MMJ, van Schaardenburg D, Reesink HW, et al. Specific autoantibodies precede the symptoms of rheumatoid arthritis: a study of serial measurements in blood donors. Arthritis Rheum 2004;50(2):380–6.

12. Shmerling RH, Delbanco TL. The rheumatoid factor: an analysis of clinical utility. Am J Med 1991;91(5):528–34.

13. Fathi NA, Ezz-Eldin AM, Mosad E, et al. Diagnostic performance and predictive value of rheumatoid factor, anti-cyclic-citrullinated peptide antibodies and HLA-DRB1 locus genes in rheumatoid arthritis. Int Arch Med 2008;1(1):20.

14. Chang P-Y, Yang C-T, Cheng C-H, et al. Diagnostic performance of anti-cyclic citrullinated peptide and rheumatoid factor in patients with rheumatoid arthritis. Int J Rheum Dis 2016;19(9):880–6.

15. Sun P, Wang W, Chen L, et al. Diagnostic value of autoantibodies combined detection for rheumatoid arthritis. J Clin Lab Anal 2017;31(5). https://doi.org/10.1002/jcla.22086.

16. Sakthiswary R, Shaharir SS, Mohd Said MS, et al. IgA rheumatoid factor as a serological predictor of poor response to tumour necrosis factor α inhibitors in rheumatoid arthritis. Int J Rheum Dis 2014;17(8):872–7.

17. Aleyd E, Al M, Tuk CW, et al. IgA complexes in plasma and synovial fluid of patients with rheumatoid arthritis induce neutrophil extracellular traps via FcαRI. J Immunol 2016;197(12):4552–9.

18. Ingegnoli F, Castelli R, Gualtierotti R. Rheumatoid factors: clinical applications. Dis Markers 2013;35(6):727–34.

19. Gorevic PD. Rheumatoid factor, complement, and mixed cryoglobulinemia. Clin Dev Immunol 2012;2012:439018.

20. Shen L, Suresh L. Autoantibodies, detection methods and panels for diagnosis of Sjögren's syndrome. Clin Immunol 2017;182:24–9.

21. Huo A-P, Lin K-C, Chou C-T. Predictive and prognostic value of antinuclear antibodies and rheumatoid factor in primary Sjogren's syndrome. Int J Rheum Dis 2010;13(1):39–47.

22. Sasso EH. The rheumatoid factor response in the etiology of mixed cryoglobulins associated with hepatitis C virus infection. Ann Med Interne 2000;151(1):30–40.

23. Nielsen SF, Bojesen SE, Schnohr P, et al. Elevated rheumatoid factor and long term risk of rheumatoid arthritis: a prospective cohort study. BMJ 2012;345:e5244.

24. Børretzen M, Chapman C, Natvig JB, et al. Differences in mutational patterns between rheumatoid factors in health and disease are related to variable heavy chain family and germ-line gene usage. Eur J Immunol 1997;27(3):735–41.

25. Tan EM, Feltkamp TE, Smolen JS, et al. Range of antinuclear antibodies in "healthy" individuals. Arthritis Rheum 1997;40(9):1601–11.

26. Agmon-Levin N, Damoiseaux J, Kallenberg C, et al. International recommendations for the assessment of autoantibodies to cellular antigens referred to as anti-nuclear antibodies. Ann Rheum Dis 2014;73(1):17–23.

27. Arbuckle MR, McClain MT, Rubertone MV, et al. Development of autoantibodies before the clinical onset of systemic lupus erythematosus. N Engl J Med 2003;349(16):1526–33.

28. Young KA, Munroe ME, Guthridge JM, et al. Screening characteristics for enrichment of individuals at higher risk for transitioning to classified SLE. Lupus 2019; 28(5):597–606.

29. Kang I, Siperstein R, Quan T, et al. Utility of age, gender, ANA titer and pattern as predictors of anti-ENA and -dsDNA antibodies. Clin Rheumatol 2004;23(6): 509–15.

30. Keech CL, Howarth S, Coates T, et al. Rapid and sensitive detection of anti-Ro (SS-A) antibodies by indirect immunofluorescence of 60kDa Ro HEp-2 transfectants. Pathology 1996;28(1):54–7.

31. Pollock W, Toh BH. Routine immunofluorescence detection of Ro/SS-A autoantibody using HEp-2 cells transfected with human 60 kDa Ro/SS-A. J Clin Pathol 1999;52(9):684–7.

32. Mahler M, Ngo JT, Schulte-Pelkum J, et al. Limited reliability of the indirect immunofluorescence technique for the detection of anti-Rib-P antibodies. Arthritis Res Ther 2008;10(6):R131.

33. Musset L, Miyara M, Benveniste O, et al. Analysis of autoantibodies to 3-hydroxy-3-methylglutaryl-coenzyme A reductase using different technologies. J Immunol Res 2014;2014:405956.

34. Palterer B, Vitiello G, Carraresi A, et al. Bench to bedside review of myositis autoantibodies. Clin Mol Allergy 2018;16:5.

35. Sciascia S, Amigo M-C, Roccatello D, et al. Diagnosing antiphospholipid syndrome: "extra-criteria" manifestations and technical advances. Nat Rev Rheumatol 2017;13(9):548–60.

36. Favaloro EJ. Variability and diagnostic utility of antiphospholipid antibodies including lupus anticoagulants. Int J Lab Hematol 2013;35(3):269–74.

37. de Laat B, Derksen RHWM, Urbanus RT, et al. IgG antibodies that recognize epitope Gly40-Arg43 in domain I of beta 2-glycoprotein I cause LAC, and their presence correlates strongly with thrombosis. Blood 2005;105(4):1540–5.

38. Pengo V, Ruffatti A, Tonello M, et al. Antiphospholipid syndrome: antibodies to Domain 1 of β2-glycoprotein 1 correctly classify patients at risk. J Thromb Haemost 2015;13(5):782–7.

39. Kelchtermans H, Pelkmans L, de Laat B, et al. IgG/IgM antiphospholipid antibodies present in the classification criteria for the antiphospholipid syndrome: a critical review of their association with thrombosis. J Thromb Haemost 2016; 14(8):1530–48.

40. Abdel-Wahab N, Lopez-Olivo MA, Pinto-Patarroyo GP, et al. Systematic review of case reports of antiphospholipid syndrome following infection. Lupus 2016; 25(14):1520–31.

41. Abdel-Wahab N, Talathi S, Lopez-Olivo MA, et al. Risk of developing antiphospholipid antibodies following viral infection: a systematic review and meta-analysis. Lupus 2018;27(4):572–83.

42. Roubey RAS. Risky business: the interpretation, use, and abuse of antiphospholipid antibody tests in clinical practice. Lupus 2010;19(4):440–5.

43. Miyakis S, Lockshin MD, Atsumi T, et al. International consensus statement on an update of the classification criteria for definite antiphospholipid syndrome (APS). J Thromb Haemost 2006;4(2):295–306.

44. Nakazawa D, Masuda S, Tomaru U, et al. Pathogenesis and therapeutic interventions for ANCA-associated vasculitis. Nat Rev Rheumatol 2019;15(2):91–101.

45. Jennette JC, Falk RJ, Bacon PA, et al. 2012 revised international Chapel Hill consensus conference nomenclature of vasculitides. Arthritis Rheum 2013; 65(1):1–11.

46. Stone JH, Merkel PA, Spiera R, et al. Rituximab versus cyclophosphamide for ANCA-associated vasculitis. N Engl J Med 2010;363(3):221–32.

47. Cornec D, Berti A, Hummel A, et al. Identification and phenotyping of circulating autoreactive proteinase 3-specific B cells in patients with PR3-ANCA associated vasculitis and healthy controls. J Autoimmun 2017;84:122–31.

48. Dumoitier N, Terrier B, London J, et al. Implication of B lymphocytes in the pathogenesis of ANCA-associated vasculitides. Autoimmun Rev 2015;14(11): 996–1004.

49. Xiao H, Heeringa P, Hu P, et al. Antineutrophil cytoplasmic autoantibodies specific for myeloperoxidase cause glomerulonephritis and vasculitis in mice. J Clin Invest 2002;110(7):955–63.

50. Little MA, Smyth L, Salama AD, et al. Experimental autoimmune vasculitis: an animal model of anti-neutrophil cytoplasmic autoantibody-associated systemic vasculitis. Am J Pathol 2009;174(4):1212–20.

51. Falk RJ, Terrell RS, Charles LA, et al. Anti-neutrophil cytoplasmic autoantibodies induce neutrophils to degranulate and produce oxygen radicals in vitro. Proc Natl Acad Sci U S A 1990;87(11):4115–9.

52. Kessenbrock K, Krumbholz M, Schönermarck U, et al. Netting neutrophils in autoimmune small-vessel vasculitis. Nat Med 2009;15(6):623–5.

53. Stone JH, Talor M, Stebbing J, et al. Test characteristics of immunofluorescence and ELISA tests in 856 consecutive patients with possible ANCA-associated conditions. Arthritis Care Res 2000;13(6):424–34.

54. Romero-Sánchez C, Benavides-Solarte M, Galindo-Ibáñez I, et al. Frequency of positive ANCA test in a population with clinical symptoms suggestive of autoimmune disease and the interference of ANA in its interpretation. Reumatol Clin 2019. https://doi.org/10.1016/j.reuma.2018.09.007.

55. Moodie FD, Leaker B, Cambridge G, et al. Alpha-enolase: a novel cytosolic autoantigen in ANCA positive vasculitis. Kidney Int 1993;43(3):675–81.

56. Talor MV, Stone JH, Stebbing J, et al. Antibodies to selected minor target antigens in patients with anti-neutrophil cytoplasmic antibodies (ANCA). Clin Exp Immunol 2007;150(1):42–8.

57. Kain R, Tadema H, McKinney EF, et al. High prevalence of autoantibodies to hLAMP-2 in anti-neutrophil cytoplasmic antibody-associated vasculitis. J Am Soc Nephrol 2012;23(3):556–66.

58. Pendergraft WF 3rd, Niles JL. Trojan horses: drug culprits associated with anti-neutrophil cytoplasmic autoantibody (ANCA) vasculitis. Curr Opin Rheumatol 2014;26(1):42–9.

59. Aeddula NR, Pathireddy S, Ansari A, et al. Hydralazine-associated antineutrophil cytoplasmic antibody vasculitis with pulmonary-renal syndrome. BMJ Case Rep 2018;2018. https://doi.org/10.1136/bcr-2018-227161.

60. Garg L, Gupta S, Swami A, et al. Levamisole/cocaine induced systemic vasculitis and immune complex glomerulonephritis. Case Rep Nephrol Urol 2015;2015: 372413.

61. Chen B, Yang X, Sun S, et al. Propylthiouracil-induced vasculitis with alveolar hemorrhage confirmed by clinical, laboratory, computed tomography, and bronchoscopy findings: a case report and literature review. Iran Red Crescent Med J 2016;18(4):e23320.

62. McGrath MM, Isakova T, Rennke HG, et al. Contaminated cocaine and antineutrophil cytoplasmic antibody-associated disease. Clin J Am Soc Nephrol 2011; 6(12):2799–805.

63. Kamisawa T, Zen Y, Pillai S, et al. IgG4-related disease. Lancet 2015;385(9976): 1460–71.
64. Deshpande V, Zen Y, Chan JK, et al. Consensus statement on the pathology of IgG4-related disease. Mod Pathol 2012;25(9):1181–92.
65. Wallace ZS, Deshpande V, Mattoo H, et al. IgG4-Related disease: clinical and laboratory features in one hundred twenty-five patients. Arthritis Rheumatol 2015;67(9):2466–75.
66. Wallace ZS, Mattoo H, Mahajan VS, et al. Predictors of disease relapse in IgG4-related disease following rituximab. Rheumatology (Oxford) 2016;55(6):1000–8.
67. Du H, Shi L, Chen P, et al. Prohibitin is involved in patients with IgG4 related disease. PLoS One 2015;10(5):e0125331.
68. Shiokawa M, Kodama Y, Kuriyama K, et al. Pathogenicity of IgG in patients with IgG4-related disease. Gut 2016;65(8):1322–32.
69. Hubers LM, Vos H, Schuurman AR, et al. Annexin A11 is targeted by IgG4 and IgG1 autoantibodies in IgG4-related disease. Gut 2018;67(4):728–35.
70. Perugino CA, AlSalem SB, Mattoo H, et al. Identification of galectin-3 as an autoantigen in patients with IgG4-related disease. J Allergy Clin Immunol 2019; 143(2):736–45.e6.
71. Shiokawa M, Kodama Y, Sekiguchi K, et al. Laminin 511 is a target antigen in autoimmune pancreatitis. Sci Transl Med 2018;10(453). https://doi.org/10.1126/scitranslmed.aaq0997.
72. Aalberse RC, Stapel SO, Schuurman J, et al. Immunoglobulin G4: an odd antibody. Clin Exp Allergy 2009;39(4):469–77.
73. Aalberse RC, van der Gaag R, van Leeuwen J. Serologic aspects of IgG4 antibodies. I. Prolonged immunization results in an IgG4-restricted response. J Immunol 1983;130(2):722–6.
74. Nouri-Aria KT, Wachholz PA, Francis JN, et al. Grass pollen immunotherapy induces mucosal and peripheral IL-10 responses and blocking IgG activity. J Immunol 2004;172(5):3252–9.
75. Carruthers MN, Khosroshahi A, Augustin T, et al. The diagnostic utility of serum IgG4 concentrations in IgG4-related disease. Ann Rheum Dis 2015;74(1):14–8.
76. Strehl JD, Hartmann A, Agaimy A. Numerous IgG4-positive plasma cells are ubiquitous in diverse localised non-specific chronic inflammatory conditions and need to be distinguished from IgG4-related systemic disorders. J Clin Pathol 2011;64(3):237–43.
77. Chang SY, Keogh KA, Lewis JE, et al. IgG4-positive plasma cells in granulomatosis with polyangiitis (Wegener's): a clinicopathologic and immunohistochemical study on 43 granulomatosis with polyangiitis and 20 control cases. Hum Pathol 2013;44(11):2432–7.
78. Igawa T, Hayashi T, Ishiguro K, et al. IgG4-producing lymphoma arising in a patient with IgG4-related disease. Med Mol Morphol 2016;49(4):243–9.
79. Jurado RL, Campbell J, Martin PD. Prozone phenomenon in secondary syphilis. Has its time arrived? Arch Intern Med 1993;153(21):2496–8.
80. Khosroshahi A, Cheryk LA, Carruthers MN, et al. Brief Report: spuriously low serum IgG4 concentrations caused by the prozone phenomenon in patients with IgG4-related disease. Arthritis Rheumatol 2014;66(1):213–7.

Analysis of the Complement System in the Clinical Immunology Laboratory

Morris Ling, MD[a,b,c,d],*, Mandakolathur Murali, MD[a,c,d]

KEYWORDS

- Complement • CH50 • C3 • C4 • Classical pathway • Lectin pathway
- Alternative pathway • Membrane attack complex

KEY POINTS

- The initial steps in the complement cascade are triggered by (1) antigen-antibody complexes (classical pathway), (2) lectin binding (lectin pathway), or (3) accelerated C3 tick-over (alternative pathway).
- Formation of the C3 and C5 convertases results in production of anaphylatoxins (C3a and C5a) and the downstream formation of the membrane attack complex.
- Complement receptors are G-protein-coupled receptors expressed on various immune cells and rarely on other cells. These receptors are activated by complement protein fragments that are generated in the plasma during complement activation.
- Fluid phase and membrane-bound regulators promote effective host defense against infection and immune homeostasis and prevent inappropriate complement activation.
- Functional complement activity and quantitation of individual complement components facilitates the diagnosis of diseases of complement deficiency, exuberant complement activation, and complement dysregulation.

HISTORY AND INTRODUCTION

The discovery of complement dates to the late 1800s, when Jules Bordet identified an unknown heat-labile lytic substance in blood that possessed activity against various forms of bacteria. This heat-labile mediator appeared to promote nonspecific antimicrobial activity, complementing the function of heat-stable serum proteins

Disclosure Statement: The authors have nothing to disclose.
[a] Division of Rheumatology, Allergy and Immunology, Department of Medicine, Massachusetts General Hospital, 55 Fruit Street, Cox 201, Boston, MA 02114, USA; [b] Center for Immunology and Inflammatory Diseases, Massachusetts General Hospital, 55 Fruit Street, Cox 201, Boston, MA 02114, USA; [c] Department of Pathology, Massachusetts General Hospital, 55 Fruit Street, Cox 201, Boston, MA 02114, USA; [d] Department of Medicine, Harvard Medical School, 55 Fruit Street, Cox 201, Boston, MA 02114, USA
* Corresponding author. Division of Rheumatology, Allergy and Immunology, Department of Medicine, Massachusetts General Hospital, 55 Fruit Street, Cox 201, Boston, MA 02114.
E-mail address: mling@mgh.harvard.edu

Clin Lab Med 39 (2019) 579–590
https://doi.org/10.1016/j.cll.2019.07.006
0272-2712/19/© 2019 Elsevier Inc. All rights reserved.

(ie, antibodies). This component was thus termed "complement" by Paul Ehrlich in 1899.[1] The complement system is now known to be a key component of the innate immune system. Activation of complement involves a complex cascade of proteases, providing a first line of defense against pathogens as well as playing a role in eliminating cellular debris. Its function complements that of antibodies and phagocytes by (1) eliminating microbes (through cytolytic membrane attack by disrupting bacterial cell walls), (2) removing apoptotic cells and debris (through opsonization of antigens to promote phagocytosis), (3) augmenting inflammation (through chemoattraction and activation of leukocytes, particularly macrophages and neutrophils), and (4) acting as costimulators of B-cell activation and antibody production and thereby augmenting innate and adaptive immune responses (eg, via C3d).[2] Normal host (self) cells express regulatory proteins that protect against complement-mediated attack, whereas foreign pathogens (non-self) and altered host cells are susceptible to such attack, leading to opsonization of pathogens and autoreactive cells.

Soluble proteins of the complement system are synthesized by the liver and circulate initially as inactive pro-enzymes that become functionally active on cleavage by a protease. In the setting of infection or inflammation, the production of certain complement proteins and other acute phase reactants is augmented by inflammatory cytokines, such as tumor necrosis factorα, interleukin (IL)-1, and IL-6, which are produced by leukocytes (eg, macrophages and neutrophils).[2] The initial steps in the complement cascade are triggered by (1) antigen-antibody complexes (*classical pathway*), (2) lectin binding (*lectin pathway*), or (3) accelerated C3 tick-over (*alternative pathway*) (**Fig. 1**). After this initial activation, protease-mediated cleavage of complement proteins leads to activation of the aforementioned complement-mediated functions and downstream activation of adaptive immune responses. The other role for complement is immune homeostasis as clearance of apoptotic cells and debris removes self-antigens from the circulation, which reduces the risk of developing autoimmunity.

CLASSICAL PATHWAY

The classical pathway is initiated by C1q. When C1q recognizes certain target molecules (eg, immune complexes or surface-bound pentraxins), a conformational change occurs, allowing C1q to interact with C1r and C1s and form activated $C1qr_2s_2$.[3] The active enzymatic site is on C1s. Subsequently, activated $C1qr_2s_2$ cleaves C4, then C2, to generate the classical pathway C3 convertase, C4b2a. C4b2a is then able to induce proteolytic activity and activate the common terminal pathway.[4]

LECTIN PATHWAY

The lectin pathway can be triggered by circulating pattern recognition receptors (PRRs) that recognize carbohydrates on microbial surfaces. These include (1) mannose binding lectin (MBL), a "collectin"; and (2) ficolins. Ficolins are PRRs with a fibrinogen-like domain, for example, M-ficolin (ficolin-1, secreted by lung and blood cells), L-ficolin (ficolin-2), and H-ficolin (ficolin-3); the latter two are synthesized in the liver and circulate in blood. MBL-associated serine proteases (MASP-1 and MASP-2) are evolutionarily related to C1r and C1s, and function similarly.[5] MBL complexes with MASPs, which then cleave C4 and C2 to form the lectin pathway C3 convertase, C4b2a.

ALTERNATIVE PATHWAY

The alternative pathway is activated by augmentation of C3 tick-over, which is the spontaneous hydrolysis of the thioester bond of C3 that occurs at a low level

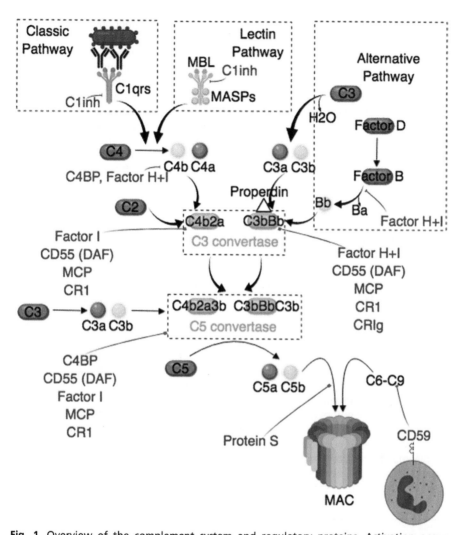

Fig. 1. Overview of the complement system and regulatory proteins. Activation occurs through 3 different pathways: the classical, lectin, and alternative pathways. The classical pathway is initiated through the activated C1 complex (C1qrs), and the lectin pathway is triggered by a number of PRRs, including MBL and MASPs 1 and 2. The alternative pathway can be activated by spontaneous hydrolysis of C3 (tick-over) or by C3 formed via the classical and lectin pathways. Activation of complement results in the production of the classical and lectin pathway C3 convertase (C4b2a) and the alternative pathway C3 convertase (C3bBb), which have proteolytic activity for C3 and form their respective C5 convertases by generation of more C3b (C4b2a3b and C3bBbC3b). Cleavage of C5 leads onward to the common terminal pathway, which produces the cytolytic MAC. Regulatory proteins are present both in the fluid phase or bound to the cell surface. The major fluid phase regulators include the serum C1INH, C4BP, protein S, factor H, factor I, and an AI, whereas the major cell-bound regulators include CD55 (DAF), CD59 (MAC-IP, or protectin), MCP (or CD46), CR1 (or CD35), and CRIg. (Figure created with BioRender.)

constitutively, but does not proceed further if C3b does not encounter its stabilizing counterpart, Bb.[6,7] Bb is a proteolytic fragment formed as a result of factor D-dependent cleavage of factor B. The alternative pathway C3 convertase, C3bBb, is formed when C3b binds to Bb. The activity of C3bBb is stabilized by properdin, which is found on activated surfaces with decreased sialic acid content (eg, foreign cell membranes), but not on host cell membranes rich in sialic acid. The labile thioester group on C3b is also able to covalently and stably bind exposed amino or hydroxyl groups on the neighboring cell surfaces of pathogens or altered host cell membranes. This process augments C3 tick-over while also promoting subsequent complement activation on the surfaces of targeted pathogens or altered self-structures.[8] The alternative pathway can also be activated or augmented by C3b generated by the classical or lectin pathways.

COMMON TERMINAL PATHWAY

After formation of the C3 convertase, C4b2a via the classical and/or lectin pathways, or C3bBb via the alternative pathway, the complement cascade proceeds due to the proteolytic activity of the C3 convertase on C3, which produces an inflammatory mediator or "anaphylatoxin" (C3a) and an enzymatic cleavage component (C3b). This leads to the formation of their respective C5 convertases (C4b2a3b and C3bBbC3b).[3] Subsequent cleavage of C5 by the C5 convertase also produces an inflammatory mediator or "anaphylatoxin" (C5a) and an enzymatic cleavage component (C5b). The anaphylatoxins C3a, C4a, and C5a activate mast cells and the resulting mediators contribute to the vascular phase of inflammation. C5a is also a chemoattractant that recruits neutrophils and monocytes, contributing to the cellular phase of inflammation. C5b initiates the common terminal pathway and, after complexing with C6, C7, C8, and C9, forms the cytolytic membrane attack complex (MAC).

Complement receptors are G-protein-coupled receptors expressed on various immune cells and rarely on other cells (**Table 1**). These receptors are activated by complement protein fragments, principally those derived from C3, which are generated in the plasma during complement activation.[9] C3a is recognized by C3aR, which is expressed on mast cells and basophils and functions as a potent anaphylatoxin. The ligand for complement receptor 1 (CR1) is C3b, which is expressed on red blood

Table 1
Complement receptors

Ligand	Receptor	Cells of Distribution	Function
C3a[a]	C3aR	Mast cells, basophils	Anaphylatoxin
C3b[a]	CR1 (CD35)	RBCs, WBCs, monocytes, DCs, podocytes	Immune complex clearance, phagocytosis
C3d[a]	CR2 (CD21)	B cells	Costimulation
iC3b[a]	CR3 (CD11b/CD18)	Phagocytic cells	Phagocytosis
C3dg[a]	CR4 (CD11c/CD18)	?NK cells, monocytes, DCs	?Phagocytosis
C5a	C5aR (CD88)	WBCs, monocytes, DCs, certain tissues	Anaphylatoxin
C5a	C5L2 (intracellular, not functionally a GPCR)	WBCs, monocytes, DCs, certain tissues	?Decoy receptor

Abbreviations: DC, dendritic cell; GPCR, G protein-coupled receptor; NK, natural killer; RBC, red blood cell; WBC, white blood cell.
[a] Fragments of C3.

cells (RBCs), white blood cells (WBCs), monocytes, dendritic cells (DCs), and podocytes. Its functions include immune complex clearance and phagocytosis. The ligand for CR2 is C3d, which is expressed on B cells and functions in costimulation. The ligand for CR3 is iC3b, which is expressed on phagocytic cells and is important in phagocytosis. Finally, CR4 recognizes C3dg, which is expressed on natural killer cells, monocytes, and DCs and may play a role on phagocytosis as well. **Table 1** also summarizes the role of C5a receptors.[10]

FLUID PHASE REGULATORS

To promote effective host defense against infection and immune homeostasis and to prevent inappropriate complement activation, regulatory proteins play an important role, whether present in the fluid phase or bound to the cell surface. The major fluid phase regulators include the serum C1 inhibitor (C1INH), C4 binding protein (C4BP), protein S, factor H, factor I, and an anaphylatoxin inhibitor (AI).[11]

C1 INH is a member of the serpin family of serine protease inhibitors and is an important fluid phase regulator as it inhibits several circulating complement proteases (C1r, C1s, and the MASPs), contact system proteases (HMW kininogen, kallikrein, factor XIa, and factor XIIa), and fibrinolytics (plasmin).[12] When these proteolytic cascades are activated by C1q, bradykinin (derived from contact activation of factor XII) and several other vasoactive substances are generated, resulting in increased vascular permeability.

C4BP binds and degrades C4b to form C4c and C4d.[13] C4d does not have protease activity; rather, its production limits amplification of complement activation via the classical and lectin pathways.

Protein S, a cofactor for activated protein C (APC) in the coagulation cascade, binds to the C5bC6C7 complex to prevent insertion into the cell membrane and subsequent formation of a cytolytic complex with C8 and C9.[14] Protein S can also bind C4BP to influence the coagulation cascade, which highlights the close association between the coagulation and complement systems.[15]

Serum regulatory protein factor H is able to bind C3b and interfere with the ability of C3b to cleave C5 and factor B on cell surfaces, which would in turn inhibit the formation of C3 and C5 convertases. Factor H also acts as an essential cofactor for factor I, another fluid phase regulator that mediates proteolytic degradation of plasma C3b. The importance of factor H is highlighted by disorders that arise from certain mutations or single nucleotide polymorphisms in the gene, including age-related macular degeneration (AMD) and atypical hemolytic uremic syndrome (aHUS).[16]

MEMBRANE-BOUND REGULATORS

The major cell-bound regulators include CD55 (delay accelerating factor, or DAF), CD59 (MAC-inhibitory protein, or MAC-IP, or protectin), membrane cofactor protein (MCP, or CD46), CR1 (or CD35), and CRIg (complement receptor of the immunoglobulin superfamily).[11]

CD55 (or DAF) is a membrane-bound glycoprotein that promotes the decay dissociation of C4b2a and thus interrupts formation of the classical and lectin pathway C3 convertases. By limiting C3b formation, CD55 also inhibits signal amplification by C3b via the alternative pathway.[17]

CD59 is a membrane-bound glycoprotein that can hinder the polymerization of C9 and thereby inhibit the formation of the MAC and cytolysis.[18]

Similar to factor H, MCP (CD46) can serve as a cofactor for factor I-mediated proteolysis of plasma C3b.[19]

Membrane-bound CR1 is a complement receptor that also binds to C3b in immune complexes and serves as a cofactor for factor I-mediated degradation of C3b.

CRIg is a complement receptor on tissue-resident macrophages that recognizes C3b-opsonized surfaces and plays a role in immune clearance. However, the extracellular domain of CRIg binds to C3b in such a way that it interferes with substrate binding, limiting C3b-mediated activation of C3 and C5, thus inhibiting the alternative pathway.[20]

LABORATORY TESTING

Complement assays are performed on serum samples received in gold or red top tubes transported on ice to limit ex vivo tick-over. Improper handling and/or prolonged transport time at room temperature may affect the interpretation of antigenic and functional assays. On receipt, the sample is centrifuged and the serum is aliquoted and stored at $-70°C$.

Methods of Complement Testing

Functional complement activity is traditionally assessed using a hemolytic assay. To evaluate classical pathway activation, serial dilutions of the sample are made and incubated with antibody-sensitized sheep erythrocytes. The CH50 is the reciprocal of the dilution at which 50% hemolysis is seen. Similarly, alternative pathway activation can be assessed using rabbit (or guinea pig) erythrocytes, which specifically activate the alternative pathway due to decreased sialic acid content. The AH50 is the reciprocal dilution at which 50% hemolysis is seen. Alternatively, quantitation of classical pathway activation can be performed using nephelometric, turbidimetric, or enzyme-linked immunosorbent assay–based assays of formation of the neoantigen MAC complex, which is a less time-consuming assay that can be automated, and has been demonstrated to have excellent concordance with the hemolytic assay.

Individual complement components, quantitated in the past by immunodiffusion, is now measured by nephelometry or turbidometry,[21] with the caveat that the selection of antibodies may affect the interpretation of the assay depending on what epitopes are recognized by the antibodies (ie, intact protein only, soluble fragments after proteolysis only, or both). Most assays for C3 and C4 quantitate intact proteins as well as the major soluble fragments formed during activation. However, interpretation may be complicated by limited detection of certain proteolytic products. Membrane-bound regulatory proteins such as CD55, CD59, and CD35 (CR1) can be assessed using flow cytometry.[22]

Diagnostic Considerations and Laboratory Testing for Complement Deficiency

Fig. 2 highlights a suggested algorithm for determining the possible cause of complement deficiency. If CH50 is low and AH50 is normal, this finding points to a likely deficiency in a complement protein or regulatory protein involving the classical pathway. Factors that should be considered for quantitative and functional testing include C1, C2, and C4. C1 inhibitor deficiency evaluation should be considered in patients with nonpruritic angioedema without urticaria. If a single component is abnormal, the defect may either be hereditary or functional; genetic testing may be helpful to sort this out. However, if there are abnormalities in multiple components of the classical pathway, the problem is likely one of complement consumption as can be seen in immune complex diseases such as systemic lupus erythematosus (SLE), Sjögren's syndrome, rheumatoid arthritis, and cryoglobulinemia.

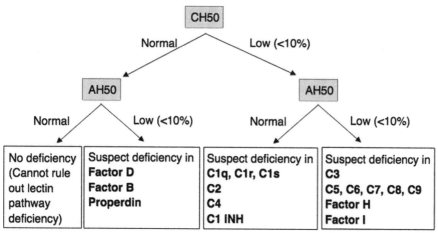

Fig. 2. Algorithm for laboratory testing of complement deficiency. When a disorder of complement is suspected, measurement of CH50 and AH50 is a recommended starting point for laboratory testing of complement deficiency and dysregulation. Antigenic or functional deficiency can be confirmed through the addition of individual purified components with correction of CH50 or AH50. When a particular factor is implicated, it may be appropriate to assess antigen levels of the factor as well as associated regulatory proteins to differentiate antigenic deficiency from functional deficiency.

If CH50 is normal and AH50 is low, this is consistent with a likely deficiency in a complement protein or regulatory protein involving the alternative pathway. Factors that should be considered for quantitative and functional testing include properdin, and antigen levels should be considered for factor B, factor D, factor H, and factor I, and MCP. Deficiencies of properdin and factor B/D are associated with Neisserial and pneumococcal infections. Factor H/I and MCP haploinsufficiency are seen in aHUS. Factor H abnormalities have also been associated with membranoproliferative glomerulonephritis and AMD.[23,24] Abnormalities may indicate a hereditary deficiency of one or more of these regulatory factors. Rarely, gram-negative sepsis, Henoch-Schönlein purpura, IgA nephropathy, and complement factor-mediated glomerulonephritis (C3 nephritic factor) may be associated with a decrease in alternative pathway activation (low AH50) with preservation of normal classical pathway function (normal CH50). C3 nephritic factor is an immunoglobulin (Ig)G antibody that stabilizes C3bBb, promoting C5 activation and MAC-mediated glomerulonephritis (aka type II membranoproliferative glomerulonephritis).

If CH50 and AH50 are both low, this is consistent with a likely deficiency in a complement protein or regulatory protein involving the terminal pathway. Factors that should be considered for quantitative and functional testing include C3, C5, C6, C7, C8, and C9, and antigen levels should be considered for factor H and factor I. If a single component is abnormal, the deficiency may be hereditary, and genetic testing may be helpful. However, if there are abnormalities in multiple components of the terminal pathway, the problem is likely one of complement consumption (eg, SLE, other immune complex disease, or shock).

If CH50 and AH50 are both normal but there is high clinical suspicion for complement deficiency, the defect may be in the lectin pathway. In this case, measurement of MBL may be helpful. However, it is unlikely that a systemic disease causing complement consumption would specifically target the lectin pathway while leaving the classical and alternative pathways intact.

Diagnostic Considerations and Laboratory Testing for Complement Dysregulation

Table 2 highlights laboratory test patterns of complement activation in systemic disease. Activation of the classical pathway would typically manifest as low CH50, low C3, low C4, and normal factor B. Relevant conditions in which such a pattern could be seen include warm autoimmune hemolytic anemia, SLE, Sjögren syndrome, rheumatoid arthritis, and cryoglobulinemia.

With regard to the alternative pathway, activation would typically manifest as low CH50, low C3, normal C4, and low factor B. Relevant conditions in which such a pattern could be seen include aHUS and C3 nephritic factor glomerulonephritis (C3 NF GN). Typical hemolytic uremic syndrome (HUS) presents as a clinical triad of nonimmune hemolytic anemia, thrombocytopenia, and renal impairment, but in the absence of a known bacterial trigger, this syndrome is termed aHUS, which comprises approximately 10% of total cases and has a poor prognosis.[25–27] Approximately 50% to 60% of familial and sporadic aHUS cases are linked to various mutations of the complement pathway.[28,29] The etiology of aHUS is quite heterogeneous, as complete or partial factor H deficiency (the most common),[30–32] deficiency in MCP (CD46) (second most common, seen in 10%–15% of patients with aHUS),[33–35] and many other mutations have been described (for example, gain of function mutations of factor B and C3, and loss of function mutations of factor I, MCP, thrombomodulin, and CFHR1/3 [complement factor H-related pseudogenes]).[33,36–38] Patients with aHUS exhibit low C3, high levels of activated complement components (C3b, C3c, C3d), and normal C4, which suggests selective activation of the alternative pathway.[30] The C3 convertases of the classical and lectin pathways are formed by C2 and C4 proteolysis, whereas the alternative pathway convertase cleaves C3 and bypasses C4.[39]

Activation of the terminal pathway would typically manifest as low CH50, low C3, normal C4, and normal factor B. This can be seen in conditions such as paroxysmal nocturnal hemoglobinuria (PNH). Patients with PNH present with the clinical triad of hemolytic anemia, bone marrow failure, and thrombosis.[40] On a baseline of chronic low-level hemolysis, patients often experience episodic severe hemolysis triggered by perturbations, such as surgery, infection, or inflammation. PNH arises from an expanded clonal proliferation of hematopoietic cells with somatic mutations in phosphatidylinositol glycan class A (PIGA), a gene involved in glycosylphosphatidylinositol (GPI) anchor biosynthesis.[41–44] Both CD55 (DAF) and CD59 (MAC-IP) are GPI-anchored proteins with a crucial role in complement regulation. Global deficiency of CD55 and CD59 results in dysregulated complement activation, leading to complement-mediated intravascular hemolysis of erythrocytes as well as activation of other hematopoietic cells. PNH is a clinical diagnosis (one may observe intravascular hemolysis, thrombosis, bleeding diathesis, and/or recurrent infections) that can be confirmed by findings of low CH50 and low AH50, flow cytometry

Table 2
Laboratory test patterns of complement activation

Profiles of Activation	CH50	C3	C4	Factor B
Classical	↓	↓	↓	Normal
Alternative	↓	↓	Normal	↓
Terminal	↓	↓	Normal	Normal
Fluid phase (classical)	↓	Normal	↓	Normal
Acute phase	↑	↑	↑	↑

↑ (or ↓) indicate increase (or decrease) of the indicated complement component or factor.

demonstrating CD55 and CD59 deficiency, and genetic testing (if needed). Although the Ham test (which involves assessing RBC fragility in a mild acid) was once used for this condition, it is now considered obsolete due to low sensitivity and specificity. Eculizumab is a promising therapeutic for the treatment of both aHUS and PNH; it specifically binds to the terminal complement component C5, inhibiting its cleavage by the C5 convertase.[45] Due the potent effect of eculizumab in blocking MAC formation, meningococcal vaccination is imperative to reduce the risk of invasive meningococcal disease, though even this measure does not completely mitigate the risk.[46]

Activation of the fluid phase components of the classical pathway would typically manifest as low CH50, normal C3, low C4, and normal factor B. Relevant conditions in which such a pattern could be seen include hereditary and acquired C1 inhibitor deficiency or dysfunction. Hereditary angioedema (HAE) is an autosomal dominant disease that usually presents before age 20 to 30 and is characterized by recurrent episodes of subcutaneous and/or submucosal edema involving the face, extremities, and/or abdomen. Oropharyngeal edema may be life-threatening. Pruritus and urticaria are not typically seen. There is often a family history, but 20% to 25% of cases arise from new mutations. Triggers of angioedema include trauma, infection, dental procedures, or emotional stress, with a potential increasing frequency and severity of episodes with puberty, menses, and ovulation. In type I HAE or C1 inhibitor deficiency, there is a low C1 inhibitor level and function. In type II HAE or C1 inhibitor dysfunction, the C1 inhibitor level is usually normal or high, but the C1 inhibitor function is abnormal. In type III HAE or HAE with normal C1 inhibitor, there is normal C1 inhibitor level and function, complicating the diagnosis. A subset of these patients may have mutations in factor XII, resulting in abnormal production of bradykinin.[47–49] In all 3 situations, bradykinin has been demonstrated to be the main mediator of the angioedema. Most patients with HAE have a persistently low C4 with normal C1q and C3.[50] However, in rare cases, the C4 level can be normal between attacks.[51] HAE can be differentiated from acquired C1 inhibitor deficiency (also called acquired angioedema [AAE]), by measuring C1q, which is low in AAE but not in HAE. AAE may be seen in patients with chronic lymphoproliferative disorders, such as multiple myeloma as well as rare cases of SLE that may have an autoantibody to C1 inhibitor.[52]

Acute and chronic inflammation may lead to an increase in complement proteins, which are among the acute phase reactants synthesized by the liver in response to inflammatory cytokines.

SUMMARY

The delicate balance between complement activation and regulation thus plays a key role in innate immunity and autoimmunity. Understanding the pathways involved in complement activation and function, how the complement system is regulated, and how complement laboratory tests are interpreted will aid in the appropriate diagnosis of disorders of complement deficiency and dysregulation.

REFERENCES

1. Chaplin H Jr. Review: the burgeoning history of the complement system 1888-2005. Immunohematology 2005;21(3):85–93.

2. Holers VM. Complement and its receptors: new insights into human disease. Annu Rev Immunol 2014;32:433–59.

3. Carroll MC. The role of complement and complement receptors in induction and regulation of immunity. Annu Rev Immunol 1998;16:545–68.

4. Sim RB, Tsiftsoglou SA. Proteases of the complement system. Biochem Soc Trans 2004;32(Pt 1):21–7.
5. Garred P, Genster N, Pilely K, et al. A journey through the lectin pathway of complement-MBL and beyond. Immunol Rev 2016;274(1):74–97.
6. Merle NS, Church SE, Fremeaux-Bacchi V, et al. Complement system part I - molecular mechanisms of activation and regulation. Front Immunol 2015;6:262.
7. Nilsson B, Nilsson Ekdahl K. The tick-over theory revisited: is C3 a contact-activated protein? Immunobiology 2012;217(11):1106–10.
8. Muller-Eberhard HJ, Gotze O. C3 proactivator convertase and its mode of action. J Exp Med 1972;135(4):1003–8.
9. Dierich MP, Schulz TF, Eigentler A, et al. Structural and functional relationships among receptors and regulators of the complement system. Mol Immunol 1988;25(11):1043–51.
10. Ward PA. Functions of C5a receptors. J Mol Med (Berl) 2009;87(4):375–8.
11. Campbell RD, Law SK, Reid KB, et al. Structure, organization, and regulation of the complement genes. Annu Rev Immunol 1988;6:161–95.
12. Davis AE 3rd. C1 inhibitor and hereditary angioneurotic edema. Annu Rev Immunol 1988;6:595–628.
13. Gigli I, Fujita T, Nussenzweig V. Modulation of the classical pathway C3 convertase by plasma proteins C4 binding protein and C3b inactivator. Proc Natl Acad Sci U S A 1979;76(12):6596–600.
14. Podack ER, Kolb WP, Muller-Eberhard HJ. The SC5b-7 complex: formation, isolation, properties, and subunit composition. J Immunol 1977;119(6):2024–9.
15. Blom AM, Villoutreix BO, Dahlback B. Complement inhibitor C4b-binding protein-friend or foe in the innate immune system? Mol Immunol 2004;40(18):1333–46.
16. Skerka C, Chen Q, Fremeaux-Bacchi V, et al. Complement factor H related proteins (CFHRs). Mol Immunol 2013;56(3):170–80.
17. Medof ME, Kinoshita T, Nussenzweig V. Inhibition of complement activation on the surface of cells after incorporation of decay-accelerating factor (DAF) into their membranes. J Exp Med 1984;160(5):1558–78.
18. Rollins SA, Sims PJ. The complement-inhibitory activity of CD59 resides in its capacity to block incorporation of C9 into membrane C5b-9. J Immunol 1990; 144(9):3478–83.
19. Liszewski MK, Leung M, Cui W, et al. Dissecting sites important for complement regulatory activity in membrane cofactor protein (MCP; CD46). J Biol Chem 2000; 275(48):37692–701.
20. Wiesmann C, Katschke KJ, Yin J, et al. Structure of C3b in complex with CRIg gives insights into regulation of complement activation. Nature 2006;444(7116): 217–20.
21. Mollnes TE, Jokiranta TS, Truedsson L, et al. Complement analysis in the 21st century. Mol Immunol 2007;44(16):3838–49.
22. Terstappen LW, Nguyen M, Lazarus HM, et al. Expression of the DAF (CD55) and CD59 antigens during normal hematopoietic cell differentiation. J Leukoc Biol 1992;52(6):652–60.
23. Noris M, Remuzzi G. Translational mini-review series on complement factor H: therapies of renal diseases associated with complement factor H abnormalities: atypical haemolytic uraemic syndrome and membranoproliferative glomerulonephritis. Clin Exp Immunol 2008;151(2):199–209.
24. Zipfel PF, Lauer N, Skerka C. The role of complement in AMD. Adv Exp Med Biol 2010;703:9–24.

25. Constantinescu AR, Bitzan M, Weiss LS, et al. Non-enteropathic hemolytic uremic syndrome: causes and short-term course. Am J Kidney Dis 2004;43(6):976–82.

26. Kaplan BS, Meyers KE, Schulman SL. The pathogenesis and treatment of hemolytic uremic syndrome. J Am Soc Nephrol 1998;9(6):1126–33.

27. Noris M, Remuzzi G. Hemolytic uremic syndrome. J Am Soc Nephrol 2005;16(4): 1035–50.

28. Noris M, Remuzzi G. Atypical hemolytic-uremic syndrome. N Engl J Med 2009; 361(17):1676–87.

29. Warwicker P, Goodship TH, Donne RL, et al. Genetic studies into inherited and sporadic hemolytic uremic syndrome. Kidney Int 1998;53(4):836–44.

30. Noris M, Ruggenenti P, Perna A, et al. Hypocomplementemia discloses genetic predisposition to hemolytic uremic syndrome and thrombotic thrombocytopenic purpura: role of factor H abnormalities. Italian Registry of Familial and Recurrent Hemolytic Uremic Syndrome/Thrombotic Thrombocytopenic Purpura. J Am Soc Nephrol 1999;10(2):281–93.

31. Richards A, Buddles MR, Donne RL, et al. Factor H mutations in hemolytic uremic syndrome cluster in exons 18-20, a domain important for host cell recognition. Am J Hum Genet 2001;68(2):485–90.

32. Rougier N, Kazatchkine MD, Rougier JP, et al. Human complement factor H deficiency associated with hemolytic uremic syndrome. J Am Soc Nephrol 1998; 9(12):2318–26.

33. Caprioli J, Noris M, Brioschi S, et al. Genetics of HUS: the impact of MCP, CFH, and IF mutations on clinical presentation, response to treatment, and outcome. Blood 2006;108(4):1267–79.

34. Noris M, Brioschi S, Caprioli J, et al. Familial haemolytic uraemic syndrome and an MCP mutation. Lancet 2003;362(9395):1542–7.

35. Richards A, Kemp EJ, Liszewski MK, et al. Mutations in human complement regulator, membrane cofactor protein (CD46), predispose to development of familial hemolytic uremic syndrome. Proc Natl Acad Sci U S A 2003;100(22):12966–71.

36. Delvaeye M, Noris M, De Vriese A, et al. Thrombomodulin mutations in atypical hemolytic-uremic syndrome. N Engl J Med 2009;361(4):345–57.

37. Fremeaux-Bacchi V, Miller EC, Liszewski MK, et al. Mutations in complement C3 predispose to development of atypical hemolytic uremic syndrome. Blood 2008; 112(13):4948–52.

38. Kavanagh D, Kemp EJ, Mayland E, et al. Mutations in complement factor I predispose to development of atypical hemolytic uremic syndrome. J Am Soc Nephrol 2005;16(7):2150–5.

39. Walport MJ. Complement. First of two parts. N Engl J Med 2001;344(14): 1058–66.

40. Socie G, Mary JY, de Gramont A, et al. Paroxysmal nocturnal haemoglobinuria: long-term follow-up and prognostic factors. French Society of Haematology. Lancet 1996;348(9027):573–7.

41. Bessler M, Mason PJ, Hillmen P, et al. Paroxysmal nocturnal haemoglobinuria (PNH) is caused by somatic mutations in the PIG-A gene. EMBO J 1994;13(1): 110–7.

42. Miyata T, Takeda J, Iida Y, et al. The cloning of PIG-A, a component in the early step of GPI-anchor biosynthesis. Science 1993;259(5099):1318–20.

43. Nafa K, Mason PJ, Hillmen P, et al. Mutations in the PIG-A gene causing paroxysmal nocturnal hemoglobinuria are mainly of the frameshift type. Blood 1995; 86(12):4650–5.

44. Takeda J, Miyata T, Kawagoe K, et al. Deficiency of the GPI anchor caused by a somatic mutation of the PIG-A gene in paroxysmal nocturnal hemoglobinuria. Cell 1993;73(4):703–11.
45. Wong EK, Kavanagh D. Anticomplement C5 therapy with eculizumab for the treatment of paroxysmal nocturnal hemoglobinuria and atypical hemolytic uremic syndrome. Transl Res 2015;165(2):306–20.
46. McNamara LA, Topaz N, Wang X, et al. High risk for invasive meningococcal disease among patients receiving eculizumab (Soliris) despite receipt of meningococcal vaccine. MMWR Morb Mortal Wkly Rep 2017;66(27):734–7.
47. Bork K, Barnstedt SE, Koch P, et al. Hereditary angioedema with normal C1-inhibitor activity in women. Lancet 2000;356(9225):213–7.
48. Cichon S, Martin L, Hennies HC, et al. Increased activity of coagulation factor XII (Hageman factor) causes hereditary angioedema type III. Am J Hum Genet 2006; 79(6):1098–104.
49. Dewald G, Bork K. Missense mutations in the coagulation factor XII (Hageman factor) gene in hereditary angioedema with normal C1 inhibitor. Biochem Biophys Res Commun 2006;343(4):1286–9.
50. Pappalardo E, Cicardi M, Duponchel C, et al. Frequent de novo mutations and exon deletions in the C1inhibitor gene of patients with angioedema. J Allergy Clin Immunol 2000;106(6):1147–54.
51. Zuraw BL, Sugimoto S, Curd JG. The value of rocket immunoelectrophoresis for C4 activation in the evaluation of patients with angioedema or C1-inhibitor deficiency. J Allergy Clin Immunol 1986;78(6):1115–20.
52. Meszaros T, Fust G, Farkas H, et al. C1-inhibitor autoantibodies in SLE. Lupus 2010;19(5):634–8.

Flow Cytometry as a Diagnostic Tool in Primary and Secondary Immune Deficiencies

Jocelyn R. Farmer, MD, PhD[a,b,*], Michelle DeLelys, MLA[c,d]

KEYWORDS

- Flow cytometry • Lymphocytes • Primary immune deficiency
- Secondary immune deficiency

KEY POINTS

- Flow cytometry is a widely used time-effective and cost-effective method for diagnosing and monitoring primary and secondary immune deficiencies.
- Design of a clinical flow cytometric assay involves consideration of specimen collection, marker and fluorochrome selection, antibody titration, instrument setup, compensation, gating, reference ranges, and cross validation.
- Flow cytometry is essential in the diagnostic workup of severe primary immune deficiencies, including severe combined immune deficiency and congenital agammaglobulinemia.
- Flow cytometry can be used diagnostically (eg, human immunodeficiency virus) and for therapeutic monitoring (eg, B-cell depletion therapy) in the context of secondary immune deficiencies.

INTRODUCTION

Flow cytometry is an incredibly powerful diagnostic tool, one that can assess the number, activation status, and maturation potential of individual immune cells in a sampled specimen. The technology can aid in the diagnosis of immune disorders, such as

Disclosure Statement: This work was supported by the National Institutes of Health (T32-HL116275 to J.R. Farmer).
[a] Division of Rheumatology, Allergy and Immunology, Massachusetts General Hospital, COX 201, MGH, 55 Fruit Street, Boston, MA 02114, USA; [b] Ragon Institute of MGH, MIT and Harvard, Cambridge, MA, USA; [c] Cellular Therapeutics and Transplantation/Flow Cytometry, Department of Pathology, Massachusetts General Hospital, WRN 506, MGH, 55 Fruit Street, Boston, MA 02114, USA; [d] Cellular Therapeutics and Transplantation/Flow Cytometry, Department of Cancer Center, Massachusetts General Hospital, WRN 506, MGH, 55 Fruit Street, Boston, MA 02114, USA
* Corresponding author. COX 201, MGH, 55 Fruit Street, Boston, MA 02114.
E-mail address: jrfarmer@partners.org

primary immune deficiencies and hematopoietic malignancies, and can also be used to monitor the immune system's response to therapeutic intervention or acute disease state. Flow cytometry is most often performed on peripheral blood mononuclear cells, but other specimen types (eg, lymph nodes or bone marrow) also can be analyzed depending on the unique clinical question at hand. Standard flow cytometry tests can have a processing turnaround time of less than 1 hour and use relatively inexpensive reagents, making flow cytometry an accessible clinical resource. In this article, we review commonly used methods in the clinical flow cytometry laboratory for the analysis of peripheral blood lymphocytes, specifically, as well as the applicability of these techniques in the diagnosis and management of inherited and acquired forms of immune deficiency.

TECHNICAL CONCEPTS

Flow cytometry is the measurement of optical characteristics of single cells (or other particles of a similar size) as they pass through a fluid stream in single file. Conventional flow cytometry relies on the use of fluorophore-conjugated primary antibodies that specifically recognize and bind to proteins on or within cells. These fluorescent dye-conjugated antibodies are excited when the cells pass one-by-one through a laser. The unique light emission from each fluorochrome is captured and used to approximate levels of target protein in cells of interest. In addition, measures of forward and side scatter of light are captured, which approximate parameters of cell size and internal complexity, respectively. Flow cytometers can analyze multiple fluorescently tagged proteins on a single cell and currently, many clinical laboratories routinely run 8 to 12 color flow cytometric assays.

ASSAY DESIGN AND SETUP

Considerations for designing and validating a new flow cytometry assay include: acceptable specimen types and specimen preparation, use of anticoagulant, cell marker and fluorochrome selection, antibody titration, instrument setup, compensation, gating strategy, development of normal reference ranges, and cross validation.

Specimen conditions are crucial to the successful implementation of a flow cytometric test in a clinical laboratory. Most flow cytometry analyses are performed on fresh anticoagulated peripheral blood. If absolute cell counts are to be reported and calculated using a separate white blood cell count, cell counts should be measured before manipulation of the specimen for flow cytometry. Each laboratory must perform a validation to determine the acceptable specimen age, storage temperature, and anticoagulant for a flow cytometric assay, as the analysis can be compromised by a loss in cell viability. Cell viability in a specimen can be assessed using a membrane-impermeable DNA-binding dye, such as 7-AAD, but specimen age limits in most clinical flow cytometry laboratories preclude analysis 4 days after collection. Room temperature versus refrigerated storage should be validated by the testing site. The most frequent anticoagulant types used in the clinical flow cytometry laboratory are EDTA, Acid Citrate Dextrose, and sodium heparin. and should be validated based on the specific flow cytometric test being performed.[1]

Selection of appropriate cell markers and the corresponding fluorochrome-antibody conjugates is a critical step in flow cytometry assay design. Cell markers must be selected such that they can reliably identify the population(s) of interest in a typical sample. One of the most widely used markers in human flow cytometric analyses of leukocytes is CD45, which stains all white blood cells. The use of CD45 in flow cytometric assays allows the incorporation of a "clean-up" step to distinguish

CD45+ white blood cells from CD45- debris and red blood cells, which can bind to antibodies nonspecifically. When designing a flow cytometry panel, antigens that are expressed at the lowest density on or within the cell should be detected using the most reliable fluorochromes with the highest staining index. Conversely, antigens that are expressed at the highest density on or within the cell should be detected using fluorochromes with the lowest staining index.[2] For example, CD8 is a marker that is highly expressed on cytotoxic T cells. When using CD8 to analyze cytotoxic T cells, this marker should be paired with a low stain index fluorochrome.

A critical aspect of assay design is the titration of antibody concentration. Although commercially produced reagents generally provide a "manufacturer's recommended volume" to be used in the analysis, this recommendation always should be verified and/or modified to produce results with the optimal signal to noise ratio in staining intensity. Antibody titration should ideally be performed on the sample type and disease condition that will be eventually tested. The staining intensity plateaus with increasing volumes of the reagent, indicating the saturation of all antibody binding sites (**Fig. 1**). Although a range of reagent staining concentration may be acceptable, a consistent staining concentration should be decided on for routine testing.

Flow cytometric surface staining involves a brief incubation of fluorochrome-conjugated antibodies with the cells of interest followed by removal of excess unbound antibodies, typically using centrifugation. If red blood cells are not being assayed, they are removed before or after antibody staining using a lysing solution. Once the cells of interest are stained, the stained specimen can be stabilized using a fixative (eg, paraformaldehyde). Intracellular staining involves an additional permeabilization step, to allow fluorescent-conjugated primary antibodies to pass through cellular membranes. Data collection on a flow cytometry instrument is rapid; hundreds to thousands of cells can be analyzed per second if the cells are adequately concentrated in the stained sample. Some clinical assays can detect incredibly rare populations of cells (eg, as low as 0.001% of all events), but the total number of cells collected should be adjusted as needed for the appropriate level of statistical significance. Spectral overlap between fluorochromes can result in spillover between fluorescence channels. However, this can be algebraically deconvoluted and accounted for using compensation, which uses measurements of singly labeled beads or cells. Recommendations for compensation vary between manufacturers. This process should be verified and validated using manufacturer and institutional guidelines.[2]

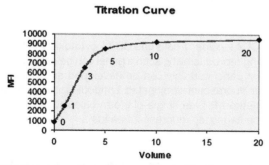

Fig. 1. Antibody titration curve. To perform antibody titration, an increasing amount of antibody is added to a known concentration of cells of interest. The median fluorescence intensity (MFI) for the negative population is subtracted from the MFI for the positive population and graphed to determine the point of saturation, which is the optimal reagent volume to perform testing.

Flow cytometry data can be acquired and analyzed using a variety of software packages. Flow cytometry analysis relies heavily on the use of "gating" of cell populations and subpopulations defined by specific combinations of antibody markers. Although this step is performed manually, approaches to automated analysis are being developed. The best markers exhibit a bimodal expression pattern and clearly delineate positive and negative cell populations. Other markers may require a staining control to determine the threshold for positive staining. Flow cytometric data can be reported qualitatively, by describing the fluorescent patterns identified on cell populations of interest, but also quantitatively, by reporting numerical values associated with each sampled gate.

Validation of a clinical flow cytometry assay involves verification of the numerical output of the test against a previously validated flow cytometry assay, reference material, or by using results from a different testing method.[3] Test sensitivity, specificity, precision, and accuracy should be included in the validation if possible. In addition, reference ranges obtained from age-matched healthy controls should be determined and included in the report. Laboratories performing clinical flow cytometry testing should ensure that the appropriate quality control measures are implemented. Flow cytometer performance needs to be monitored using calibration reagents to ensure that the lasers and detectors are functioning properly and are stable. In addition, each flow cytometer should have digital fluorescent compensation performed on a routine schedule. Enrollment in proficiency testing is highly recommended, but interlaboratory or intralaboratory concordance assessment is also an acceptable alternative. Although the large variety of flow cytometry instruments and fluorochrome-conjugates presents a significant challenge, there are growing efforts to standardize antibody staining panels and gating formats. This is further helped by the availability of monoclonal antibodies against most clinically significant markers.

COMMON LYMPHOCYTE TESTING PANELS

The following panels are commonly used in clinical laboratories for the analysis of lymphocyte subsets.

Lymphocyte Subset Panel

A lymphocyte subset panel is routinely performed in most clinical flow cytometry laboratories and provides a basic quantitative assessment of cells present in the patient's adaptive immune system. A lymphocyte subset panel includes staining for T cells (CD3+), B cells (CD19+), and natural killer (NK) cells (CD3-CD[16 + 56]+). T-cell subsets can be further included, adding additional information on the percentages and absolute counts of CD4+ helper T cells and CD8+ cytotoxic T cells (**Fig. 2A**). Because of their robust staining reproducibility, such a panel can be easily automated. Although a lymphocyte subset panel certainly can be developed and validated by combining multiple single-color fluorescent-conjugated antibodies, it is often offered as a kit, which contains a method for the single-platform calculations of absolute counts in addition to cell percentages (eg, fluorescent beads).

Naïve/Memory T-Cell Panel

Although there are many panels in use to distinguish subpopulations of naïve and memory T cells, almost all rely on CD45RA (naïve) and CD45RO (memory) (**Fig. 2B**). Additional functional trafficking markers (eg, CCR7 or CD62L) can be used to further distinguish T cell central memory (CD45RO+ CCR7+) and T cell effector memory (CD45RO+ CCR7−) subpopulations.

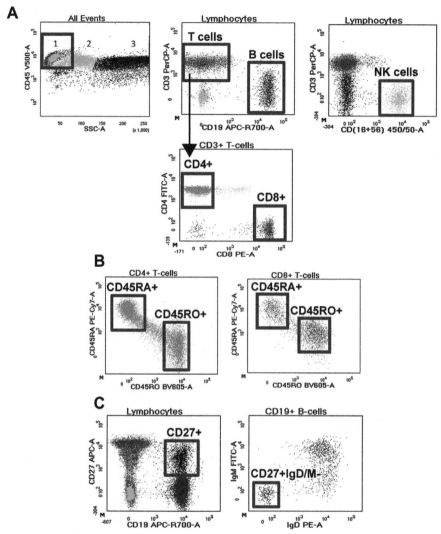

Fig. 2. Commonly used lymphocyte panels. Peripheral healthy control donor blood analyzed by flow cytometry using the (*A*) lymphocyte subset panel, (*B*) naïve/memory T-cell panel, and (*C*) memory B-cell panel. Lymphocyte subset panel shown by dot plots as total lymphocyte gate ("1" *top, left*), B-cell and T-cell subsets (*top, middle*), and NK-cell subset (*top, right*) with further division to CD4+ and CD8+ T-cell subsets from the total CD3+ gate (*bottom*). Naïve/Memory T-cell panel shown by dot plots as total CD4+ T-cell gate (*left*) and total CD8+ T-cell gate (*right*), with naïve (CD45RA+) and memory (CD45RO+) T-cell populations indicated. Memory B-cell panel shown by dot plots to indicate total CD27+ memory B cells (*left*) and CD27+IgD/M- class-switched memory B cells (*right*). Commonly quantitated lymphocyte populations highlighted in red.

Memory B-Cell Panel

Analysis of memory B-cell subsets is often ordered in patients with suspected or diagnosed primary or secondary humoral immune deficiencies. This test is well established and often uses a combination of CD19, CD27, immunoglobulin (Ig)M, and IgD to identify naïve (CD27−IgD/M+), marginal zone (CD27+IgD/M+), and class-switched memory (CD27+IgD/M−) B-cell subsets (**Fig. 2**C). As this test involves staining for immunoglobulin heavy chains, IgM and IgD, peripheral blood specimens must be washed thoroughly before combining with antibodies to prevent plasma immunoglobulins from "soaking up" staining antibodies before they are able to bind to their respective targets on the cell surface.

Double-Negative T-Cell Panel

If abundant double-negative T cells (CD4−CD8−) are identified on the initial lymphocyte subset panel, a specific double-negative T-cell panel may be considered. The following markers are run in conjunction: CD45, CD3, CD4, CD8, T-cell receptor (TCR)-alpha/beta (α/β), and TCR-gamma/delta (γ/δ). An expansion of TCR-α/β double-negative T cells has been described in severe immune dysregulatory conditions, including autoimmune lymphoproliferative syndrome (ALPS), in which a pathologic expansion of double-negative T cells has been defined as CD3+CD4−CD8−TCR-α/β+ cells >1.5% of total lymphocytes or >2.5% of total T cells (**Fig. 3**).[4] The murine marker B220, an isoform of CD45R, also can be included in this panel, as double-negative T cells in humans stain positively for this marker. In ALPS, B220+ staining on double-negative T cells has been described in patients with *FAS* and *FASLG* mutations, specifically.[5]

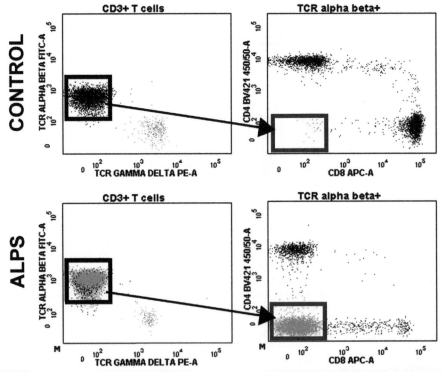

Fig. 3. Analysis by double-negative T-cell panel of peripheral blood from healthy control (*top*) versus patient with ALPS (*bottom*). Total CD3+ T-cell gate (*left*) and TCR-α/β CD3+ T-cell gate (*right*) shown by dot plots with atypical population of double-negative (CD4-CD8-) T cells in the patient with ALPS colored in green and highlighted in red.

Plasmablast Panel

A higher than normal percentage of plasmablasts can correlate with the diagnosis of autoimmune disease, and increased plasmablasts in peripheral circulation has been described as a biomarker of IgG4-related disease (IgG4-RD) activity, specifically (**Fig. 4**).[6] A plasmablast flow cytometry panel includes a minimum staining for CD19, CD20, CD27, and CD38, as plasmablasts have been defined in the literature as CD19+CD20-CD27+CD38++ cells.[7] In principle, this panel can be combined with the memory B-cell panel if adequate fluorochrome options exist.

Lymphoma Panel

Flow cytometry is widely used in the diagnosis of lymphomas. However, this topic has been extensively reviewed in a recent volume of *Clinics in Laboratory Medicine* (Volume 37 issue 4.pages:697-964.) and is outside the scope of this article.

APPLICATION TO PRIMARY IMMUNE DEFICIENCIES

In the workup of primary immune deficiencies, peripheral flow cytometry classically has been used in patients who present with a spectrum of atypical, frequent, and/or multiorgan infections.[8] More recently, the definition of primary immune deficiency was broadened to include "primary immune dysregulation," whereby patients may

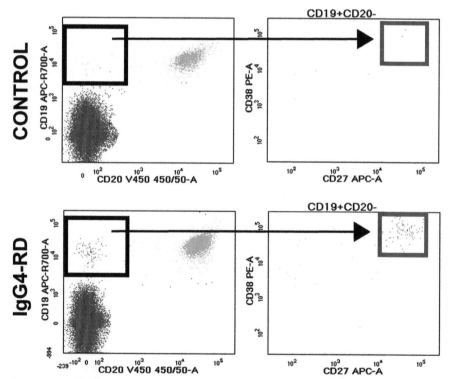

Fig. 4. Analysis by plasmablast panel of peripheral blood from healthy control (*top*) versus patient with IgG4-RD (*bottom*). Total lymphocyte gate (*left*) and CD19+CD20- B-cell gate (*right*) shown by dot plots with atypical population of plasmablasts in patient with IgG4-RD colored in purple and highlighted in red.

additionally or alternatively present with autoimmune disease, end-organ lymphoproliferation, lymphocytic malignancies, or even severe forms of atopy as the primary clinical presentations.[9–11] In the workup of an underlying primary immune deficiency, peripheral flow cytometry is an essential diagnostic tool that can facilitate an accurate assessment of circulating lymphocyte counts, as well as B-cell and T-cell maturation potential, as described in the preceding sections.

Low Lymphocytes (CD45+)

Primary immune deficiencies are a rare cause of absolute lymphocytopenia. In total, primary immune deficiencies have been estimated to have a worldwide prevalence of 1% to 2%.[12] However, in its most severe form (ie, severe combined immune deficiency [SCID]), a missed diagnosis of primary immune deficiency can be fatal within the first few years on life. Concern for missed SCID diagnoses in infancy ultimately prompted the onset of newborn screening by T-cell receptor excision circle (TREC) assay, first introduced in the United States as a statewide initiative in Wisconsin in 2008.[13] As of 2018, an estimated 92% of American infants underwent newborn screening for SCID.[14] Despite this progress, peripheral blood flow cytometry remains a central and cost-effective diagnostic tool in the evaluation of primary immune deficiency diseases. First, for all patients born outside of the geographic or temporal window of newborn screening, peripheral flow cytometry is frequently the first direct analysis of lymphocyte subsets in the patient. Second, for all patients found to have abnormally low TRECs on newborn screening, peripheral flow cytometry remains the recommended next-line diagnostic test and includes a minimum flow panel to assess numbers of B cells, NK cells, and CD4+/CD8+ T cells (as well as CD45RA and CD45RO staining within the respective T-cell compartments to determine absolute counts of naïve T cells).[15] As curative treatment for SCID is recommended if an infant is found to have a persistently low T-cell count (<300 cells/µL of autologous T cells),[15] peripheral flow cytometry has direct impact on patient care, specifically the urgent consideration of bone marrow transplantation[8] or more recently, gene editing.[16] Finally, by defining the affected lineages (B cells, T cells, and/or NK cells), peripheral flow cytometry can aid in refining the SCID diagnosis toward potential gene candidates and/or specific therapeutic options (eg, considering congenital adenosine deaminase deficiency and enzyme replacement therapy in a patient with B-T-NK-SCID[17]).

Low T Cells (CD3+)

Results of the first 7 years of newborn screening by TREC assay in California identified severe T-cell lymphocytopenia at a rate of 1 in 15,300 live births with the major etiologies identified being SCID, atypical SCID, and complete DiGeorge syndrome (a condition of congenital thymic absence prohibiting T-cell development).[18] In all cases of low TRECs, flow cytometry was the next-line diagnostic test used to confirm the presence of CD3+ T-cell lymphocytopenia. Prompt hematopoietic stem cell transplantation and thymic transplant in cases of SCID and complete DiGeorge syndrome, respectively, resulted in an overall survival rate of 94% in this cohort.[18] Thus, rapid assessment of peripheral lymphocyte counts by flow cytometry will continue to be an invaluable tool in the workup of congenital T-cell lymphocytopenia. Isolated idiopathic CD4+ T-cell lymphocytopenia (ICL) has also been described, although the prevalence is rare.[19–21] Unfortunately, outcomes have historically been unfavorable in ICL because of frequent, severe, and atypical infections.[22] It is unclear how the onset of newborn screening may alter the natural history of ICL moving forward. In addition, isolated CD8+ T-cell lymphocytopenia can be seen in the setting of rare primary immune deficiency disorders. This includes CD8-alpha deficiency, MHC I deficiency, forms of Omenn syndrome, and ZAP-70 deficiency.[8] CD8+ T-cell lymphocytopenia typically presents with a milder clinical course than CD4+ T-cell lymphocytopenia, with most patients developing recurrent sinopulmonary infections in adulthood.

Low B Cells (CD19+)

Although B-cell and T-cell lymphocytopenia co-occurs frequently in SCID, primary isolated B-cell lymphocytopenia has also been described. The initial description of this condition was a case of x-linked agammaglobulinemia by Dr Bruton in 1952,[23] ultimately identified as inherited Bruton tyrosine kinase deficiency.[24,25] Subsequently, autosomal-recessive forms of primary B-cell lymphocytopenia were described, centering around congenital defects in B-cell receptor production and downstream signaling.[8] Patients with primary B-cell lymphocytopenia have severe and early-onset recurrent sinopulmonary infections. As these patients are currently not identified via newborn screening, analysis of peripheral lymphocyte counts by flow cytometry with a minimal assessment of B cells, NK cells, and CD4+/CD8+ T cells is recommended in all patients who present with agammaglobulinemia. Consideration is under way to initiate B-cell lymphocytopenia screening more directly via analysis of kappa-deleting recombination excision circles.[26]

Low Natural Killer Cells (CD3-CD[16+56]+)

Isolated low NK-cell counts also can be primary. Classic NK-cell deficiency is defined by an absence of NK cells (present at ≤1% of circulating lymphocytes) and their function in the peripheral blood.[27] Patients with classic NK-cell deficiency present with early-onset and severe viral pathogens as a predominant feature, and monogenic causes have been described.[28] Initial evaluation should include flow cytometry to assess peripheral lymphocyte counts, including NK cells, as well as B cells and CD4+/CD8+ T cells, as NK-cell deficiency can co-occur with severe and combined immune deficiencies, as detailed in the preceding sections. An entity of functional NK-cell deficiency, in which NK-cell counts are normal yet function is impaired, has also been described.[29] These disorders will be discussed in greater depth in the Sara Barmettler's article, "Laboratory Assays of Immune Cell Function in Immunodeficiencies," on functional flow cytometry elsewhere in this issue.

APPLICATION TO SECONDARY IMMUNE DEFICIENCIES

In the workup of secondary immune deficiencies, peripheral flow cytometry is frequently used both diagnostically and in the context of therapeutic monitoring. As an example of diagnostic utility, the CD4+ T-cell count during chronic human immunodeficiency virus (HIV) infection is required to accurately diagnose the level of acquired immune dysfunction and inform the appropriate prophylactic therapy for the patient.[30] As an example of therapeutic monitoring, in patients receiving B-cell depletion therapy (eg, the anti-CD20 monoclonal antibody, Rituximab), systematic monitoring of CD19+ B cells in the periphery can inform both when the patient may be at highest risk for immunosuppression and secondary infections (time of B-cell nadir) as well as when the patient may be at highest risk for autoimmune disease flare (time of B-cell reconstitution). This therapeutic monitoring strategy can ultimately be used to optimize a patient's B-cell deletion regimen.[31-33]

Low Lymphocytes (CD45+)

Low absolute lymphocyte counts are most commonly seen in states of acquired immune deficiency. In a retrospective study of 1042 hospitalized patients, lymphocytopenia was most commonly due to sepsis (24%), postoperative state (22%), malignancy (17%), use of systemic or inhaled corticosteroids (15%), posttransplantation (10%), use of chemotherapy and/or radiation (9%), trauma or hemorrhage (8%), viral infection (2.5%), or HIV infection, specifically (1.2%).[34] Age-related declines in lymphocyte counts have also been described,[35] with potential contributions from loss of bone marrow precursor production and thymic output.[36,37] The decision to pursue additional peripheral flow cytometry testing in the clinical context of lymphocytopenia is driven by factors that include severity and duration of the lymphocytopenia, known comorbidities (eg, HIV infection status), concurrent laboratory abnormalities (eg, multilineage cytopenias) and/or clinical condition of the patient. Flow cytometry may be of particular utility in cases in which there is concern for malignancy (eg, lymphoma, in which flow cytometry can provide a rapid and cost-effective assessment of atypical lymphocyte surface marker expression and clonality[38]) and/or known comorbidities (eg, HIV infection, in which flow cytometry can provide a rapid and cost-effective assessment of CD4+ T-cell counts[30]).

Low T Cells (CD3+)

Low absolute CD3+ T-cell counts are most commonly seen in states of acquired immune deficiency. Global CD3+ T-cell lymphocytopenia will present with a preserved CD4:CD8 cell ratio of 2:1. If this ratio is skewed, specific evaluation for causes of isolated CD4+ or CD8+ T-cell lymphocytopenia should be undertaken. Screening for preexisting HIV infection is essential in the workup of isolated CD4+ T-cell lymphocytopenia, as the natural history of HIV-induced lymphocytopenia is severe, progressive, and specific for CD4+ T cells (can skew the CD4:CD8 ratio to <1:1[39]). Fortunately, CD4+ T-cell counts can be recovered with antiretroviral therapy.[40] Thus, peripheral lymphocyte flow cytometry continues to be essential in the care of patients with chronic HIV infection, informing both degree of acquired immune deficiency at diagnosis as well as during therapeutic antiretroviral intervention. Outside of HIV, low CD4+ and CD8+ T-cell counts can occur coincident with chronic illness, including end-stage renal disease,[41] protein-wasting enteropathy,[42] and cirrhosis.[43] Finally, there are numerous iatrogenic causes of T-cell lymphocytopenia. Most notably, systemic high-dose corticosteroid therapy has been shown to preferentially deplete CD4+ T-cell counts in the peripheral blood of healthy control subjects as early as 4 hours posttreatment.[44]

Low B Cells (CD19+)

With the onset of anti-CD20 depletion therapy in the management of B-cell malignancies and systemic autoantibody diseases, secondary isolated B-cell lymphocytopenia is becoming more prevalent. Best studied to date is the anti-CD20 monoclonal antibody, rituximab, whereby B-cell lymphocytopenia is anticipated up to 9 months posttreatment when given as a single agent and up to 24 months posttreatment when given in combination with chemotherapy (**Fig. 5**).[45] However, patients with failed peripheral B-cell recovery more than 24 months post-rituximab therapy, in terms of total B-cell counts, B-cell maturation potential, and/or antibody responses, have been described.[46,47] This patient subset may represent an underlying genetic predisposition to humoral immune dysfunction. Unfortunately, detailed evaluation of antibody levels, B-cell counts, and peripheral B-cell maturation is not routinely undertaken

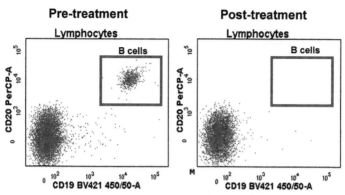

Fig. 5. Peripheral human blood before and after B-cell depletion therapy. Gating of total lymphocytes shown by dot plot of the B-cell markers CD19 and CD20. Loss of total B cells highlighted in the posttreatment sample in red.

across the disciplines of hematology/oncology and rheumatology before the initiation of B-cell depletion therapy in most cases.[47] Other secondary causes of B-cell predominant lymphocytopenia include infections[48] and thymic neoplasms (Good syndrome).[49]

Low Natural Killer Cells (CD3-CD[16+56]+)

NK-cell counts as well as function may be compromised in acute states of immune activation, including infections and autoimmune disease.[50] As the markers CD16 and CD56 also can be found on a subset of NK T cells, care should be taken to exclude this population by gating for only CD3−CD(16+ 56)+ cells when analyzing NK cells by flow cytometry.

APPLICATION TO IMMUNE DYSREGULATION
Loss of Class-Switched Memory (CD27+IgD−) B Cells

Presence of class-switched memory B cells in the peripheral blood is a marker of intact B-cell differentiation, an indicator that B cells have successfully received T-cell help and are thus primed for effective anti-pathogen antibody production. As mentioned in the preceding section, loss of B-cell maturation can be iatrogenic, best described in a prolonged state in a subset of patients following B-cell depletion therapy.[46] Alternatively, loss of CD27+IgD− B cells is well described in common variable immune deficiency (CVID) (**Fig. 6**A), which is the most common symptomatic primary immune deficiency worldwide.[51] Unlike B-cell lymphocytopenia causing agammaglobulinemia, patients with CVID typically present with mildly low immunoglobulin levels and adult-onset infections. Within the broad categorization of CVID, patients with low class-switched memory B cells (<2% total CD19+ B cells) have been shown to be at increased risk for autoimmune and lymphoproliferative end-organ sequalae.[52] Thus, detailed B-cell profiling, including a minimum analysis of CD27 and IgD staining within the CD19+ B-cell compartment, is recommended at the time of CVID diagnosis.[51]

Loss of Naïve (CD45RA+) T Cells

Infants are born with a predominance of naïve (CD45RA+) T cells in the periphery, which slowly shift toward an increasing ratio of memory (CD45RO+) T cells in circulation with age.[53] In the workup of newborn SCID, loss of naïve T cells within the

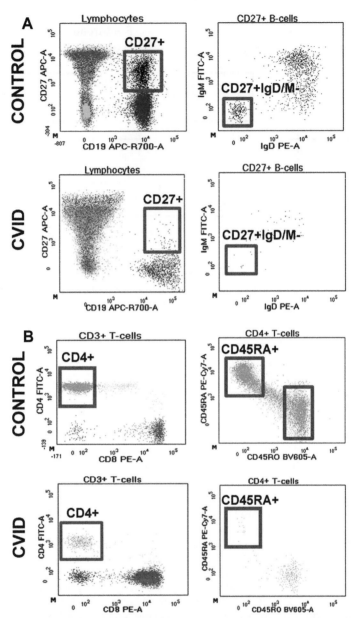

Fig. 6. Flow cytometric abnormalities observed in CVID. (*A*) Memory B-cell panel shown by dot plots in healthy control (*top*) versus patient with CVID (*bottom*) demonstrating loss of memory (CD27+) and class-switched memory (CD27+IgD/M−) B-cell populations in the patient. (*B*) Naïve/memory T-cell panel shown by dot plots in healthy control (*top*) versus patient with CVID (*bottom*) demonstrating loss of total CD4+ T cells in addition to shift toward a memory CD45RO+T-cell phenotype in the patient.

CD4+ compartment (CD45RO+ >80%[54]) is highly concerning for maternal engraftment and should prompt expedited evaluation independent of normal total CD4+ T-cell counts.[54] Thus, follow-up screening of a newborn with low TRECs must include at a minimum CD45RA/CD45RO staining within the CD4+ T-cell compartment.[8] In addition, loss of naïve CD4+ T cells has been described in adult-onset primary immune deficiencies, including CVID specifically (**Fig. 6**B).[55] Within the broad categorization of CVID, patients with low naïve CD4+ T-cell counts (<20% total CD4+ T cells) have been shown to be at increased risk for autoimmune and lymphoproliferative end-organ sequalae.[56]

Expansion of Double-Negative (CD4−CD8−) T Cells

ALPS is a rare, often inherited disorder of dysregulated lymphocyte apoptosis, which can be diagnosed in part by simple flow cytometric evaluation of the patient's peripheral blood. Expansion of double-negative T cells, whereby CD3+CD4−CD8−TCR-α/β+ T cells are found at more than 1.5% of total lymphocytes or more than 2.5% of total T cells, is a diagnostic criterion for the disease.[4] As double-negative T-cell expansion can be observed in other states of immune dysregulation,[57,58] additional testing for defective lymphocyte apoptosis and/or somatic or germline mutations in *FAS*, *FASLG*, and *CASP10* is recommended in the diagnostic workup for ALPS.[4] These tests can be performed secondarily if the initial flow cytometric evaluation is concerning.

Expansion of Plasmablasts (CD20−CD27+CD38++) B Cells

Short-lived plasmablasts are seen physiologically in the peripheral blood during states of acute immune activation, such as viral infections.[59] These cells also have been described in the pathologic context of chronic autoimmune diseases, including systemic lupus erythematosus[60] and more recently, IgG4-RD.[61] For IgG4-RD specifically, utility has been demonstrated in the analysis of plasmablast expansion during autoimmune disease flare and subsequent contraction during therapeutic intervention.[6,62] However, routine testing for circulating plasmablast counts is not required for IgG4-RD diagnosis at the present time.

LIMITATIONS AND CHALLENGES

Flow cytometry has far-reaching diagnostic utility, yet many limitations remain, ranging from technical to regulatory. As many clinical flow cytometry laboratories are located in large urban areas, space is a limitation in terms of both instrumentation and personnel. Flow cytometers have become slightly reduced in size, but to keep up with the demand for increasing fluorochrome options (thus requiring more lasers), more and more components are being added to the instruments. Although certain types of flow cytometers have reached the ability to assess up to 40 different parameters (eg, mass cytometry using heavy metal ion tags instead of fluorochromes), these instruments have not yet been approved for use in clinical laboratories. Currently, the maximum number is 10 to 12 color flow cytometers. Finally, approaches for data acquisition, analysis, and reporting vary widely between institutions. There is an unmet need for consensus guidelines for panel design, analysis, and reporting. One major concern about flow cytometric consensus guidelines, however, is that they often do not evolve concurrent with the technology.

FUTURE DIRECTIONS

Flow cytometry has come a long way since its inception in the 1960s. It has progressed from single-color to multicolor analyses. It has been streamlined in terms of cost and efficiency, such that flow cytometry is now used all over the world in both the clinical and research arenas. With the coming opportunity to expand to 40 or more marker analyses in the clinical flow cytometry laboratory, the potential for single-tube analyses is on the horizon. This will offer clinicians unparalleled insights into highly specialized cell subsets of the immune system as well as offer the clinical flow cytometry laboratory the novel potential to create large standardized panels, as virtually any combination of markers could be assessed simultaneously. However, mass data acquisition will undoubtedly bring about new challenges, specifically data analysis and reporting. For now, highly multiplexed flow cytometry requires trained bioinformaticians to aid in data interpretation and is limited to the research setting.

REFERENCES

1. Davis BH, Dasgupta A, Kussick S, et al. Validation of cell-based fluorescence assays: practice guidelines from the ICSH and ICCS - part II - preanalytical issues. Cytometry B Clin Cytom 2013;84(5):286–90.
2. Tanqri S, Vall H, Kaplan D, et al. Validation of cell-based fluorescence assays: practice guidelines from the ICSH and ICCS - part III - analytical issues. Cytometry B Clin Cytom 2013;84(5):291–308.
3. Wood B, Jevremovic D, Bene MC, et al. Validation of cell-based fluorescence assays: practice guidelines from the ICSH and ICCS - part V - assay performance criteria. Cytometry B Clin Cytom 2013;84(5):315–23.
4. Oliveira JB, Bleesing JJ, Dianzani U, et al. Revised diagnostic criteria and classification for the autoimmune lymphoproliferative syndrome (ALPS): report from the 2009 NIH International Workshop. Blood 2010;116(14):e35–40.
5. Bleesing JJ, Brown MR, Dale JK, et al. TcR-alpha/beta(+) CD4(−)CD8(−) T cells in humans with the autoimmune lymphoproliferative syndrome express a novel CD45 isoform that is analogous to murine B220 and represents a marker of altered O-glycan biosynthesis. Clin Immunol 2001;100(3):314–24.
6. Wallace ZS, Mattoo H, Carruthers M, et al. Plasmablasts as a biomarker for IgG4-related disease, independent of serum IgG4 concentrations. Ann Rheum Dis 2015;74(1):190–5.
7. Kaminski DA, Wei C, Qian Y, et al. Advances in human B cell phenotypic profiling. Front Immunol 2012;3:302.
8. Bonilla FA, Khan DA, Ballas ZK, et al. Practice parameter for the diagnosis and management of primary immunodeficiency. J Allergy Clin Immunol 2015;136(5):1186–205.e1–78.
9. Bussone G, Mouthon L. Autoimmune manifestations in primary immune deficiencies. Autoimmun Rev 2009;8(4):332–6.
10. Mayor PC, Eng KH, Singel KL, et al. Cancer in primary immunodeficiency diseases: cancer incidence in the United States immune deficiency network registry. J Allergy Clin Immunol 2018;141(3):1028–35.
11. Sokol K, Milner JD. The overlap between allergy and immunodeficiency. Curr Opin Pediatr 2018;30(6):848–54.
12. Modell V, Knaus M, Modell F, et al. Global overview of primary immunodeficiencies: a report from Jeffrey Modell Centers worldwide focused on diagnosis, treatment, and discovery. Immunol Res 2014;60(1):132–44.
13. Routes JM, Grossman WJ, Verbsky J, et al. Statewide newborn screening for severe T-cell lymphopenia. JAMA 2009;302(22):2465–70.
14. King JR, Hammarstrom L. Newborn screening for primary immunodeficiency diseases: history, current and future practice. J Clin Immunol 2018;38(1):56–66.

15. Thakar MS, Hintermeyer MK, Gries MG, et al. A practical approach to newborn screening for severe combined immunodeficiency using the T cell receptor excision circle assay. Front Immunol 2017;8:1470.

16. Mamcarz E, Zhou S, Lockey T, et al. Lentiviral gene therapy combined with low-dose Busulfan in infants with SCID-X1. N Engl J Med 2019;380(16):1525–34.

17. Curtis MG, Walker B, Denny TN. Flow cytometric methods for prenatal and neonatal diagnosis. J Immunol Methods 2011;363(2):198–209.

18. Amatuni GS, Currier RJ, Church JA, et al. Newborn screening for severe combined immunodeficiency and T-cell lymphopenia in California, 2010-2017. Pediatrics 2019;143(2) [pii:e20182300].

19. Smith DK, Neal JJ, Holmberg SD. Unexplained opportunistic infections and CD4+ T-lymphocytopenia without HIV infection. An investigation of cases in the United States. The Centers for Disease Control idiopathic CD4+ T-lymphocytopenia task force. N Engl J Med 1993;328(6):373–9.

20. Brooks JP, Ghaffari G. Idiopathic CD4 lymphocytopenia. Allergy Asthma Proc 2016;37(6):501–4.

21. Des Jarlais DC, Friedman SR, Marmor M, et al. CD4 lymphocytopenia among injecting drug users in New York City. J Acquir Immune Defic Syndr 1993;6(7):820–2.

22. Yarmohammadi H, Cunningham-Rundles C. Idiopathic CD4 lymphocytopenia: pathogenesis, etiologies, clinical presentations and treatment strategies. Ann Allergy Asthma Immunol 2017;119(4):374–8.

23. Bruton OC. Agammaglobulinemia. Pediatrics 1952;9(6):722–8.

24. Thomas JD, Sideras P, Smith CI, et al. Colocalization of X-linked agammaglobulinemia and X-linked immunodeficiency genes. Science 1993;261(5119):355–8.

25. Rawlings DJ, Saffran DC, Tsukada S, et al. Mutation of unique region of Bruton's tyrosine kinase in immunodeficient XID mice. Science 1993;261(5119):358–61.

26. Nakagawa N, Imai K, Kanegane H, et al. Quantification of kappa-deleting recombination excision circles in Guthrie cards for the identification of early B-cell maturation defects. J Allergy Clin Immunol 2011;128(1):223–5.e2.

27. Orange JS. Natural killer cell deficiency. J Allergy Clin Immunol 2013;132(3):515–25.

28. Mace EM, Orange JS. Genetic causes of human NK cell deficiency and their effect on NK cell subsets. Front Immunol 2016;7:545.

29. Risma KA, Frayer RW, Filipovich AH, et al. Aberrant maturation of mutant perforin underlies the clinical diversity of hemophagocytic lymphohistiocytosis. J Clin Invest 2006;116(1):182–92.

30. Kagan JM, Sanchez AM, Landay A, et al. A brief chronicle of CD4 as a biomarker for HIV/AIDS: a tribute to the memory of John L. Fahey. For Immunopathol Dis Therap 2015;6(1–2):55–64.

31. Trouvin AP, Jacquot S, Grigioni S, et al. Usefulness of monitoring of B cell depletion in rituximab-treated rheumatoid arthritis patients in order to predict clinical relapse: a prospective observational study. Clin Exp Immunol 2015;180(1):11–8.

32. Thiel J, Rizzi M, Engesser M, et al. B cell repopulation kinetics after rituximab treatment in ANCA-associated vasculitides compared to rheumatoid arthritis, and connective tissue diseases: a longitudinal observational study on 120 patients. Arthritis Res Ther 2017;19(1):101.

33. Ellwardt E, Ellwardt L, Bittner S, et al. Monitoring B-cell repopulation after depletion therapy in neurologic patients. Neurol Neuroimmunol Neuroinflamm 2018;5(4):e463.

34. Castelino DJ, McNair P, Kay TW. Lymphocytopenia in a hospital population–what does it signify? Aust N Z J Med 1997;27(2):170–4.
35. Tavares SM, Junior Wde L, Lopes ESMR. Normal lymphocyte immunophenotype in an elderly population. Rev Bras Hematol Hemoter 2014;36(3):180–3.
36. Palmer DB. The effect of age on thymic function. Front Immunol 2013;4:316.
37. Cancro MP, Hao Y, Scholz JL, et al. B cells and aging: molecules and mechanisms. Trends Immunol 2009;30(7):313–8.
38. Kaleem Z. Flow cytometric analysis of lymphomas: current status and usefulness. Arch Pathol Lab Med 2006;130(12):1850–8.
39. Laurence J. T-cell subsets in health, infectious disease, and idiopathic CD4+ T lymphocytopenia. Ann Intern Med 1993;119(1):55–62.
40. Lok JJ, Bosch RJ, Benson CA, et al. Long-term increase in CD4+ T-cell counts during combination antiretroviral therapy for HIV-1 infection. AIDS 2010;24(12): 1867–76.
41. Yoon JW, Gollapudi S, Pahl MV, et al. Naive and central memory T-cell lymphopenia in end-stage renal disease. Kidney Int 2006;70(2):371–6.
42. Magdo HS, Stillwell TL, Greenhawt MJ, et al. Immune abnormalities in Fontan protein-losing enteropathy: a case-control study. J Pediatr 2015;167(2):331–7.
43. Gandhi RT. Cirrhosis is associated with low CD4+ T cell counts: implications for HIV-infected patients with liver disease. Clin Infect Dis 2007;44(3):438–40.
44. Olnes MJ, Kotliarov Y, Biancotto A, et al. Effects of systemically administered hydrocortisone on the human immunome. Sci Rep 2016;6:23002.
45. Kimby E. Tolerability and safety of rituximab (MabThera). Cancer Treat Rev 2005; 31(6):456–73.
46. Sacco KA, Abraham RS. Consequences of B-cell-depleting therapy: hypogammaglobulinemia and impaired B-cell reconstitution. Immunotherapy 2018;10(8): 713–28.
47. Barmettler S, Ong MS, Farmer JR, et al. Association of immunoglobulin levels, infectious risk, and mortality with rituximab and hypogammaglobulinemia. JAMA Netw Open 2018;1(7):e184169.
48. Martire B, Foti C, Cassano N, et al. Persistent B-cell lymphopenia, multiorgan disease, and erythema multiforme caused by *Mycoplasma pneumoniae* infection. Pediatr Dermatol 2005;22(6):558–60.
49. Montella L, Masci AM, Merkabaoui G, et al. B-cell lymphopenia and hypogammaglobulinemia in thymoma patients. Ann Hematol 2003;82(6):343–7.
50. Fogel LA, Yokoyama WM, French AR. Natural killer cells in human autoimmune disorders. Arthritis Res Ther 2013;15(4):216.
51. Bonilla FA, Barlan I, Chapel H, et al. International consensus document (ICON): common variable immunodeficiency disorders. J Allergy Clin Immunol Pract 2016;4(1):38–59.
52. Wehr C, Kivioja T, Schmitt C, et al. The EUROclass trial: defining subgroups in common variable immunodeficiency. Blood 2008;111(1):77–85.
53. Kverneland AH, Streitz M, Geissler E, et al. Age and gender leucocytes variances and references values generated using the standardized ONE-Study protocol. Cytometry A 2016;89(6):543–64.
54. Shearer WT, Dunn E, Notarangelo LD, et al. Establishing diagnostic criteria for severe combined immunodeficiency disease (SCID), leaky SCID, and Omenn syndrome: the Primary Immune Deficiency Treatment Consortium experience. J Allergy Clin Immunol 2014;133(4):1092–8.

55. Malphettes M, Gerard L, Carmagnat M, et al. Late-onset combined immune deficiency: a subset of common variable immunodeficiency with severe T cell defect. Clin Infect Dis 2009;49(9):1329–38.
56. Farmer JR, Ong MS, Barmettler S, et al. Common variable immunodeficiency non-infectious disease endotypes redefined using unbiased network clustering in large electronic datasets. Front Immunol 2017;8:1740.
57. Russell TB, Kurre P. Double-negative T cells are non-ALPS-specific markers of immune dysregulation found in patients with aplastic anemia. Blood 2010;116(23): 5072–3.
58. Juvet SC, Zhang L. Double negative regulatory T cells in transplantation and autoimmunity: recent progress and future directions. J Mol Cell Biol 2012;4(1):48–58.
59. Fink K. Origin and function of circulating plasmablasts during acute viral infections. Front Immunol 2012;3:78.
60. Malkiel S, Barlev AN, Atisha-Fregoso Y, et al. Plasma cell differentiation pathways in systemic lupus erythematosus. Front Immunol 2018;9:427.
61. Mattoo H, Mahajan VS, Della-Torre E, et al. De novo oligoclonal expansions of circulating plasmablasts in active and relapsing IgG4-related disease. J Allergy Clin Immunol 2014;134(3):679–87.
62. Lin W, Zhang P, Chen H, et al. Circulating plasmablasts/plasma cells: a potential biomarker for IgG4-related disease. Arthritis Res Ther 2017;19(1):25.

Laboratory Assays of Immune Cell Function in Immunodeficiencies

Sara Barmettler, MD

KEYWORDS

• Immunodeficiency • Laboratory assay • Immune cell function

KEY POINTS

- Laboratory assays of the function of immune cells are essential for assessing and diagnosing immune deficiencies.
- Laboratory assessments of immune cell function should be performed in conjunction with a detailed history and physical examination, which should guide the evaluation of patients with a suspected immune deficiency.
- As genetic sequencing becomes more readily available, laboratory assays of immune cell function will be critical for assessing and demonstrating the functional impact of genetic mutations.

DEFECTS IN T-CELL FUNCTION

One of the most common types of laboratory assay for immune cell function is flow cytometry. Please see Jocelyn R. Farmer and Michelle DeLelys's article, "Flow Cytometry as a Diagnostic Tool in Primary and Secondary Immune Deficiencies," in this issue, for additional information regarding the use of flow cytometry for enumeration of immune cells and immunophenotyping to identify quantitative abnormalities in T, B, or natural killer (NK) cells.

T lymphocytes, or T cells, are essential for cell-mediated immunity, and are an important component of the adaptive immune system.[1] In addition to cellular immune defects, T-cell dysfunction can affect B-cell function, leading to humoral defects. Lymphocyte enumeration by flow cytometry is important for quantifying T cells, including total T cells (cluster of differentiation [CD] 3+), helper T cells (CD4+), and killer T cells (CD8+), as well as B (CD19+) and NK (CD16+56+) cells, but should also be accompanied by functional assays for better characterization of immune defects.

Disclosure: The author has nothing to disclose.
Allergy and Immunology Unit, Division of Rheumatology, Allergy and Immunology, Massachusetts General Hospital, 55 Fruit Street, MGH Allergy Associates, COX 201, Boston, MA 02114, USA
E-mail address: sbarmettler@mgh.harvard.edu

Clin Lab Med 39 (2019) 609–623
https://doi.org/10.1016/j.cll.2019.07.008
0272-2712/19/© 2019 Elsevier Inc. All rights reserved.

Severe Combined Immunodeficiency

Severe combined immunodeficiency (SCID) is characterized by markedly low T-cell levels (CD3+ count <300 cells/μL), susceptibility to severe and recurrent infections, chronic diarrhea, and failure to thrive.[2] Newborn screening (NBS) for SCID is increasingly being implemented across the United States[3] and around the world.[4] NBS for SCID measures T-cell receptor excision circles (TRECs) as a biomarker for naive T cells. TRECs have been shown to be sensitive, specific, and cost-effective.[5–7] Patients with SCID have impaired T-cell development and function, with primary or secondary B-cell defects. For patients with low TREC levels identified on NBS or with a clinical concern for SCID, flow cytometry evaluating T, B, and NK cells is performed to classify the nature of the defect. The function of T cells is evaluated by lymphocyte proliferation assays.

Lymphocyte proliferation assays

Lymphocyte proliferation assays are used to assess the function of T cells by measuring peripheral blood T-cell proliferation in response to different stimuli (mitogens or antigens).[8] In the lymphocyte proliferation assays, peripheral blood mononuclear cells (PBMCs) are purified from whole blood (usually approximately 10 mL of whole blood) and cultured in standard media in the presence or absence of a stimulus. Frequently used stimuli include mitogens (plant lectins that bind to the carbohydrate component of lymphocyte surface glycoproteins, including antigen receptors, and activate intracellular signaling pathways, leading to polyclonal cell stimulation and division) or antigens (processed and presented by accessory cells and stimulate only antigen-specific T cells).[8] Examples of mitogens are phytohemagglutinin, concanavalin A, and anti-CD3, which predominantly activate T cells. Pokeweed mitogen stimulates both B and T cells. Recall antigens include tetanus toxoid, diphtheria toxoid, or *Candida* antigen. After culture for approximately 3 days with mitogens, or 5 to 7 days with antigens, tritiated thymidine is added to the culture for an additional 10 to 24 hours. The radioactive thymidine is incorporated into DNA as the cells divide, and this allows an indirect measure of cell division. The cells are collected, and the incorporated radioactivity is measured. Control PBMCs are used as a technical and reference control, and are usually analyzed in parallel with the patient specimen or can be analyzed on a regular basis by the laboratory. The data are reported as counts per minute (CPM) of radioactivity incorporated during the culture period and compared with the normal control. A stimulation index may also be reported, which is the ratio of CPM obtained with and without the stimulus.[8] Mitogen proliferation tests may be performed at any age, including newborns.[9] Antigen proliferation tests require prior antigen exposure, and are limited in utility in patients less than 6 months to 1 year of age, and in patients who have not received immunizations.[8]

There are several factors that can cause decreased T-cell responsiveness, including medications and infections. Medications such as steroids can decrease mitogen responsiveness; however, there is evidence in 1 cohort to suggest that 24 hours after a dose of steroids, T-cell proliferation was normal.[10] Infections can also decrease lymphocyte responsiveness, and these include human immunodeficiency virus, measles, cytomegalovirus, malaria, and trypanosomes.[8]

Cutaneous delayed-type hypersensitivity

Another measure of T-cell function is delayed hypersensitivity skin testing.[11] Delayed hypersensitivity skin testing uses intradermal injection of an antigen to assess the in vivo T cell–specific antigen response. Given that the test measures recall response to an antigen, this requires that the patient has been exposed to the antigen, and is often of low utility in patients less than 1 year of age.[11–13] The method is similar to the purified protein derivative (Mantoux) test, in which the recall antigen (0.1 mL of antigen) is injected into the superficial layers of the dermis, usually on the ventral surface of the forearm. A distance of at least 3 cm between antigen injection sites is preferable. This test elicits induration and erythema, which are measured at 48 to 72 hours using the largest diameter of induration. The most commonly used recall antigens include the *Candida*, *Trichophyton*, and tuberculin skin testing antigens. Other options include the mumps skin test antigen.[11] A normal response is considered to be at least 2 to 5 mm of induration.[12] Although it can be performed more quickly and is less expensive than in vitro assays of T-cell proliferation, there are many disease states that can affect testing, including malnutrition, immunosuppression, and infections,[11] and negative responses should be interpreted with caution.

Hyperimmunoglobulin M Syndrome

Hyperimmunoglobulin M (hyper-IgM) syndrome is characterized by normal or high immunoglobulin (Ig) M levels, recurrent infections, and low IgG, immunoglobulin, and IgE levels.[14] X-linked hyper-IgM is the most common form of hyper-IgM syndrome, and is caused by mutations in CD40 ligand (CD40L). CD40L is expressed on CD4+ T cells and interacts with CD40 on B cells, which leads to B-cell activation, proliferation, class switch recombination, and affinity maturation.[14,15] Flow cytometry can be used to assess surface expression of CD40L on activated CD4+ T cells.[16] This method involves activation of T cells, often with phytohemagglutinin and phorbol myristate acetate (PMA), followed by flow cytometric analysis.[14] Other markers of T-cell activation are used as controls, such as CD25 or CD69 expression.[17] If CD40L expression is absent or reduced on activated cells, this can help with the diagnosis of X-linked hyper-IgM. This assay is useful in mutations that result in a lack of protein expression on the cell surface; however, other types of mutations, such as some splice site and cytoplasmic tail mutations, may not result in abnormal expression.[14] A functional assessment of CD40L can be performed using the soluble form of the receptor (CD40-μIg).[18] Hyper-IgM syndrome can also be caused by autosomal recessive defects, including mutations in the CD40 gene. This condition can cause defective CD40 expression on B cells, which can be analyzed by flow cytometry.[14] Autosomal recessive hyper-IgM syndrome can also be caused by mutations in uracil nucleoside glycosylase (UNG) and activation-induced cytidine deaminase (AID).[14] CD40L gene sequencing is the gold standard for diagnosing CD40L deficiency in patients with suggestive symptoms and abnormal CD40 ligand protein expression by flow cytometry. Similarly, genetic testing for CD40, AID, and UNG mutations is recommended for the diagnosis of hyper-IgM syndrome.

Autoimmune Lymphoproliferative Syndrome

Autoimmune lymphoproliferative syndrome (ALPS) is characterized by dysregulation of lymphocyte apoptosis, which leads to lymphoproliferation, including lymphadenopathy and hepatosplenomegaly, autoimmune cytopenias, and increased risk for lymphoma.[19] ALPS can be caused by defects in proteins involved in the Fas-mediated apoptotic pathway. There are several gene defects associated with ALPS, including Fas/CD95, Fas ligand (FasL), caspase10, and caspase8. These defects lead to increased levels of double-negative T cells (DNTs), which are cells that express the T-cell receptor (TCR) alpha and beta chains but do not express the CD4+ or CD8+ coreceptors. The criteria for ALPS include increased DNT levels, in the context of normal or increased total lymphocyte counts. Double-negative T cells are assessed using antibodies to αβ-TCR, because most double-negative T cells are γδ-TCR+. In addition, defective in vitro Fas receptor–mediated lymphocyte apoptosis has been described in patients with ALPS.[19,20] Apoptosis assays can be performed on Epstein-Barr virus (EBV) transformed lymphocytes, where apoptosis is induced with APO-1 anti-Fas antibody.[19] The apoptosis assays are laborious and often require several days to weeks of cell culture but are critical for the proper diagnosis of ALPS when mutations in ALPS-linked genes cannot be identified.

Hyperimmunoglobulin E Syndrome

Hyperimmunoglobulin E syndrome (hyper-IgE syndrome [HIES]) is characterized by recurrent pulmonary infections, staphylococcal abscesses, eczema, bone/connective tissue defects, and increased IgE levels.[21] Autosomal dominant HIES is caused by missense mutations in signal transducer and activator of transcription (STAT) 3. STAT3 is a transcription factor and is required for induction of CD4+ T cells to produce interleukin (IL)-17a. Impaired T-helper (Th) 17 cell differentiation has been described in patients with autosomal dominant HIES.[22] A flow cytometry–based functional assay can be used to assess the ability of T cells to synthesize IL-17a. In this assay, PBMCs are stimulated with a phorbol ester ([PMA) and ionomycin in the presence of molecules that prevent exocytosis of IL-17a (eg, brefeldin A) for 4 hours, then fixed and stained for intracellular cytokines.[22] Flow cytometry can be used to detect phosphorylated STAT3. PBMCs are incubated with stimuli or with IL-6, and then fixed, permeabilized, and stained. A conjugated phospho-STAT3 antibody against phospho-S727 is used to identify intracellular or intranuclear phospho-STAT3.[23] In patients with STAT3 mutations that affect the SH2 or transactivation domains of the protein, STAT3 phosphorylation is abnormal. However, STAT3 mutations that affect the DNA-binding domain of the protein show normal STAT3 phosphorylation. The gold standard for confirming the diagnosis of AD-HIES is STAT3 gene sequencing.

Dedicator of cytokinesis 8 (DOCK8) deficiency is a combined immunodeficiency that was previously classified as a subtype of autosomal recessive HIES.[24] DOCK8 is characterized by recurrent sinopulmonary infections, skin and systemic viral infections, and eczema.[25] DOCK8 protein expression can be assessed using intracellular staining for DOCK8 on mononuclear cells from peripheral blood.[25] DOCK8 deficiency is an autosomal recessive condition, so confirmation of the diagnosis requires biallelic mutations in the DOCK8 gene.

Wiskott-Aldrich Syndrome

Wiskott-Aldrich syndrome (WAS) is an X-linked disease characterized by eczema, thrombocytopenia, and immunodeficiency, caused by mutations in the WAS gene.[26] Patients with WAS have thrombocytopenia with small platelet size. The WAS gene product is a cytoplasmic protein involved in signaling and regulation of the actin cytoskeleton.[26] Flow cytometry can be used to assess the WAS protein (WASp), using an anti-WASp antibody.[27,28] A complete absence of WASp is associated with a more severe WAS phenotype. Of note, there are patients with missense mutations in WAS that express a normal amount of nonfunctional WASp. The gold standard for confirming a diagnosis of WAS in a patient with suggestive clinical symptoms is WAS gene sequencing.

Ataxia-Telangiectasia

Ataxia-telangiectasia (AT) is an autosomal recessive disorder caused by mutations in the ATM gene, characterized by progressive cerebellar ataxia, oculocutaneous telangiectasias, abnormal eye movements, neurologic abnormalities, and immune deficiency.[29] Patients can have both humoral and cell-mediated immune deficiency. Patients with AT with profoundly decreased circulative naive T cells can be identified on the newborn screen for SCID using quantification of TRECs.[30] There are functional and molecular assays that have been used to assist in the diagnosis of ATM.[31] Rapid immunoblotting assay for ATM protein shows depleted protein in most patients with ATM.[32] Patients with ATM show radiation sensitivity.[33] Normally, DNA mechanisms induce phosphorylation of H2AX to γ-H2AX after exposure to ionizing radiation. Phosphorylation of H2AX does not occur in patients with ATM gene defects,[34] and thus flow cytometry can also be used to quantify γ-H2AX in T-cell lines, lymphoblastoid cell lines, and PBMCs.[35]

DEFECTS IN B-CELL FUNCTION

Humoral immunodeficiency is often evaluated using quantitative assays for total immunoglobulins (IgG, IgA, and IgM) in addition to measurement of specific antibody responses. The assessment of B-cell function in conjunction with assessment of immunoglobulin levels is critical, because there are some patients in whom production of functional antibodies is low despite normal serum immunoglobulin levels.[12,36] In contrast, assessment of functional antibody levels is important in cases of low total immunoglobulin levels, because some patients have normal responses to immunization, suggesting B-cell function is (at least partially) preserved. Specific antibody responses can be evaluated by measuring natural antibodies (eg, isohemagglutinins) or by measuring specific antibody production in response to immunization.

Common Variable Immunodeficiency

Common variable immunodeficiency (CVID) is characterized by recurrent sinopulmonary infections, low age-adjusted IgG level with low IgA and/or IgM levels, impaired specific antibody responses following immunization, and exclusion of other causes of hypogammaglobulinemia in patients more than 2 years old.[37] In addition to recurrent infections, a subset of patients with CVID have inflammatory, lymphoproliferative, and autoimmune complications.[38] In addition to measuring serum immunoglobulin levels, assessment of the specific antibody titers and the response to immunizations is critical in the diagnosis of CVID. Some patients with CVID have reduced levels of circulating memory B cells (CD27+ B cells) and especially low levels of isotype switched memory B cells (CD27+ IgD− IgM−).[39,40] There is evidence of T-cell dysregulation in a subset of patients with CVID, with a reduced CD4+/CD8+ ratio and reduced percentage of CD4+ T cells expressing CD45RA+.[37,41] There have been an increasing number of genetic mutations associated with CVID, which include ICOS, TNFRSF13B (TACI), TNFRSF13C (BAFF-R), TNFSF12 (TWEAK), CD19, CD81, CR2 (CD21), MS4A1 (CD20), TNFRSF7 (CD27), IL21, IL21R, LRBA (lipopolysaccharide-responsive vesicle trafficking, beach-containing and anchor-containing), CTLA4, PRKCD, PLCG2, NFKB1, NFKB2, PIK3CD, PIK3R1, VAV1, RAC2, BLK, IKZF1 (IKAROS), and IRF2BP2.[42]

Natural antibodies assessment

Specific antibody responses can be evaluated by measuring levels of natural antibodies such as isohemagglutinins. Isohemagglutinins are antibodies that are spontaneously generated in response to polysaccharides present in gut flora that cross-react with A or B blood group erythrocyte antigens.[43,44] They generally appear in the blood by 6 months of age but are not present in patients with blood type AB. Isohemagglutinin testing is usually performed by blood banks.

Specific antibody responses to immunization

Vaccine-induced antibody titers can be used to evaluate specific responses to protein and polysaccharide antigens. IgG antibodies to tetanus and diphtheria toxoids provide an evaluation of the response to T cell–dependent protein antigens. IgG antibodies to *Streptococcus pneumoniae* and meningococcal polysaccharide vaccines assess the T-independent antibody response. Polysaccharide vaccine antigens activate B cells directly, and do not require T-cell help.

Protective levels are often considered to be greater than or equal to 1.0 μg/mL for the *Haemophilus influenzae* B conjugate vaccine, greater than or equal to 2.0 μg/mL for the meningococcal conjugate and polysaccharide vaccines, greater than or equal to 0.15 IU/mL for tetanus, and greater than or equal to 5 IU for the rabies vaccine.[45]

For the pneumococcal antibody assessment, there are some controversies regarding the definition of a protective titer. Many immunologists consider a serotype-specific IgG concentration of greater than or equal to 1.3 μg/mL to be protective against invasive pneumococcal disease.[12,45] In children aged 2 to 5 years, an adequate response is considered to be at least 50% of the vaccine serotypes tested. If the initial evaluation does now show adequate titers to at least 50% of the serotypes, the polysaccharide pneumococcal vaccine (23-valent pneumococcal polysaccharide vaccine [PPV-23]) should be given and the serotypes should be reassessed in 4 to 6 weeks.[45] In older children (>6 years old) and adults, an adequate response is considered to be at least 70% of the serotypes.[12,45] If this is not the case, the PPV-23 should be administered and the titers should be reassessed 4 to 6 weeks after vaccination. For prevaccination titers greater than or equal to 1.3 μg/mL, a 2-fold increase after vaccination is considered adequate.[45]

In patients receiving immunoglobulin replacement, assessment of specific antibody production is difficult because the serologies are not necessarily reflective of the native antibody production in the patient. Patients must be taken off immunoglobulin replacement for at least 3 to 4 months before testing can be considered to be reliable. Research protocols have been developed to use neoantigens, which include bacteriophage ΦX174[45]; however, these are not commercially available. The rabies vaccine and the *Salmonella typhi* Vi vaccine are also being investigated for potential use.[45]

Specific Antibody Deficiency

Specific antibody deficiency is characterized by recurrent sinopulmonary infections, normal immunoglobulin levels (IgG, IgA, IgM), and selectively diminished antibody responses to polysaccharide antigens following vaccination.[36] Response to protein antigens and all other parameters of immune function are normal. The interpretation of protective antibody response to pneumococcal polysaccharide vaccines was discussed earlier.

X-Linked Agammaglobulinemia

X-linked agammaglobulinemia (XLA) is characterized by recurrent infections, including sinopulmonary infections, gastrointestinal infections, skin infections, arthritis, inflammatory bowel disease, and hypogammaglobulinemia.[2,46,47] Laboratory findings include decreased to absent peripheral B cells and profoundly decreased serum immunoglobulin levels, with low/absent specific antibody titers. Patients often present around 6 months of age, with the waning of protective maternal antibodies. In XLA, mutations in Bruton tyrosine kinase (*BTK*) result in defective tonic pre-BCR signaling, impaired B-cell survival, and arrest in maturation at the pre–B-cell stage. The protein encoded by BTK plays a crucial role in B-cell development. The BTK protein can be evaluated using flow cytometry.[18] BTK protein expression is evaluated in either monocytes or platelets, because patients with XLA generally have very few B cells.[48,49] An anti-BTK monoclonal antibody can be used to assess expression of intracytoplasmic BTK protein.[49] Absent or reduced BTK protein expression is observed in approximately 95% of patients with XLA, but 5% may have normal protein expression with abnormal function.[18] The gold standard for XLA diagnosis is BTK gene sequencing.

Congenital Agammaglobulinemia

Other forms of congenital agammaglobulinemia can be caused by autosomal recessive or autosomal dominant mutations involved in B-cell function and maturation. The clinical and laboratory features of these disorders resemble XLA; however, the patterns of inheritance differ and this has implications for genetic counseling. Genetic studies are recommended to test for mutations associated with congenital agammaglobulinemia. Autosomal recessive agammaglobulinemia can be caused by mutations in IGHM, CD79A, CLNK, CD79B, and IGLL1.[50–55] Autosomal dominant agammaglobulinemia can be caused by mutations in TCF3 and LRRC8.[56,57]

Lipopolysaccharide-Responsive Vesicle Trafficking, Beach-Containing and Anchor-Containing Deficiency

LRBA deficiency is caused by biallelic loss-of-function mutations in the gene LRBA.[58] LRBA deficiency is characterized by early-onset hypogammaglobulinemia, autoimmunity, and inflammatory bowel disease.[59] LRBA protein is normally expressed intracellularly in B cells, T cells, monocytes, and NK cells. LRBA protein expression can be assessed by flow cytometry after stimulation.[18,60] Several stimuli can be used, including antigen stimulation, mitogens, bacterial superantigens, cytokines, and toll-like receptor (TLR) agonists; however, the most efficient activation condition for PBMCs was found to be stimulation with phytohemagglutinin for 4 days followed by stimulation with anti-CD3/anti-CD28 for 48 hours.[60] Genetic testing for biallelic mutations in LRBA is necessary for a definitive diagnosis.

DEFECTS IN NATURAL KILLER CELL FUNCTION

NK cells are a component of the innate immune system that play a role in controlling microbial infections and certain types of tumors.[61] NK cell deficiencies or dysfunction have been described in patients with recurrent herpes virus family infections, as well as conditions such as hemophagocytic lymphohistiocytosis (HLH).[62]

Hemophagocytic Lymphohistiocytosis

HLH is a life-threatening disorder characterized by uncontrolled, excessive cytotoxic lymphocyte and macrophage activation, with accompanying massive inflammatory cytokine release.[63] Primary HLH is caused by mutations in proteins involved in cytotoxic lymphocyte degranulation, including perforin (PRF1), UNC13D, STXBP2, STX11, RAB27A, LYST, and AP3B1.[64] Secondary HLH occurs in the setting of infection, malignancy, and rheumatologic or other conditions.[63] Evaluation includes immunophenotyping to test for the presence or absence of NK cells and cytotoxic T cells. Cytotoxicity assays can be used to measure the effector function of these cells.[64] In these assays, PBMCs are cultured with labeled target cells, and levels of markers of apoptosis (eg, annexin V, 7-AAD) or cell death (release of radiolabeled chromium) are measured.[65] Flow cytometry can be used to assess CD107a mobilization.[64,66] Lysosome-associated membrane protein-1 (LAMP1 or CD107a) is a marker of degranulation and is normally expressed on the luminal surface of cytotoxic cell granules. These granules are transported to the cell surface and fuse with the cell membrane to release perforin and granzyme, exposing CD107a. CD107a expression can be assessed by flow cytometry using anti-CD107a antibodies in the presence of K562 target cells to induce degranulation.[64] Perforin and granzyme B expression can also be assessed by flow cytometry.[67,68] Perforin and CD107a tests have been shown to be more sensitive and no less specific than NK cytotoxicity testing for screening patients with genetic causes of HLH.[64]

X-Linked Lymphoproliferative Disease

X-linked lymphoproliferative disease (XLP) is characterized by uncontrolled lymphopro-liferation following EBV infection. Patients also have fulminant infectious mononucleosis, dysgammaglobulinemia and increased risk of lymphoma.[69] XLP-1 is caused by muta-tions in the signaling lymphocyte activation molecule (SLAM)–associated protein (SAP) gene. XLP-2 is caused by X-linked inhibitor of apoptosis (XIAP) deficiency. Intracellular flow cytometry can be used to evaluate for the absence of the SAP protein in XLP1 and XIAP protein in XLP2.[70–73] Genetic testing is the gold standard for diagnosing XLP.

DEFECTS IN INNATE IMMUNITY
Leukocyte Adhesion Deficiency

Leukocyte adhesion deficiency (LAD) syndromes are characterized by defects in leukocyte chemotaxis (particularly neutrophils). There are 3 LAD syndromes that have been described.[74] LAD-I is caused by mutations in the beta-2 integrin gene, with absent or decreased expression of the neutrophil adhesion molecule CD18,[75] which causes defective adhesion of leukocytes to the endothelium. LAD-I is charac-terized by recurrent bacterial infections, delayed separation of the umbilical cord, ab-sent pus formation, impaired wound healing, and leukocytosis. LAD-II is caused by mutations in the fucose transporter that lead to absent fucosylated carbohydrate ligands for selectins. In patients with LAD2, CD15 (sialyl-Lewis X) expression is absent on neutrophils.[75] LAD-II is characterized by less severe infections than patients with LAD-I. Patients with LAD-II may have severe intellectual disabilities, short stature, and microcephaly. In addition, LAD-II is associated with the Bombay (hh) blood phenotype, with red blood cells lacking A, B, and H antigens. LAD-III is caused by mu-tations in kindlin-3, which is an essential component of integrin activation. LAD-III is characterized by severe infections, delayed separation of the umbilical cord, bleeding complications, and marked leukocytosis.

To diagnose LAD-I, flow cytometry can be performed using CD11 and CD18 mono-clonal antibodies to show the absence of functional CD18 and the associated alpha subunit molecules CD11a, CD11b, and CD11c on the surface of leukocytes.[75] There are some cases in which abnormal CD18 can be expressed, so CD11a should also be assessed.[76] In LAD-II, the defect in fucose metabolism leads to the absence of sialyl-Lewis X (CD15a), which is a carbohydrate ligand on the cell surface of neutrophils. LAD-II can be diagnosed by evaluating CD15 expression on neutrophils by flow cytometry.[75] In LAD-III, integrin expression is intact, but there is impaired integrin acti-vation.[77] Genetic sequencing for LAD mutations (beta-2 subunit in LAD-I, the gene encoding GDP-fucose transporter in LAD-III, the kindlin-3 gene in LAD-III) is recom-mended to confirm the diagnosis.

Chronic Granulomatous Disease

Chronic granulomatous disease (CGD) is a phagocyte disorder caused by mutations in nicotinamide dinucleotide phosphate (NADPH) oxidase subunits. Patients with CGD typically present with increased susceptibility to bacterial (*Staphylococcus aureus, Pseudomonas aeruginosa, Nocardia asteroides, Salmonella typhi*) and fungal infections (*Candida* and *Aspergillus*). Defects in the genes encoding subunits of the NADPH oxidase complex result in decreased or absent oxidative burst and reactive oxygen intermediate production. The NADPH oxidase complex is encoded by 5 genes: CYBB (which encodes gp91^{phox}), CYBA (which encodes p22^{phox}), NCF1 (which encodes 47^{phox}), NCF2 (which encodes p67^{phox}), and NCF4 (which encodes p40^{phox}). CYBB is located on the X chromosome, and X-linked CGD accounts for about two-thirds of cases in the United States.

The neutrophil oxidative burst pathway can be evaluated using the nitroblue tetrazolium (NBT) test and the dihydrorhodamine-123 (DHR) flow assay. Both of these tests are abnormal in patients with CGD; however, the DHR flow assay is considered to be a more sensitive test.[78] In the nitroblue tetrazolium test, neutrophils are activated to produce superoxide, which oxidizes NBT from a yellow water-soluble compound to a dark-blue insoluble formazan.[79] In patients with CGD, this change is not observed.[80] The DHR flow cytometric assay measures the change in fluorescence of DHR-loaded granulocytes after PMA stimulation.[81] Activated neutrophils normally produce superoxides that oxidize DHR, resulting in increased fluorescence. Cells from patients with CGD cannot generate an oxidative burst and do not oxidize DHR.[34] Carriers of X-linked CGD show a bimodal pattern of induction of neutrophil oxidative burst caused by random X inactivation.[34]

Defects in the Interleukin-12/23–Interferon-Gamma Pathways

Mendelian susceptibility to mycobacterial diseases are a group of diseases characterized by defects in the genetic components of the IL-12/23–IFN-gamma pathways, which can lead to invasive infections caused by low-virulence mycobacterial and *Salmonella* species.[82] Mutations have been described in INF-gamma receptor 1 and 2 (IFNγR1 and 2), IL-12 receptor beta-1 (IL12RB1), IL12B, and the STAT1 genes. Western blotting and flow cytometry can be used to identify the specific defects. IL12RB1 and IFNγR1 defects typically result in absent cell-surface protein expression, which can be assessed by using flow cytometry with monoclonal reagents specific for these two proteins.[62,83] However, IFNγR1 surface expression is increased on blood mononuclear cells in the autosomal dominant form of IFNγR1 deficiency because of the accumulation of the nonfunctional mutant form of this receptor.[84] Abnormalities in IFNγR2 or STAT1 can be evaluated by monocyte STAT1 phosphorylation in response to IFN-γ, which can be done by flow cytometry or Western blotting.[85] Decreased STAT1 phosphorylation suggests a possible defect in STAT1, IFNγR1, or IFNγR2.[34]

Toll-Like Receptor Pathway Defects

The TLRs are a group of pattern recognition receptors that recognize specific molecular components of microorganisms and initiate signals to initiate cytokine synthesis. Defects in TLRs can cause increased susceptibility to infections, and these include IL-1 receptor–associated kinase 4 (IRAK4), myeloid differentiation primary response gene 88 defect (MYD88), nuclear factor kappa-B essential modulator defect (NEMO), TLR3 receptor defects, and unc-93 homolog (UNC93B) defects. Mutations in TLR3 and UNC93B have been associated with herpes simplex encephalitis.[86] Flow cytometry assays can be used to assess the TLRs. In these assays, mononuclear cells can be stimulated with TLR-specific ligands, and cytokine production is measured by an enzyme-linked immunosorbent assay.[62,87] The specific molecules used to induce the TLRs may include Pam3CSK4 to activate TLRs 1 and 2, zymosan to activate TLR2 and TLR6, poly(I:C) for TLR3, ultrapure lipopolysaccharide for TLR4, flagellin for TLR5, loxoribine for TLR7, and oligodinucleotide 2216 for TLR9.[87] Abnormal tests should be confirmed by repeat testing because the TLR testing is sensitive to the condition of the cells and illness. Persistently abnormal testing should prompt genetic testing.

SECONDARY IMMUNE DISORDERS

Secondary immune disorders are far more common than primary immunodeficiencies. Secondary immune disorders can be caused by several disease states, including infections, malignancy, medications, surgeries, or environmental exposures.[88] These disorders can lead to increased susceptibility to infection, malignancy, and autoimmune disease. A detailed clinical history and physical examination is critical for identifying potential causes, such as infection, malnutrition, extremes of age, metabolic or neoplastic diseases, use of immunosuppressive medications, surgery and trauma, and exposure to environmental conditions.[88] This history and examination can lead to targeted laboratory evaluation based on these findings to confirm these potential diagnoses. The immune impairment usually improves with the resolution of the primary condition.

There are some cases in which a primary immunodeficiency presents with immune dysregulation, and may be uncovered by the use of an immunosuppressive agent or concomitant disease state. One such example is the use of biologic agents such as rituximab, which is an anti-CD20 monoclonal antibody used in several subspecialties for rheumatologic, hematologic, oncologic, and renal indications. There is a subset of patients who develop prolonged, symptomatic hypogammaglobulinemia following rituximab therapy who may have underlying immune deficiency or immune dysregulation.[89–92] Evaluation of serum immunoglobulins and B-cell flow cytometry may be helpful in these cases, both before use of this biologic agent and following its use to assess immune recovery.[89] Similarly, evaluation of T-cell and B-cell function by T-cell proliferation and assessment of antibody titers, respectively, may be helpful in evaluating the extent of immune dysfunction.

SUMMARY

Laboratory assays of immune cell functions are essential in assessing and diagnosing immune deficiencies. The quantification of immune cells is critical in the initial assessment of immune defects; however, functional assessment is also of utmost importance. Functional testing must be used in conjunction with genetic testing to understand the type and impact of genetic defects. Advances in diagnostic techniques continue to expand the ability of clinicians and researchers to understand the complex immune pathophysiology that underlies these disorders.

REFERENCES

1. Larosa DF, Orange JS. 1. Lymphocytes. J Allergy Clin Immunol 2008;121(2 Suppl):S364–9 [quiz: S412].
2. Picard C, Bobby Gaspar H, Al-Herz W, et al. International Union of Immunological Societies: 2017 primary immunodeficiency diseases committee report on inborn errors of immunity. J Clin Immunol 2018;38(1):96–128.
3. Dorsey M, Puck J. Newborn screening for severe combined immunodeficiency in the US: current status and approach to management. Int J Neonatal Screen 2017;3(2):15.

4. Therrell BL, Padilla CD, Loeber JG, et al. Current status of newborn screening worldwide: 2015. Semin Perinatol 2015;39(3):171–87.
5. Puck JM. Laboratory technology for population-based screening for severe combined immunodeficiency in neonates: the winner is T-cell receptor excision circles. J Allergy Clin Immunol 2012;129(3):607–16.
6. Chan K, Puck JM. Development of population-based newborn screening for severe combined immunodeficiency. J Allergy Clin Immunol 2005;115(2):391–8.
7. Morinishi Y, Imai K, Nakagawa N, et al. Identification of severe combined immunodeficiency by T-cell receptor excision circles quantification using neonatal guthrie cards. J Pediatr 2009;155(6):829–33.
8. Bonilla FA. Interpretation of lymphocyte proliferation tests. Ann Allergy Asthma Immunol 2008;101(1):101–4.
9. Hicks MJ, Jones JF, Thies AC, et al. Age-related changes in mitogen-induced lymphocyte function from birth to old age. Am J Clin Pathol 1983;80(2):159–63.
10. Chiang JL, Patterson R, McGillen JJ, et al. Long-term corticosteroid effect on lymphocyte and polymorphonuclear cell function in asthmatics. J Allergy Clin Immunol 1980;65(4):263–8.
11. Ahmed AR, Blose DA. Delayed-type hypersensitivity skin testing. A review. Arch Dermatol 1983;119(11):934–45.
12. Bonilla FA, Khan DA, Ballas ZK, et al. Practice parameter for the diagnosis and management of primary immunodeficiency. J Allergy Clin Immunol 2015;136(5): 1186–205.e1-78.
13. Franz ML, Carella JA, Galant SP. Cutaneous delayed hypersensitivity in a healthy pediatric population: diagnostic value of diptheriatetanus toxoids. J Pediatr 1976; 88(6):975–7.
14. Davies EG, Thrasher AJ. Update on the hyper immunoglobulin M syndromes. Br J Haematol 2010;149(2):167–80.
15. Vargas-Hernández A, Berrón-Ruiz L, Staines-Boone T, et al. Clinical and genetic analysis of patients with X-linked hyper-IgM syndrome. Clin Genet 2013;83(6): 585–7.
16. O'Gorman MR, Zaas D, Paniagua M, et al. Development of a rapid whole blood flow cytometry procedure for the diagnosis of X-linked hyper-IgM syndrome patients and carriers. Clin Immunol Immunopathol 1997;85(2):172–81.
17. Gilmour KC, Walshe D, Heath S, et al. Immunological and genetic analysis of 65 patients with a clinical suspicion of X linked hyper-IgM. Mol Pathol 2003;56(5): 256–62.
18. Abraham RS, Aubert G. Flow cytometry, a versatile tool for diagnosis and monitoring of primary immunodeficiencies. Clin Vaccin Immunol 2016;23(4):254–71.
19. Bleesing JJ, Brown MR, Straus SE, et al. Immunophenotypic profiles in families with autoimmune lymphoproliferative syndrome. Blood 2001;98(8):2466–73.
20. Lim MS, Straus SE, Dale JK, et al. Pathological findings in human autoimmune lymphoproliferative syndrome. Am J Pathol 1998;153(5):1541–50.
21. Freeman AF, Holland SM. The hyper IgE syndromes. Immunol Allergy Clin North Am 2008;28(2):277–91, viii.
22. Milner JD, Brenchley JM, Laurence A, et al. Impaired T(H)17 cell differentiation in subjects with autosomal dominant hyper-IgE syndrome. Nature 2008;452(7188): 773–6.
23. Holland SM, DeLeo FR, Elloumi HZ, et al. STAT3 mutations in the hyper-IgE syndrome. N Engl J Med 2007;357(16):1608–19.
24. Zhang Q, Davis JC, Lamborn IT, et al. Combined immunodeficiency associated with DOCK8 mutations. N Engl J Med 2009;361(21):2046–55.

25. Pai S-Y, de Boer H, Massaad MJ, et al. Flow cytometry diagnosis of dedicator of cytokinesis 8 (DOCK8) deficiency. J Allergy Clin Immunol 2014;134(1):221–3.

26. Blundell MP, Worth A, Bouma G, et al. The Wiskott-Aldrich syndrome: the actin cytoskeleton and immune cell function. Dis Markers 2010;29(3–4):157–75.

27. Yamada M, Ohtsu M, Kobayashi I, et al. Flow cytometric analysis of Wiskott-Aldrich syndrome (WAS) protein in lymphocytes from WAS patients and their familial carriers. Blood 1999;93(2):756–7.

28. Chiang SCC, Vergamini SM, Husami A, et al. Screening for Wiskott-Aldrich syndrome by flow cytometry. J Allergy Clin Immunol 2018;142(1):333–5.e8.

29. Gatti R, Perlman S. Ataxia-telangiectasia. In: Adam MP, Ardinger HH, Pagon RA, et al, editors. GeneReviews®. Seattle (WA): University of Washington, Seattle; 1993. Available at: http://www.ncbi.nlm.nih.gov/books/NBK26468/. Accessed January 13, 2019.

30. Mallott J, Kwan A, Church J, et al. Newborn screening for SCID identifies patients with ataxia telangiectasia. J Clin Immunol 2013;33(3):540–9.

31. Cousin MA, Smith MJ, Sigafoos AN, et al. Utility of DNA, RNA, protein, and functional approaches to solve cryptic immunodeficiencies. J Clin Immunol 2018; 38(3):307–19.

32. Chun HH, Sun X, Nahas SA, et al. Improved diagnostic testing for ataxia-telangiectasia by immunoblotting of nuclear lysates for ATM protein expression. Mol Genet Metab 2003;80(4):437–43.

33. Hannan MA, Hellani A, Al-Khodairy FM, et al. Deficiency in the repair of UV-induced DNA damage in human skin fibroblasts compromised for the ATM gene. Carcinogenesis 2002;23(10):1617–24.

34. Locke BA, Dasu T, Verbsky JW. Laboratory diagnosis of primary immunodeficiencies. Clin Rev Allergy Immunol 2014;46(2):154–68.

35. Porcedda P, Turinetto V, Brusco A, et al. A rapid flow cytometry test based on histone H2AX phosphorylation for the sensitive and specific diagnosis of ataxia telangiectasia. Cytometry A 2008;73(6):508–16.

36. Perez E, Bonilla FA, Orange JS, et al. Specific antibody deficiency: controversies in diagnosis and management. Front Immunol 2017;8. https://doi.org/10.3389/fimmu.2017.00586.

37. Bonilla FA, Barlan I, Chapel H, et al. International Consensus Document (ICON): common variable immunodeficiency disorders. J Allergy Clin Immunol Pract 2016;4(1):38–59.

38. Farmer JR, Ong M-S, Barmettler S, et al. Common variable immunodeficiency non-infectious disease endotypes redefined using unbiased network clustering in large electronic Datasets. Front Immunol 2017;8:1740.

39. Wehr C, Kivioja T, Schmitt C, et al. The EUROclass trial: defining subgroups in common variable immunodeficiency. Blood 2008;111(1):77–85.

40. Quinti I, Soresina A, Spadaro G, et al. Long-term follow-up and outcome of a large cohort of patients with common variable immunodeficiency. J Clin Immunol 2007;27(3):308–16.

41. Baumert E, Wolff-Vorbeck G, Schlesier M, et al. Immunophenotypical alterations in a subset of patients with common variable immunodeficiency (CVID). Clin Exp Immunol 1992;90(1):25–30.

42. Bogaert DJA, Dullaers M, Lambrecht BN, et al. Genes associated with common variable immunodeficiency: one diagnosis to rule them all? J Med Genet 2016; 53(9):575–90.

43. Fong SW, Qaqundah BY, Taylor WF. Developmental patterns of ABO isoagglutinins in normal children correlated with the effects of age, sex, and maternal isoagglutinins. Transfusion 1974;14(6):551–9.
44. Paris K, Sorensen RU. Assessment and clinical interpretation of polysaccharide antibody responses. Ann Allergy Asthma Immunol 2007;99(5):462–4.
45. Orange JS, Ballow M, Stiehm ER, et al. Use and interpretation of diagnostic vaccination in primary immunodeficiency: a working group report of the basic and clinical immunology interest section of the American Academy of Allergy, Asthma & Immunology. J Allergy Clin Immunol 2012;130(3 Suppl):S1–24.
46. Bruton OC. Agammaglobulinemia. Pediatrics 1952;9(6):722–8.
47. Barmettler S, Otani IM, Minhas J, et al. Gastrointestinal manifestations in X-linked agammaglobulinemia. J Clin Immunol 2017;37(3):287–94.
48. Kanegane H, Futatani T, Wang Y, et al. Clinical and mutational characteristics of X-linked agammaglobulinemia and its carrier identified by flow cytometric assessment combined with genetic analysis. J Allergy Clin Immunol 2001; 108(6):1012–20.
49. Futatani T, Miyawaki T, Tsukada S, et al. Deficient expression of Bruton's tyrosine kinase in monocytes from X-linked agammaglobulinemia as evaluated by a flow cytometric analysis and its clinical application to carrier detection. Blood 1998; 91(2):595–602.
50. Conley ME, Dobbs AK, Farmer DM, et al. Primary B cell immunodeficiencies: comparisons and contrasts. Annu Rev Immunol 2009;27:199–227.
51. Yel L, Minegishi Y, Coustan-Smith E, et al. Mutations in the mu heavy-chain gene in patients with agammaglobulinemia. N Engl J Med 1996;335(20):1486–93.
52. Khalili A, Plebani A, Vitali M, et al. Autosomal recessive agammaglobulinemia: a novel non-sense mutation in CD79a. J Clin Immunol 2014;34(2):138–41.
53. Minegishi Y, Coustan-Smith E, Wang YH, et al. Mutations in the human lambda5/ 14.1 gene result in B cell deficiency and agammaglobulinemia. J Exp Med 1998; 187(1):71–7.
54. Lougaris V, Vitali M, Baronio M, et al. Autosomal recessive agammaglobulinemia: the third case of Igβ deficiency due to a novel non-sense mutation. J Clin Immunol 2014;34(4):425–7.
55. Gemayel KT, Litman GW, Sriaroon P. Autosomal recessive agammaglobulinemia associated with an IGLL1 gene missense mutation. Ann Allergy Asthma Immunol 2016;117(4):439–41.
56. Boisson B, Wang Y-D, Bosompem A, et al. A recurrent dominant negative E47 mutation causes agammaglobulinemia and BCR(-) B cells. J Clin Invest 2013; 123(11):4781–5.
57. Kubota K, Kim JY, Sawada A, et al. LRRC8 involved in B cell development belongs to a novel family of leucine-rich repeat proteins. FEBS Lett 2004; 564(1–2):147–52.
58. Lo B, Fritz JM, Su HC, et al. CHAI and LATAIE: new genetic diseases of CTLA-4 checkpoint insufficiency. Blood 2016;128(8):1037–42.
59. Lopez-Herrera G, Tampella G, Pan-Hammarström Q, et al. Deleterious mutations in LRBA are associated with a syndrome of immune deficiency and autoimmunity. Am J Hum Genet 2012;90(6):986–1001.
60. Gámez-Díaz L, Sigmund EC, Reiser V, et al. Rapid flow cytometry-based test for the diagnosis of lipopolysaccharide responsive Beige-like anchor (LRBA) deficiency. Front Immunol 2018;9:720.
61. Vivier E, Tomasello E, Baratin M, et al. Functions of natural killer cells. Nat Immunol 2008;9(5):503–10.

62. Oliveira JB, Fleisher TA. Laboratory evaluation of primary immunodeficiencies. J Allergy Clin Immunol 2010;125(2 Suppl 2):S297–305.

63. Janka GE. Familial and acquired hemophagocytic lymphohistiocytosis. Annu Rev Med 2012;63:233–46.

64. Rubin TS, Zhang K, Gifford C, et al. Perforin and CD107a testing is superior to NK cell function testing for screening patients for genetic HLH. Blood 2017;129(22): 2993–9.

65. Bradley TP, Bonavida B. Mechanism of cell-mediated cytotoxicity at the single cell level. IV. Natural killing and antibody-dependent cellular cytotoxicity can be mediated by the same human effector cell as determined by the two-target conjugate assay. J Immunol 1982;129(5):2260–5.

66. Alter G, Malenfant JM, Altfeld M. CD107a as a functional marker for the identification of natural killer cell activity. J Immunol Methods 2004;294(1–2):15–22.

67. Gupta S, Weitzman S. Primary and secondary hemophagocytic lymphohistiocytosis: clinical features, pathogenesis and therapy. Expert Rev Clin Immunol 2010;6(1):137–54.

68. Molleran Lee S, Villanueva J, Sumegi J, et al. Characterisation of diverse PRF1 mutations leading to decreased natural killer cell activity in North American families with haemophagocytic lymphohistiocytosis. J Med Genet 2004;41(2): 137–44.

69. Filipovich AH, Zhang K, Snow AL, et al. X-linked lymphoproliferative syndromes: brothers or distant cousins? Blood 2010;116(18):3398–408.

70. Marcenaro S, Gallo F, Martini S, et al. Analysis of natural killer-cell function in familial hemophagocytic lymphohistiocytosis (FHL): defective CD107a surface expression heralds Munc13-4 defect and discriminates between genetic subtypes of the disease. Blood 2006;108(7):2316–23.

71. Shinozaki K, Kanegane H, Matsukura H, et al. Activation-dependent T cell expression of the X-linked lymphoproliferative disease gene product SLAM-associated protein and its assessment for patient detection. Int Immunol 2002;14(10): 1215–23.

72. Tabata Y, Villanueva J, Lee SM, et al. Rapid detection of intracellular SH2D1A protein in cytotoxic lymphocytes from patients with X-linked lymphoproliferative disease and their family members. Blood 2005;105(8):3066–71.

73. Gifford CE, Weingartner E, Villanueva J, et al. Clinical flow cytometric screening of SAP and XIAP expression accurately identifies patients with SH2D1A and XIAP/ BIRC4 mutations. Cytometry B Clin Cytom 2014;86(4):263–71.

74. Hanna S, Etzioni A. Leukocyte adhesion deficiencies. Ann N Y Acad Sci 2012; 1250:50–5.

75. Etzioni A. Leukocyte adhesion deficiencies: molecular basis, clinical findings, and therapeutic options. Adv Exp Med Biol 2007;601:51–60.

76. Levy-Mendelovich S, Rechavi E, Abuzaitoun O, et al. Highlighting the problematic reliance on CD18 for diagnosing leukocyte adhesion deficiency type 1. Immunol Res 2016;64(2):476–82.

77. O'Gorman MRG. Recent developments related to the laboratory diagnosis of primary immunodeficiency diseases. Curr Opin Pediatr 2008;20(6):688–97.

78. Elloumi HZ, Holland SM. Diagnostic assays for chronic granulomatous disease and other neutrophil disorders. Methods Mol Biol 2007;412:505–23.

79. Freeman R, King B. Technique for the performance of the nitro-blue tetrazolium (NBT) test. J Clin Pathol 1972;25(10):912–4.

80. Nathan DG, Baehner RL, Weaver DK. Failure of nitro blue tetrazolium reduction in the phagocytic vacuoles of leukocytes in chronic granulomatous disease. J Clin Invest 1969;48(10):1895–904.
81. Jirapongsananuruk O, Malech HL, Kuhns DB, et al. Diagnostic paradigm for evaluation of male patients with chronic granulomatous disease, based on the dihydrorhodamine 123 assay. J Allergy Clin Immunol 2003;111(2):374–9.
82. Bustamante J, Boisson-Dupuis S, Abel L, et al. Mendelian susceptibility to mycobacterial disease: genetic, immunological, and clinical features of inborn errors of IFN-γ immunity. Semin Immunol 2014;26(6):454–70.
83. Filipe-Santos O, Bustamante J, Chapgier A, et al. Inborn errors of IL-12/23- and IFN-gamma-mediated immunity: molecular, cellular, and clinical features. Semin Immunol 2006;18(6):347–61.
84. Jouanguy E, Lamhamedi-Cherradi S, Lammas D, et al. A human IFNGR1 small deletion hotspot associated with dominant susceptibility to mycobacterial infection. Nat Genet 1999;21(4):370–8.
85. Fleisher TA, Dorman SE, Anderson JA, et al. Detection of intracellular phosphorylated STAT-1 by flow cytometry. Clin Immunol 1999;90(3):425–30.
86. Zhang S-Y, Casanova J-L. Inborn errors underlying herpes simplex encephalitis: from TLR3 to IRF3. J Exp Med 2015;212(9):1342–3.
87. Deering RP, Orange JS. Development of a clinical assay to evaluate toll-like receptor function. Clin Vaccin Immunol 2006;13(1):68–76.
88. Chinen J, Shearer WT. Secondary immunodeficiencies, including HIV infection. J Allergy Clin Immunol 2010;125(2 Suppl 2):S195–203.
89. Barmettler S, Ong M-S, Farmer JR, et al. Association of immunoglobulin levels, infectious risk, and mortality with rituximab and hypogammaglobulinemia. JAMA Netw Open 2018;1(7):e184169.
90. Casulo C, Maragulia J, Zelenetz AD. Incidence of hypogammaglobulinemia in patients receiving rituximab and the use of intravenous immunoglobulin for recurrent infections. Clin Lymphoma Myeloma Leuk 2013;13(2):106–11.
91. Makatsori M, Kiani-Alikhan S, Manson AL, et al. Hypogammaglobulinaemia after rituximab treatment-incidence and outcomes. QJM 2014;107(10):821–8.
92. Diwakar L, Gorrie S, Richter A, et al. Does rituximab aggravate pre-existing hypogammaglobulinaemia? J Clin Pathol 2010;63(3):275–7.

Food Allergy Testing

Nicole A. LaHood, MD[a], Sarita U. Patil, MD[b,c,d],*

KEYWORDS

- Food allergy • Immunoglobulin E • Skin testing • Oral food challenge
- Component testing

KEY POINTS

- Serum-specific immunoglobulin E (IgE) measurement can be helpful in the diagnosis of IgE-mediated food allergies, and clinically useful values vary by individual foods.
- Skin prick testing using whole-food allergen extracts provides an in vivo surrogate of IgE sensitization, and clinically useful values have been defined for various foods.
- For particular foods, component-specific IgE testing to particular protein components can provide additional diagnostic discrimination.

INTRODUCTION

Food allergy is "an adverse health effect arising from a specific immune response that occurs reproducibly on exposure to a given food."[1] The gold standard for diagnosis of food allergy is an oral food challenge (OFC) to the culprit allergen that elicits reproducible clinical symptoms. Whether open, blinded, or placebo controlled, OFCs can occur in the outpatient setting under close clinical observation by trained providers who are equipped to manage potential reactions, including anaphylaxis. In an OFC, the potential food is ingested in predefined, incrementally increasing doses until a full serving size is ingested.[2] Objective symptoms, such as hives, swelling, vomiting, and wheezing, confirm an immunoglobulin E (IgE)-mediated allergy.

OFCs are resource intensive, however, and place patients at risk for an allergic reaction.[1,3,4] Although most individuals with IgE-mediated food allergies also have sensitization, or detectable levels of IgE, allergen-specific IgE is not sufficient for a diagnosis of food allergy. Therefore, the ability to risk stratify patients prior to OFC

Disclosure Statement: Dr. Patil is funded by NIH grant NIAID K23AI121491, and Dr. LaHood is funded by NIH grant NHLBI T32 HL116275.
^a Allergy and Immunology, Department of Medicine, Division of Rheumatology, Allergy, and Immunology, Massachusetts General Hospital, 55 Fruit Street, Cox 201, Boston, MA, USA;
^b Department of Medicine, Division of Rheumatology, Allergy, and Immunology, Massachusetts General Hospital, 55 Fruit Street, Cox 201, Boston, MA, USA; ^c Food Allergy Center, Massachusetts General Hospital for Children, Boston, MA, USA; ^d Harvard Medical School, Boston, MA, USA
* Corresponding author. 55 Fruit Street, Cox 201, Boston, MA 02114.
E-mail address: sarita.patil@mgh.harvard.edu

Clin Lab Med 39 (2019) 625–642
https://doi.org/10.1016/j.cll.2019.07.009
0272-2712/19/© 2019 Elsevier Inc. All rights reserved.

is important for patient safety. This article focuses on the various commercially available methods of testing for sensitization to aid clinicians to risk stratify and diagnose patients with IgE-mediated food allergies.

SKIN TESTING

Since the 1950s, skin prick testing (SPT) has been the preferred cutaneous method for food allergy testing.[5,6] Epicutaneous SPT technique involves application of a small amount of allergen extract and subsequent or simultaneous bloodless prick of the skin, depending on the device used. Exposure of relevant antigens to cutaneous mast cells cross-links their surface IgE and induces degranulation. The resulting local wheal and flare reaction can be measured as a surrogate of food sensitization. Local application of histamine serves as a positive control and normal saline serves as a negative control.

SPT can be performed with a variety of tools, including hypodermic or solid bore needles, or more modern devices, such as plastic or metal lancets with or without bifurcated tips and multiple head devices that simultaneously deliver up to 10 pricks. Comparison of modern skin prick devices have not found significant advantages of one over another.[5,7–9] Due to interdevice variability, however, in wheal size, technique, and acceptable control concentrations, providers should select one device for use and ensure proper training of technicians for reproducible results.[5] Testing reagents include both fresh in-office preparations and commercially available extracts, and there is no clear consensus on any individual reagent's superiority.[10–14] Although intradermal testing is used in evaluation of environmental allergies, intradermal testing to foods may increase false-positive results as well as the incidence of serious, sometimes fatal, adverse reactions and, therefore, is contraindicated.[3,15]

The sensitivity, specificity, positive predictive value (PPV), and negative predictive value (NPV) for SPT vary based on age, study design, prevalence of food allergy in the study population, SPT cutoffs, and testing techniques. Despite this variability, among study populations presenting to allergy clinics with concern for food allergy or with a clinical history consistent with IgE-mediated food allergy, the utility of SPT at various cutoffs for different age ranges has been described in several publications, as outlined in **Table 1**. Compared with the general population, these values have a higher PPV because the pretest probability is higher. Generally, a larger SPT wheal size increases specificity but decreases sensitivity across all ages. There is a higher frequency of non–IgE-mediated milk reactions in children under 2 years of age, and this should be taken into consideration when a child has a history of reaction with negative SPT to cow's milk.[16]

SERUM IMMUNOGLOBULIN E TESTING

Reliable and widely available in vitro tests for specific IgE (sIGE) to allergens were introduced in the 1990s. The first commercially available test, radioallergosorbent test, has been largely replaced by sIGE immunoenzematic assays, such as ImmunoCAP (Phadia, ThermoFisher Scientific, Uppsala, Sweden) testing, in which serum antibodies bind to allergen and are quantified with enzyme-labelled anti-IgE antibody. For the purpose of this article, only studies that use immunoenzematic testing most commonly used are discussed.

There are many factors modulating the interpretation of sIGE allergy test results to foods, because a positive value is not always predictive of clinical food allergy. Pretest probability, therefore, greatly influences test interpretation. For example, a clinical

Table 1
Skin prick testing sensitivity, specificity, positive predictive value, and negative predictive value at various cutoffs

Skin Prick Testing	Sensitivity	Specificity	Positive Predictive Value	Negative Predictive Value
Hen's egg (Challenge to raw or partially cooked egg)	Age <18[16-18,20,23,24] • 3 mm = 73%–98% • 5 mm = 74% • 6 mm = 68%–95% • 7 mm = 48%–52% • 9 mm = 22% Age <14[19,25] • 3 mm = 93% Age <2[20-22,26] • 3 mm = 79%–97% • 4 mm = 46% • 5 mm = 62% • a3 mm = 66.6%–78% • a4 mm = 26.4% • a5 mm = 4.2%	Age <18[16,20,23,24] • 3 mm = 42.9%–72% • 5 mm = 69.6%–92% • 6 mm = 70%–92% • 7 = 92.9%–100% • 9 mm = 98.2% Age <14[19,25] • 3 mm = 54%–59% Age <2[20-22,26] • 3 mm = 71%–75% • 4 mm = 93% • 5 mm = 100% • 7 mm = 100% • a3 mm = 88%–88.6% • a4 mm = 94.3% • a5 mm = 100%	Age <18[17,18,20,23,24] • 3 mm = 61%–93% • 5 mm = 81.3% • 6 mm = 95%–100% • 7 mm = 92.3%–100% • 9 mm = 95.6% Age <14[19,25] • 3 mm = 79%–80% Age <2[20-22,26] • 3 mm = 93% • 4 mm = 94%–95% • 5 mm = 100% • a3 mm = 92%–96% • a4 mm = 90.5% • a5 mm = 100%	Age <18[17,18,20,23,24] • 3 mm = 50%–90% • 5 mm = 60.0% • 6 mm = 35%–95% • 7 mm = 29%–50% • 9 mm = 41.3% Age <14[19,25] • 3 mm = 81%–83% Age <2 • 3 mm = 86% • 4 mm = 38.4%–44% • a3 mm = 50%–56.3% • a5 mm = 33.6%–42%
Hen's egg (Challenge to baked egg)	Age <18[28] • 3 mm = 100% • 4 mm = 96.2% • 11 mm = 69.2% • 25 mm = 0% Age <2[26] • 11 mm = 0%	Age <18[28] • 3 mm = 16.5% • 4 mm = 17.3% • 11 mm = 55.6% • 25 mm = 95.5% Age <2[26] • SPT 11 mm = 99%	Age <18[27,28] • 3 mm = 19% • 4 mm = 18.5% • 11 mm = 23.4% • 15 mm = 60% • 25 mm = 0% Age <2[26] • 11 mm = 82%	Age <18[28] • 3 mm = 100% • 4 mm = 95.8% • 11 mm = 90.2% • 25 mm = 83% Age <2[26] • 11 mm = 82%
Peanut	Age <18[16-18,29,30] • 3 mm = 78.9%–100% • 6 mm = 47.4%–78% • 8 mm = 31.6%–51% Age <2[20,26] • 3 mm = 100% • 4 mm = 93% • 8 mm = 54%	Age <18[16-18,29,30] • 3 mm = 29%–98.1% • 6 mm = 94%–99.8% • 8 mm = 99.9%–100% Age <2[20,26] • 3 mm = 67% • 4 mm = 100% • 8 mm = 98%	Age <18[17,18,20,29,30] • 3 mm = 28.1%–99.5% • 6 mm = 81.8%–98% • 8 mm = 85.7%–100% Age <2[20,26] • 3 mm = 94% • 4 mm = 100% • 8 mm = 96%	Age <18[16-18,20,29,30] • 3 mm = 75%–100% • 6 mm = 59%–98.9% • 8 mm = 40%–98.5% Age <2[20,26] • 3 mm = 100% • 4 mm = 75% • 8 mm = 80%

(continued on next page)

Table 1
(continued)

Skin Prick Testing	Sensitivity	Specificity	Positive Predictive Value	Negative Predictive Value
Cow's milk Challenge to raw milk	Age <18[16-18,20] • 3 mm = 74%-96% • 6 mm = 49% • 8 mm = 30% Age <14[19,25] • 3 mm = 85% Age <2[20] • 3 mm = 58% • 6 = 20% Age <1[31] • 3 mm = 72%	Age <18[16-18,20] • 3 mm = 51%-89% • 6 mm = 95% • 8 mm = 100% Age <14[19,25] • 3 mm = 70%-75% Age <2[20] • 3 mm = 91% • 6 mm = 100% Age <1[31] • 3 mm = 62%	Age <18[17,18,20] • 3 mm = 50%-75% • 6 mm = 91% • 8 mm = 100% Age <14[19,25] • 3 mm = 73%-76% Age <2[20] • 3 mm = 79% • 6 mm = 90%-100% Age <1[31] • 3 mm = 60%	Age <18[17,18,20] • 3 mm = 77%-97% • 6 mm = 64% • 8 mm = 58% Age <14[19,25] • 3 mm = 83% Age <2[20] • 3 mm = 78% • 6 mm = 68% Age <1[31] • 3 mm = 73%
Cow's milk (Challenge to baked milk)	Age <18[32] • 3 mm = 100% • 7 mm = 100% • 10 mm = 66.7% • 12 mm = 66.7% • 15 mm = 50% • 20 mm = 33.3%	Age <18[32] • 3 mm = 6.9% • 7 mm = 17.2% • 10 mm = 41.4% • 12 mm = 69% • 15 mm = 86.2% • 20 mm = 96.6%	Age <18[32] • 3 mm = 18.2% • 7 mm = 20% • 10 mm = 19% • 12 mm = 30.8% • 15 mm = 42.9% • 20 mm = 66.7%	Age <18[32] • 3 mm = 100% • 7 mm = 100% • 10 mm = 85.7% • 12 mm = 90.9% • 15 mm = 89.3% • 20 mm = 87.5%
Soy	Age <18[17,18] • 3 mm = 76%-100% Age <14[19,25] • 3 mm = 21%-29%	Age <18[17,18] • 3 mm = 47%-72% Age <14[19,25] • 3 mm = 85%-88%	Age <18[17,18] • 3 mm = 30%-35% Age <14[19,25] • 3 mm = 29%-33%	Age <18[17,18] • 3 mm = 84%-100% Age <14[19,25] • 3 mm = 82%-83%
Wheat	Age <18[17,18] • 3 mm = 75%-90% Age <14[19,25] • 3 mm = 65%-75%	Age <18[17,18] • 3 mm = 51%-97% Age <14[19,25] • 3 mm = 64%-77%	Age <18[17,18] • 3 mm = 35%-75% Age <14[19,25] • 3 mm = 49%-52%	Age <18[17,18] • 3 mm = 94%-97% Age <14[19,25] • 3 mm = 85%
Fish	Age <18[17,18] • 3 mm = 90%-100%	Age <18[17,18] • 3 mm = 57%	Age <18[17,18] • SPT 3 mm = 25%-77%	Age <18[17,18] • 3 mm = 80%-100%
Sesame	Age <2[26] • 8 mm = 48%	Age <2[26] • 8 mm = 99%	Age <2[26] • 8 mm = 95%	Age <2[26] • 8 mm = 82%

[a] SPT using egg yolk extract only. Age in years.

history of immediate hypersensitivity, young age, and relative prevalence increases pretest probability, whereas atopic dermatitis and concomitant inhalant allergies decrease pretest probability.[33] These factors can also vary based on geographic region and, therefore, should be taken into consideration when sending in vitro allergy testing.[33,34]

The sensitivity, specificity, PPV, and NPV of various sIgE cutoffs to predict positive OFC have been described in the literature (**Table 2**) and vary by individual foods. For instance, compared with peanut and milk, soy sIgE and wheat sIgE were not found as reliably correlative to clinical symptoms.[35,36] The performance of sIgE also may vary by the degree of clinical sensitivity. A subset of patients with milk and egg sensitivity may be tolerant of baked products. SPT and sIgE cutoffs, however, have less utility in evaluation of individuals who may tolerate baked milk and egg as opposed to identification of those with sensitivity to all forms of milk and egg.[27] Despite these caveats, used correctly in conjunction with SPT when possible, serum IgE testing can be a useful tool to detect clinically relevant sensitization to foods and identify high-risk individuals.

Although meat allergy is rare, alpha-gal hypersensitivity syndrome, described in 2009, occurs in individuals with tick exposure, classically to the lone star tick (*Amblyomma americanum*), resulting in sensitization to a mammalian oligosaccharide epitope, which is present in mammalian meats. Unlike most IgE-mediated reactions, clinical manifestation of alpha-gal allergy is delayed 3 hours to 6 hours after consumption of mammalian meat, and reactions range from urticaria and angioedema to life-threatening anaphylaxis with known cross-reactivity to gelatin and medications like cetuximab.[37,38] Testing for alpha-gal IgE is commercially available, and the value above which there is a 95% probability of meat allergy is 5.5 kilounits of allergen-specific IgE per liter (kU_A/L) and/or an alpha-gal IgE to total IgE ratio of 2.12%.[39]

Foods contain complex mixtures of allergenic proteins. Component testing allows assessment of sIGE to individual allergenic proteins within a food. In particular foods, studies have shown that certain protein components are linked to increased severity in clinical allergy and can indicate a higher risk of reaction to OFC.[42,43,45–53] This allows practitioners to better risk stratify whole-allergen–sensitized patients and identify those at a higher risk of severe reaction versus those who are pollen cross-sensitized, with lower risk of systemic reactions. The protein fractionation and clinical relevance of major allergens are outlined in **Table 3**.

Sensitization to certain protein components and their clinical relevance can vary by geographic region. For example, peanut sensitization in the United States occurs earlier in life and children are more likely to be sensitized to high-risk protein components like Ara h 1, Ara h 2 or Ara h 3 compared with children in other parts of the world.[34]

Pollen-food syndrome, also known as oral allergy syndrome, is the most common form of food allergy in adults, in which ingestion of certain foods, such as fresh fruits, vegetables, and nuts, leads to immediate-onset oropharyngeal symptoms. The most common cross-reactive allergens are birch, ragweed, mugwort, and grasses. Although pollen-food syndrome usually is indicative of mild limited reactions in US adults, in Mediterranean regions, certain pollen cross-reactive lipid transfer proteins have been associated with severe systemic reactions and anaphylaxis.[54]

More recently, component testing has been especially helpful in identifying pollen cross-reactive components to peanut and tree nut, notably hazelnut. The sensitivity, specificity, PPV, and NVP for various cutoffs for peanut and hazelnut are outlined in **Table 4**.

Table 2
Serum-specific immunoglobulin E sensitivity, specificity, positive predictive value, and negative predictive value at various cutoffs

Specific Immunoglobulin E Testing (ImmunoCAP)	Sensitivity	Specificity	Positive Predictive Value	Negative Predictive Value
Hen's egg white IgE (kUA/L) (Challenge to raw or partially cooked egg)	Age <18[18,23,24,35,36] • a0.35 = 97%–98% • 0.35 = 86.7% • 1.5 = 52.2% • a3.4 = 82% • a6 = 64% • a7 = 61% • 7 = 48.2% • 25 = 4.4% Age <14[25] • 0.35 = 96% Age <2[21,26] • 0.35 = 91% • 1.7 = 48%	Age <18[18,23,24,35,36] • a0.35 = 45%–51% • 0.35 = 39.6% • 1.5 = 90.6% • a3.4 = 84% • a6 = 90% • a7 = 95% • 7 = 100% • 25 = 100% Age <14[25] • 0.35 = 48% Age <2[21,26] • 0.35 = 77% • 1.7 = 98%	Age <18[18,20,23,24,35,36] • a0.35 = 80%–84% • 0.35 = 70.9% • 1.5 = 90.4% • a3.4 = 94% • a6 = 95%–96% • a7 = 98% • 7 = 100% • 25 = 100% Age <14[25] • 0.35 = 79% Age <2[20,21,26] • 0.35 = 94%–95% • 1.7 = 95%	Age <18[18,23,24,35,36] • a0.35 = 88%–89% • 0.35 = 63.6% • 1.5 = 52.7% • a3.4 = 62% • a6 = 39% • a7 = 38 • 7 = 38% • 25 = 38.1% Age <14[25] • 0.35 = 85% Age <2[21,26] • 0.35 = 68% • 1.7 = 47%
Hen's egg white IgE (kUA/L) (Challenge to baked egg)	Age <19[28,40] • 0.35 = 92.6% • 2.5 = 87% • 5 = 56% • 6 = 51.9% • 9.65 = 37% • 10 = 20% Age <2[26] • 50 = 9%	Age <19[28,40] • 0.35 = 19% • 2.5 = 48% • 5 = 69% • 6 = 85.8% • 9.65 = 95% • 10 = 94% Age <2[26] • 50 = 100%	Age <19[28,40] • 0.35 = 18% • 2.5 = 44% • 5 = 46% • 6 = 41.2% • 9.65 = 58.8% • 10 = 60% Age <2[26] • 50 = 95%	Age <19[28,40] • 0.35 = 93.1% • 2.5 = 89% • 5 = 77% • 6 = 90.3% • 9.65 = 88.7% • 10 = 71% Age <2[26] • 50 = 85%

Test				
Cow's milk IgE (kUA/L) (Challenge to raw milk)	Age <18[18,35,36] • 0.35 = 83%–100% • 5.8 = 80% • 15 = 57% • 32 = 34% Age <14[25] • 0.35 = 87% Age <1[31] • IgE 0.35 = 84% • IgE 0.7 = 74% • IgE 2.5 = 48% • IgE 5 = 30%	Age <18[18,35,36] • 0.35 = 30%–53% • 5.8 = 81% • 15 = 94% • 32 = 100% Age <14[25] • IgE 0.35 = 49% Age <1[31] • IgE 0.35 = 56% • IgE 0.7 = 71% • IgE 2.5 = 95% • IgE 5 = 99%	Age <18[18,20,35,36] • 0.35 = 57%–63% • IgE 5.8 = 80% • IgE 15 = 95% • IgE 32 = 95%–100% Age <14[25] • IgE 0.35 = 62% Age <1[31] • IgE 0.35 = 61% • IgE 0.7 = 67% • IgE 2.5 = 90% • IgE 5 = 95%	Age <18[18,35,36] • 0.35 = 76%–100% • 5.8 = 81% • 15 = 53% • 32 = 44% Age <14[25] • 0.35 = 79% Age <1[31] • 0.35 = 81% • 0.7 = 77% • 2.5 = 69% • 5 = 64%
Cow's milk IgE (kUA/L) (Challenge to baked milk)	Age <18[41] • 1.21 = 95% • 9.97 = 62% • 24.5 = 30%	Age <18[41] • 1.21 = 27% • 9.97 = 85% • 24.5 = 95%	Age <18[41] • 1.21 = 33% • 9.97 = 60% • 24.5 = 69%	Age <18[32,41] • 1.0 = >90% • 1.21 = 94% • 9.97 = 86% • 24.5 = 78%
Peanut IgE (kUA/L)	Age <18[18,30,36,42,43] • 0.35 = 87.6%–97% • 1.0 = 89.5% • 5.0 = 73.7% • 10.0 = 63.2%–76% • 15 = 57%–57.9% • 45.0 = 20% Age <2[26,44] • 0.35 = 91% • 0.4 = 90% • 2.21 = 68% • 6.20 = 44% • 14.9 = 26% • 34 = 14% • 54.2 = 3%	Age <18[18,30,36,42,43] • 0.35 = 17%–92.9% • 1.0 = 95.2% • 5.0 = 98.9% • 10.0 = 88%–99.5% • 15 = 99.8%–100% • 45.0 = 100% Age <2[26,44] • 0.35 = 68% • 0.4 = 69% • 2.21 = 90% • 6.20 = 95% • 14.9 = 98% • 34 = 99% • 54.2 = 100%	Age <18[18,20,30,36,43] • 0.35 = 31%–78% • 1.0 = 38.6% • 5.0 = 70% • 10.0 = 80%–94% • 15 = 91.7%–100% • 45.0 = 100% Age <2[26] • 34 = 95%	Age <18[18,30,36,43] • 0.35 = 59%–99.8% • 1.0 = 99.6% • 5.0 = 99.1% • 10.0 = 62%–98.8% • 15 = 36%–98.6% • 45.0 = 76% Age <2[26] • 34 = 69%

(continued on next page)

Table 2
(continued)

Specific Immunoglobulin E Testing (ImmunoCAP)	Sensitivity	Specificity	Positive Predictive Value	Negative Predictive Value
Soy IgE (kU$_A$/L)	Age <18[18,35,36] • 0.35 = 69%–94% • 5 = 68% • 30 = 44% • 65 = 24% Age <14[25] • 0.35 = 65%	Age <18[18,35,36] • 0.35 = 25%–50% • 5 = 63% • 30 = 94% • 65 = 99% Age <14[25] • 0.35 = 50%	Age <18[18,35,36] • 0.35 = 21%–22% • 5 = 28% • 30 = 73% • 65 = 50%–86% Age <14[25] • 0.35 = 22%	Age <18[18,35,36] • 0.35 = 88%–95% • 5 = 90% • 30 = 82% • 65 = 78% Age <14[25] • 0.35 = 86%
Wheat IgE (kU$_A$/L)	Age <18[18,35,36] • 0.35 = 79%–96% • 8.1 = 70% • 26 = 61% • 100 = 13% Age <14[25] • 0.35 = 82%	Age <18[18,35,36] • 0.35 = 20%–38% • 8.1 = 73% • 26 = 92% • 100 = 100% Age <14[25] • 0.35 = 34%	Age <18[18,35,36] • 0.35 = 14%–41% • 8.1 = 25% • 26 = 74% • 100 = 75%–100% Age <14[25] • 0.35 = 41%	Age <18[18,35,36] • 0.35 = 77%–97% • 8.1 = 95% • 26 = 87% • 100 = 76% Age <14[25] • 0.35 = 77%
Fish IgE (kU$_A$/L)	Age <18[18,36] • 0.35 = 94% • 1.8 = 85% • 3 = 63% • 20 = 25%	Age <18[18,36] • 0.35 = 65% • 1.8 = 88% • 3 = 91% • 20 = 100%	Age <18[18,36] • 0.35 = 49% • 1.8 = 71% • 3 = 56% • 20 = 95%–100%	Age <18[18,36] • 0.35 = 97% • 1.8 = 94% • 3 = 93% • 20 = 89%
Sesame IgE (kU$_A$/L)	Age <2[26] • 50 = 4%	Age <2[26] • 50 = 98%	Age <2[26] • 50 = 95%	Age <2[26] • 50 = 69%

[a] Hen's whole egg IgE (kUA/L). Age in years.

Table 3
Protein components of major food allergens and clinical relevance

Food	Protein Components	Components Associated with Severe Reactions/Anaphylaxis	Components Associated with Food-Pollen Allergy Syndrome
Soybean (*Glycine max*)[42]	• Gly m 3 (profilin) • Gly m 4 (pathogenesis-related protein 10/Bet v 1-like) • Gly m 5 (7s globulin, beta-conglycinin; vicilin) • Gly m 6 (11S globulin, glycerin; Irgumin) • Gly m 7 (seed biotinylated protein) • Gly m 8 (2S albumin)	• Gly m 5 • Gly m 6	• Gly m 4
Peanut (*Arachis hypogaea*)[42,43,45,46]	• Ara h 1 (7/8S globulins (vicilin) of seed transfer protein) • Ara h 2 (2S albumins (conglutin) of seed transfer protein) • Ara h 3 (11S globulins (legumins) of seed transfer protein) • Ara h 4 (11S globulins (legumins) of seed transfer protein) • Ara h 5 (profilin—Bet v 2-like) • Ara h 6 (2S albumins (conglutin) of seed transfer protein) • Ara h 7 (2S albumins (conglutin) of seed transfer protein) • Ara h 8 (pathogenesis-related protein 10/Bet v 1-like) • Ara h 9 (nonspecific lipid transfer protein) • Ara h 10 (oleosin plant lipid storage bodies) • Ara h 11 (oleosin plant lipid storage bodies) • Ara h 12 (defensin) • Ara h 13 (defensin) • Ara h 14 (oleosin plant lipid storage bodies) • Ara h 15 (oleosin plant lipid storage bodies) • Ara h 16 (nonspecific lipid transfer protein) • Ara h 17 (nonspecific lipid transfer protein)	• Ara h 1 • Ara h 2 • Ara h 3 • Ara h 6	• Ara h 8 • Ara h 9

(continued on next page)

Table 3
(continued)

Food	Protein Components	Components Associated with Severe Reactions/Anaphylaxis	Components Associated with Food-Pollen Allergy Syndrome
Cow's milk (*Bos domesticus*)[47]	• Bos d 4 (α-lactalbumin) • Bos d 5 (β-lactoglobulin) • Bos d 6 (bovine serum albumin) • Bos d 7 (lactoferrin and immunoglobulins) • Bos d 8 (whole casein) • Bos d 9 (alpha S1-casein) • Bos d 10 (alpha S2-casein) • Bos d 11 (beta-casein) • Bos d 12 (kappa-casein)	• Bos d 4 • Bos d 5 • Bos d 8	–
Hen's egg (*Gallus domesticus*)[48]	• Gal d 1 (ovomucoid) • Gal d 2 (ovalbumin), • Gal d 3 (ovotransferrin/conalbumin) • Gal d 4 (lysozyme) • Gal d 5 (alpha-livetin) • Gal d 7 (myosin light chain) • Gal d 8 (alpha-parvalbumin) • Gal d 9 (beta-enolase) • Gal d 10 (aldolase)	• Gal d 1 • Gal d 2 • Gal d 4	• Gal d 5 (bird-egg cross-reactive)
Wheat (*Triticum aestivum*)[46,49]	• Tri a 14 (nonspecific lipid transfer protein) • Tri a 17 (beta-amylase) • Tri a 18 (agglutinin isolectin 1) • Tri a 19 (omega-5 gliadin seed storage protein) • Tri a 20 (gamma gliadin) • Tri a 25 (thioredoxin) • Tri a 26 (high-molecular-weight glutenin) • Tri a 36 (low-molecular-weight glutenin GluB3-23) • Tri a 37 (alpha purothionin)	• Tri a 19	–

Food	Allergen components		
Hazelnut (*Corylus avellana*)[45,46,50,51]	• Cor a 1 (pathogenesis-related protein 10/Bet v 1-like) • Cor a 2 (profilin) • Cor a 6 (isoflavone reductase homologue) • Cor a 8 (nonspecific lipid transfer protein) • Cor a 9 (seed storage protein—11S globulin) • Cor a 10 (luminal binding protein) • Cor a 11 (7S seed storage globulin [vicilin-like]) • Cor a 12 (oleosin plant lipid storage bodies) • Cor a 13 (oleosin plant lipid storage bodies) • Cor a 14 (seed storage protein—2S albumin)	• Cor a 9 • Cor a 11 • Cor a 14	• Cor a 1
Walnut (*Juglans regia*)[51,52]	• Jug r 1 (2S albumin) • Jug r 2 (vicilin seed storage protein) • Jug r 3 (nonspecific lipid transfer protein) • Jug r 4 (11S globulin seed storage protein) • Jug r 5 (pathogenesis-related protein 10/Bet v 1-like) • Jug r 6 (vicilin-like cupin) • Jug r 7 (profilin) • Jug r 8 (nonspecific lipid transfer protein)	• Jug r 1 • Jug r 2 • Jug r 4	• Jug r 5
Cashew (*Anacardium occidentale*)[53]	• Ana o 1 (vicilin-like protein) • Ana o 2 (legume-like protein) • Ana o 3 (2S albumin)	• Ana o 3	-
Apple (*Malus domestica*)[45]	• Mal d 1 (pathogenesis-related protein 10/Bet v 1-like) • Mal d 2 (thaumatin-like protein) • Mal d 3 (nonspecific lipid transfer protein) • Mal d 4 (profilin)	• Mal d 3	• Mal d 1 • Mal d 4

(continued on next page)

Table 3
(continued)

Food	Protein Components	Components Associated with Severe Reactions/Anaphylaxis	Components Associated with Food-Pollen Allergy Syndrome
Peach (*Prunus persica*)[45]	• Pru p 1 (pathogenesis-related protein 10/Bet v 1-like) • Pru p 2 (thaumatin-like protein) • Pru p 3 (nonspecific lipid transfer protein) • Pru p 4 (profilin) • Pru p 7 (gibberellin-regulated protein) • Pru p 9 (pathogenesis-related protein 10/Bet v 1-like)	• Pru p 3 (severe reactions in Mediterranean regions/Europe)	• Pru p 1
Kiwifruit (*Actinidia deliciosa*)[45]	• Act d 1 (cysteine protease—actinidin) • Act d 2 (thaumatin-like protein) • Act d 4 (phytocystatin) • Act d 5 (kiwellin) • Act d 6 (pectin methylesterase inhibitor) • Act d 7 (pectin methylesterase) • Act d 8 (pathogenesis-related protein 10/Bet v 1-like) • Act d 9 (profilin) • Act d 10 (nonspecific lipid transfer protein) • Act d 11 (major latex protein/ripening-related protein/Bet v 1-like) • Act d 12 (cupin, 11S globulin) • Act d 13 (2S albumin)	• Act d 1	• Act d 8 • Act d 9

Table 4
Protein components sensitivity, specificity, positive negative predictive value, and negative predictive value at various cutoffs for egg, milk, peanut, and hazelnut

Immunoglobulin E Component Testing	Sensitivity	Specificity	Positive Predictive Value	Negative Predictive Value
Hen's egg • Yolk IgE (kU_A/L)	Age <18[24] • 0.35 = 55.4% • 1.0 = 26.5% Age <2[21] • 0.35 = 63%	Age <18[24] • 0.35 = 92.3% • 1.0 = 98.1% Age <2[21] • 0.35 = 93%	Age <18[24] • 0.35 = 92% • 1.0 = 95.6% Age <2[21] • 0.35 = 98%	Age <18[24] • 0.35 = 56.5% • 1.0 = 45.5% Age <2[21] • 0.35 = 37%
Hen's egg • Ovomucoid IgE (kU_A/L)	Age <19[24,28] • 0.35 = 65.5%–66.7% • 1.0 = 41.4% • 2.0 = 28.7% • 3.38 = 18.5% • 4.85 = 11.1% • 9.74 = 7.41% Age <2[21] • 0.35 = 73%	Age <19[24,28] • 0.35 = 61.3%–78.4% • 1.0 = 94.1% • 2.0 = 98% • 3.38 = 95.1% • 4.85 = 97.9% • 9.74 = 99.3% Age <2[21] • 0.35 = 82%	Age <19[24,28] • 0.35 = 24.7%–83.8% • 1.0 = 92.3% • 2.0 = 96.1% • 3.38 = 41.7% • 4.85 = 50% • 9.74 = 66.7% Age <2[21] • 0.35 = 96%	Age <19[24,28] • 0.35 = 57.1%–90.6% • 1.0 = 48.5% • 2.0 = 44.6% • 3.38 = 86% • 4.85 = 85.3% • 9.74 = 84.9% Age <2[21] • 0.35 = 35%
Hen's egg • Ovalbumin IgE (kU_A/L)	Age <18[24] • 0.35 = 87.6% • 1.3 = 55.4% • 2 = 49.4% Age <2[21] • 0.35 = 72%	Age <18[24] • 0.35 = 47.1% • 1.3 = 90.2% • 2 = 96.1% Age <2[21] • 0.35 = 83%	Age <18[24] • 0.35 = 72.7% • 1.3 = 90.2% • 2 = 95.3% Age <2[21] • 0.35 = 96%	Age <18[24] • 0.35 = 68.6% • 1.3 = 55.4% • 2 = 53.8% Age <2[21] • 0.35 = 36%
Cow's milk (baked) • Casein IgE (kU_A/L)	Age <18[41] • 0.94 = 95% • 4.95 = 74% • 20.2 = 30%	Age <18[41] • 0.94 = 32% • 4.95 = 77% • 20.2 = 95%	Age <18[41] • 0.94 = 34% • 4.95 = 54% • 20.2 = 69%	Age <18[41] • 0.94 = 96% • 4.95 = 89% • 20.2 = 78%

(continued on next page)

Table 4
(continued)

Immunoglobulin E Component Testing	Sensitivity	Specificity	Positive Predictive Value	Negative Predictive Value
Peanut • Ara h 1 IgE (kU_A/L)	Age <18[43] • 0.35 = 56%	Age <18[43] • 0.35 = 87%	Age <18[43] • 0.35 = 88%	Age <18[43] • 0.35 = 54%
Peanut • Ara h 2 IgE (kU_A/L)	Age <18[42,43] • 0.35 = 80%–100% Age <2[44] • 0.1 = 95% • 0.35 = 81% • 1.0 = 60% • 1.19 = 60% • 3.51 = 43%	Age <18[42,43] • 0.35 = 92%–96.1% Age <2[44] • 0.1 = 86% • 0.35 = 93% • 1.0 = 97% • 1.19 = 98% • 3.51 = 100%	Age <18[43] • 0.35 = 94%	Age <18[43] • 0.35 = 73%
Peanut • Ara h 3 IgE (kU_A/L)	Age <18[43] • 0.35 = 48%	Age <18[43] • 0.35 = 90%	Age <18[43] • 0.35 = 89%	Age <18[43] • 0.35 = 50%
Peanut • Ara h 8 IgE (kU_A/L)	Age <18[43] • 0.35 = 35%	Age <18[43] • 0.35 = 43%	Age <18[43] • 0.35 = 51%	Age <18[43] • 0.35 = 27%
Hazelnut • Cor a 9 IgE (kU_A/L)	Age >18[50] • 0.35 = 36% • 1.0 = 33% • 5.0 = 13% Age <18[50] • 0.35 = 83% • 1.0 = 75% • 5.0 = 48%	Age >18[50] • 0.35 = 95% • 1.0 = 100% • 5.0 = 100% Age <18[50] • 0.35 = 80% • 1.0 = 95% • 5.0 = 98%	—	—
Hazelnut • Cor a 14 IgE (kU_A/L)	Age >18[50] • 0.35 = 38% • 1.0 = 31% • 5.0 = 18% Age <18[50] • 0.35 = 70% • 1.0 = 70% • 5.0 = 60%	Age >18[50] • 0.35 = 95% • 1.0 = 98% • 5.0 = 100% Age <18[50] • 0.35 = 76% • 1.0 = 76% • 5.0 = 98%	—	—

Age in years.

Testing for sIgE components does not improve risk stratification for all foods. For instance, egg white was found to have a higher sensitivity, specificity, and PPV than other egg components like egg yolk, ovomucoid, and ovalbumin in children less than 2 years of age.[21,24]

SUMMARY

In conclusion, using both SPT and sIgE, with component testing where available, allows for more accurate assessment of food allergy and can effectively risk stratify those who may benefit from OFCs. Serial evaluation of children with IgE-mediated food allergies every 1 year to 2 years with SPT and sIgE can identify those with decreasing values who may benefit from OFC to evaluate clinical tolerance.

REFERENCES

1. Boyce JA, Assa'ad A, Burks AW, et al. Guidelines for the diagnosis and management of food allergy in the United States: summary of the NIAID-sponsored expert panel report. J Am Acad Dermatol 2011;64(1):175–92.
2. Sampson HA, Van Wijk RG, Bindslev-Jensen C, et al. Standardizing double-blind, placebo-controlled oral food challenges: American Academy of Allergy, Asthma & Immunology–European Academy of Allergy and Clinical Immunology PRACTALL consensus report. J Allergy Clin Immunol 2012;130(6): 1260–74.
3. Harris MC, Shure N. Sudden death due to allergy tests. J Allergy Clin Immunol 1950;21(3):208–16.
4. Burks AW, Sampson HA. Anaphylaxis and food allergy. Clin Rev Allergy Immunol 1999;17(3):339–60.
5. Bernstein IL, Li JT, Bernstein DI, et al. Allergy diagnostic testing: an updated practice parameter. Ann Allergy Asthma Immunol 2008;100(3):S1–48.
6. Sampson HA, Aceves S, Bock SA, et al. Food allergy: a practice parameter update—2014. J Allergy Clin Immunol 2014;134(5):1016–25.
7. Nelson HS. Variables in allergy skin testing. Allergy Proc 1994;15(6):265. Ocean-Side Publications.
8. Oppenheimer J, Nelson HS. Skin testing. Ann Allergy Asthma Immunol 2006; 96(2):S6–12.
9. Tversky JR, Chelladurai Y, McGready J, et al. Performance and pain tolerability of current diagnostic allergy skin prick test devices. J Allergy Clin Immunol Pract 2015;3(6):888–93.
10. Rance F, Juchet A, Bremont F, et al. Correlations between skin prick tests using commercial extracts and fresh foods, specific IgE, and food challenges. Allergy 1997;52(10):1031–5.
11. Ferrer Á, Huertas ÁJ, Larramendi CH, et al. Usefulness of manufactured tomato extracts in the diagnosis of tomato sensitization: comparison with the prick-prick method. Clin Mol Allergy 2008;6(1):1.
12. Łoś-Rycharska E, Sterkowicz A, Romańczuk B, et al. Comparison of results and clinical value of skin prick tests with synthetic and native food allergens in patients at the age of up to 3 years. Postepy Dermatol Alergol 2016;33(6):485.
13. Rosen JP, Selcow JE, Mendelson LM, et al. Skin testing with natural foods in patients suspected of having food allergies: is it a necessity? J Allergy Clin Immunol 1994;93(6):1068–70.

14. Sampson HA. Comparative study of commercial food antigen extracts for the diagnosis of food hypersensitivity. J Allergy Clin Immunol 1988;82(5):718–26.

15. Bock SA, Buckley J, Holst A, et al. Proper use of skin tests with food extracts in diagnosis of hypersensitivity to food in children. Clin Exp Allergy 1977;7(4): 375–83.

16. Sporik R, Hill DJ, Hosking CS. Specificity of allergen skin testing in predicting positive open food challenges to milk, egg and peanut in children. Clin Exp Allergy 2000;30(11):1541–6.

17. Sampson HA, Albergo R. Comparison of results of skin tests, RAST, and double-blind, placebo-controlled food challenges in children with atopic dermatitis. J Allergy Clin Immunol 1984;74(1):26–33.

18. Sampson HA, Ho DG. Relationship between food-specific IgE concentrations and the risk of positive food challenges in children and adolescents. J Allergy Clin Immunol 1997;100(4):444–51.

19. Verstege A, Mehl A, Rolinck-Werninghaus C, et al. The predictive value of the skin prick test weal size for the outcome of oral food challenges. Clin Exp Allergy 2005;35(9):1220–6.

20. Hill DJ, Heine RG, Hosking CS. The diagnostic value of skin prick testing in children with food allergy. Pediatr Allergy Immunol 2004;15(5):435–41.

21. Boyano-Martínez T, García-Ara C, Díaz-Pena JM, et al. Prediction of tolerance on the basis of quantification of egg white-specific IgE antibodies in children with egg allergy. J Allergy Clin Immunol 2002;110(2):304–9.

22. Monti G, Muratore MC, Peltran A, et al. High incidence of adverse reactions to egg challenge on first known exposure in young atopic dermatitis children: predictive value of skin prick test and radioallergosorbent test to egg proteins. Clin Exp Allergy 2002;32(10):1515–9.

23. Tripodi S, Di Rienzo Businco A, Alessandri C, et al. Predicting the outcome of oral food challenges with hen's egg through skin test end-point titration. Clin Exp Allergy 2009;39(8):1225–33.

24. Diéguez MC, Cerecedo I, Muriel A, et al. Utility of diagnostic tests in the follow-up of egg-allergic children. Clin Exp Allergy 2009;39(10):1575–84.

25. Mehl A, Rolinck-Werninghaus C, Staden U, et al. The atopy patch test in the diagnostic workup of suspected food-related symptoms in children. J Allergy Clin Immunol 2006;118(4):923–9.

26. Peters RL, Allen KJ, Dharmage SC, et al. Skin prick test responses and allergen-specific IgE levels as predictors of peanut, egg, and sesame allergy in infants. J Allergy Clin Immunol 2013;132(4):874–80.

27. Leonard SA. Debates in allergy medicine: baked milk and egg ingestion accelerates resolution of milk and egg allergy. World Allergy Organ J 2016;9(1):1.

28. Bartnikas LM, Sheehan WJ, Larabee KS, et al. Ovomucoid is not superior to egg white testing in predicting tolerance to baked egg. J Allergy Clin Immunol Pract 2013;1(4):354–60.

29. Pucar F, Kagan R, Lim H, et al. Peanut challenge: a retrospective study of 140 patients. Clin Exp Allergy 2001;31(1):40–6.

30. Nicolaou N, Poorafshar M, Murray C, et al. Allergy or tolerance in children sensitized to peanut: prevalence and differentiation using component-resolved diagnostics. J Allergy Clin Immunol 2010;125(1):191–7.

31. García-Ara C, Boyano-Martínez T, Díaz-Pena JM, et al. Specific IgE levels in the diagnosis of immediate hypersensitivity to cows' milk protein in the infant. J Allergy Clin Immunol 2001;107(1):185–90.

32. Bartnikas LM, Sheehan WJ, Hoffman EB, et al. Predicting food challenge outcomes for baked milk: role of specific IgE and skin prick testing. Ann Allergy Asthma Immunol 2012;109(5):309–13.
33. Santos AF, Brough HA. Making the most of in vitro tests to diagnose food allergy. J Allergy Clin Immunol Pract 2017;5(2):237–48.
34. Vereda A, van Hage M, Ahlstedt S, et al. Peanut allergy: clinical and immunologic differences among patients from 3 different geographic regions. J Allergy Clin Immunol 2011;127(3):603–7.
35. Celik-Bilgili S, Mehl A, Verstege A, et al. The predictive value of specific immunoglobulin E levels in serum for the outcome of oral food challenges. Clin Exp Allergy 2005;35(3):268–73.
36. Sampson HA. Utility of food-specific IgE concentrations in predicting symptomatic food allergy. J Allergy Clin Immunol 2001;107(5):891–6.
37. Wilson JM, Platts-Mills TA. Meat allergy and allergens. Mol Immunol 2018;100:107–12.
38. Hilger C, Fischer J, Wölbing F, et al. Role and mechanism of Galactose-alpha-1, 3-Galactose in the elicitation of delayed anaphylactic reactions to red meat. Curr Allergy Asthma Rep 2019;19(1):3.
39. Mabelane T, Basera W, Botha M, et al. Predictive values of alpha-Gal IgE levels and alpha-Gal IgE: total IgE ratio and oral food challenge-proven meat allergy in a population with a high prevalence of reported red meat allergy. Pediatr Allergy Immunol 2018;29(8):841–9.
40. Lieberman JA, Huang FR, Sampson HA, et al. Outcomes of 100 consecutive open, baked-egg oral food challenges in the allergy office. J Allergy Clin Immunol 2012;129(6):1682–4.
41. Caubet JC, Nowak-Węgrzyn A, Moshier E, et al. Utility of casein-specific IgE levels in predicting reactivity to baked milk. J Allergy Clin Immunol 2013;131(1):222–4.
42. Nicolaou N, Custovic A. Molecular diagnosis of peanut and legume allergy. Curr Opin Allergy Clin Immunol 2011;11(3):222–8.
43. Lieberman JA, Glaumann S, Batelson S, et al. The utility of peanut components in the diagnosis of IgE-mediated peanut allergy among distinct populations. J Allergy Clin Immunol Pract 2013;1(1):75–82.
44. Dang TD, Tang M, Choo S, et al. Increasing the accuracy of peanut allergy diagnosis by using Ara h 2. J Allergy Clin Immunol 2012;129(4):1056–63.
45. Hoffmann-Sommergruber K, Pfeifer S, Bublin M. Applications of molecular diagnostic testing in food allergy. Curr Allergy Asthma Rep 2015;15(9):56.
46. Hamilton RG, Kleine-Tebbe J. Molecular allergy diagnostics: analytical features that support clinical decisions. Curr Allergy Asthma Rep 2015;15(9):57.
47. Kattan JD, Cocco RR, Järvinen KM. Milk and soy allergy. Pediatr Clin North Am 2011;58(2):407–26.
48. Caubet JC, Wang J. Current understanding of egg allergy. Pediatr Clin North Am 2011;58(2):427–43.
49. Czaja-Bulsa G, Bulsa M. What do we know now about IgE-mediated wheat allergy in children? Nutrients 2017;9(1):35.
50. Masthoff LJ, Mattsson L, Zuidmeer-Jongejan L, et al. Sensitization to cor a 9 and cor a 14 is highly specific for a hazelnut allergy with objective symptoms in Dutch children and adults. J Allergy Clin Immunol 2013;132(2):393–9.
51. Valcour A, Lidholm J, Borres MP, et al. Sensitization profiles to hazelnut allergens across the United States. Ann Allergy Asthma Immunol 2019;122(1):111–6.

52. Blankestijn MA, Blom WM, Otten HG, et al. Specific IgE to Jug r 1 has no additional value compared with extract-based testing in diagnosing walnut allergy in adults. J Allergy Clin Immunol 2017;139(2):688–90.

53. Van der Valk JP, Gerth van Wijk R, Vergouwe Y, et al. sIgE Ana o 1, 2 and 3 accurately distinguish tolerant from allergic children sensitized to cashew nuts. Clin Exp Allergy 2017;47(1):113–20.

54. Katelaris CH. Food allergy and oral allergy or pollen-food syndrome. Curr Opin Allergy Clin Immunol 2010;10(3):246–51.

Immunologic Risk Assessment and Approach to Immunosuppression Regimen in Kidney Transplantation

John Choi, MD, Anil Chandraker, MD, FASN*

KEYWORDS

- Kidney transplant • Immunologic risk assessments • Immunosuppression regimen
- Transplant immunology

KEY POINTS

- Careful evaluation of immunologic risk is the key to success in kidney transplantation.
- Clinicians should understand the benefit and adverse profile of therapeutic agents to tailor the best immunosuppression regimen for each patient.
- Contemporary diagnostic tools and therapeutic agents in kidney transplantation are limited; collaborative efforts are needed to advance patient care in the era of precision medicine.

INTRODUCTION

Along with an increasing number of patients with end-stage renal disease in the United States,[1] we are also witnessing a record breaking number of kidney transplantations over the past several years.[1,2] In 2018, the United Network for Organ Sharing reported more than 21,000 kidney transplantations across the country. That is nearly 5000 more cases per year compared with 2008. In addition, the government has recently announced a policy change to incentivize kidney transplant in the care of patients with end-stage renal disease.[3] These achievements are the result of multiple efforts in the transplant community, facilitated by a better understanding of alloimmunity and effective immunosuppression practices.[4]

Immunosuppression therapy in transplantation can be categorized into 2 groups: induction therapy that is provided perioperatively and maintenance therapy for long-term allograft protection. The practice of immunosuppression in United States

Transplantation Research Center, Renal Division, Brigham and Women's Hospital, Harvard Medical School, Boston, MA, USA
* Corresponding author. Transplant Research Center, Brigham and Women's Hospital, 221 Longwood Avenue, Boston, MA 02115.
E-mail address: achandraker@bwh.harvard.edu

Clin Lab Med 39 (2019) 643–656
https://doi.org/10.1016/j.cll.2019.07.010
0272-2712/19/© 2019 Elsevier Inc. All rights reserved.

varies among centers,[5,6] and each center maintains a specific protocol considering the immunologic risks of individual patients as well as patient demographics referred to the center. In general, there has been an uptrend in the strength and dose of immunosuppressive medications in the United States.[7] This trend has translated into an overall decrease in rejection events and a higher allograft survival rate, as mentioned elsewhere in this article. However, concern among the community is increasing, because stronger immunosuppression is linked to debilitating adverse effects: opportunistic infection, malignancy, and potential harm to the kidney allograft itself. This highlights the limitations in the current practice of immunosuppression and underpins the importance of developing accurate biomarkers along with targeted therapies tailored to patient-specific immune rejection pathways.

TYPES OF REJECTION

Rejection can be defined by the timing of event. Hyperacute rejection occurs within minutes after transplantation and was most feared complication in early ages of solid organ transplantation. Hyperacute rejection is mediated by preformed antibody against the donor tissue and subsequent complement activation. Owing to improved preformed antibody screening, crossmatching strategy, and treatment options (described elsewhere in this article) this type of rejection is rare in contemporary practice. Acute rejection occurs within weeks to 1 year after transplantation, although it can occur further out. Both acute and chronic rejection are characterized by either or both lymphocyte infiltration and antibodies against the allograft.

Historically, the main goal in transplantation was to improve 1-year graft survival. Therefore, risk assessment tools were developed with a focus on avoiding hyperacute and acute rejection episodes. Despite excellent 1-year graft survival, an increasing incidence of the long-term complications of immunosuppression and chronic rejection makes it imperative to modify outcome goals and update the risk assessment process.

TRENDS IN ACUTE REJECTION AND THE PRACTICE OF IMMUNOSUPPRESSION IN UNITED STATES

The incidence of acute rejection in kidney transplantation has markedly declined over the recent decades. According to the Organ Procurement and Transplantation Network/Scientific Registry of Transplant Recipients annual outcome report from 2015 to 2016, the first year post-transplant rejection rate was only 8% in adult recipients in contemporary practice, compared with 60% and 35% in 1980 and mid 1990s, respectively.[8] This achievement, along with improvements in allograft outcomes, was a result of the introduction of induction therapy agents, better HLA matching (including availability of virtual crossmatching), and stronger maintenance immunosuppression.[7,9,10] In particular, the dramatic improvement in 1-year graft survival and the decrease in composite 1-year rejection events correlates with the introduction of calcineurin inhibitors (CNIs) and lymphodepleting agents as an induction therapy.[9] Therefore, it is not surprising that more transplantation centers in United States are incorporating induction therapy into their protocols—increasing from 45% in 1999% to 70% in 2008.[11] In addition, most centers have adopted triple therapy, composed of tacrolimus, mycophenolic acid, and steroids as an initial choice of maintenance therapy rather than single or double therapy.[6]

ADVERSE EFFECTS FROM THE TRENDS IN IMMUNOSUPPRESSION PRACTICES

Although implementing stronger immunosuppression did achieve the primary goal of improving 1-year graft survival and decreasing the rejection rate, it came with a significant cost. A prospective international study comparing antithymocyte globulin and anti–IL-2R antibody regimens showed a significant increase in overall infections with antithymocyte globulin, especially infections with bacteria and non-cytomegalovirus viruses (86% vs 75%, P-value: 0.03).[12] Notably, some studies also observed an increased association of cytomegalovirus infection with lymphodepleting agents[13–15] and CNIs.[16] In addition, the incidence of BK nephropathy has been reported to be uptrending with lymphodepleting agents and the increased popularity of CNI over mammalian target of rapamycin inhibitors in immunosuppression regimens.[17–19]

In 2003, a group analyzed the United Network for Organ Sharing database to parse out the risk factors for post-transplant lymphoproliferative disorder associated with different immunosuppressants. This study showed that exposure to monoclonal lymphodepleting agents, but not anti–IL-2R antibody had an increased tendency to develop post-transplant lymphoproliferative disorder.[20–22] Skin cancer, namely squamous cell cancer followed by basal cell cancer, is common in kidney transplantation and exposure to CNIs is a well-known risk factor.[23]

Finally, the incidence of chronic allograft nephropathy, which is highly associated with tacrolimus-induced chronic vasoconstriction, has increased proportionally with overall allograft survival, suggesting that the cumulative exposure time to tacrolimus has increased. Despite this finding, clinicians are reluctant to actively withdraw CNI when allograft function is stable, because a prior study showed an association with increased rejection rate and further prospective studies are needed.[24,25]

THE SENSITIZATION IN TRANSPLANTATION WORKING GROUP

In response to contemporary developments in molecular diagnostics, the transplant community has put forth a framework to standardize the immunologic risk assessment process.[26] The group first acknowledged current limitations in coming up with uniform guidelines owing to heterogeneity in laboratory reports (ie, mean fluorescence intensity cutoffs) and terminology, especially in published literature. Then the group suggested that alloimmune risk can be stratified based on 6 assessment criteria: complement-dependent cytotoxicity (CDC) crossmatch, flow crossmatch, single antigen bead test, history of sensitization, HLA molecular mismatch, and HLA identical. This stratification allows for the classification of patients by risk categories ranging from a low risk of de novo alloimmune response to active memory and a high risk for hyperacute rejection. In the following sections, we discuss when and how these data are collected and analyzed in contemporary practice for immunologic risk stratification. Finally, the working group concluded the importance of creating a centralized registry of patients suffering from rejection for effective research.

CURRENT FRAMEWORK FOR IMMUNOLOGIC RISK EVALUATION

In following paragraphs, we review the basic approach to immunologic risk assessment in kidney transplantation. In general, initial evaluation focuses on (1) the recipients' preexisting risk factors, (2) the use of this information to find the best matching kidney, and (3) planning ahead for induction therapy given the unpredictive nature of organ availability (**Fig. 1**A). Once the organ is offered, additional crossmatching is performed as a final checkpoint and based on variables identified during

A Pre-transplantation Evaluation

Review of History	Laboratory Test	Induction Therapy
Demographics • Age • Race • Sex • BMI	HLA & Blood Group Typing Solid Phase Assay • "Unacceptable" HLA • Calculated PRA	• Lymphodepleting agents • Immunomodulatory agents • No induction
Sensitizing events • Transfusion • Pregnancy • Previous transplant	Additional Cross-matching only if donor sample available (i.e. living donor) refer to Figure 1B.	**For Sensitized Patients** • Desensitization protocol • Exchange program (if living donor available)

B Peri-transplantation Evaluation

Tissue Typing	Peri-op factors	Maintenance Therapy
Number of HLA A-,B- and DR- Mismatch	Ischemia time • Warm Ischemia Time • Cold Ischemia Time	Standard "Triple Therapy" • Calcineurin Inhibitor or mTOR inhibitor • Antimetabolite • Steroid
Cross-matching • CDC-XM • FC-XM	Delayed Graft Function	
	Initial tolerance to immunosuppression	Early conversion to CTLA4-Ig?

Fig. 1. Immunologic risk assessment and therapeutic approach in kidney transplantation. (*A*) Pre-transplantation immunologic risk evaluation and induction therapy planning. (*B*) Peri-transplantation immunologic risks and management of maintenance immunosuppression regimen. BMI, body mass index; CDC-XM, complement-dependent cytotoxicity crossmatch; CTLA4, cytotoxic T-lymphocyte–associated protein 4; FC-XM, flow cytometry crossmatch; mTOR, mammalian target of rapamycin; PRA, panel reactive antibody.

perioperative period each center determines the appropriate choice of postoperative immunosuppression regimen (**Fig. 1**B).

Pretransplant Evaluation

Demographic factors
Basic demographic factors such as age, sex, and race can predict the of robustness of the alloimmune response. The incidence of acute rejection episodes shows a linear drop as the recipient gets older.[27] This phenomenon seems to be the result of a decreasing capacity for T-cell proliferation and B-cell activation that occurs with aging.[16] In terms of sex, male recipients who received renal allograft from a female donor were at increased risk of acute rejection compared with those who received allograft from a male donor.[28] In addition, animal studies have shown a protective effect of estradiol in chronic rejection, whereas testosterone induces an opposite effect.[29]

Racial disparity in kidney transplant outcomes[30] has been a long-standing issue in kidney transplantation. Although recent trends show overall improvement in allograft survival, African Americans are at the highest risk for acute rejection episodes.[31] Studies have yet to elucidate qualitative differences in immune mechanisms between races, and for now it is thought to be related to a combination of socioeconomic inequalities[32] as well as faster metabolism of CNI in the African American population (via CYP3A5 genotype).[33] Coding variants in APOL1 gene have been strongly linked to CKD risk and poor allograft survival in African Americans, but whether these high risk alleles have a specific immunomodulatory effect needs to be further examined. Finally, it is also noteworthy that recipient obesity is associated with a higher risk of rejection,[34,35] likely reflecting the chronic inflammatory status associated with obesity.

Donor type
Deceased donor grafts have been associated with a higher risk of acute rejection when compared with living donor grafts. Fortunately, the gap between deceased donor and living donor grafts has become significantly lower in contemporary practice; in 2014 and 2015, acute rejection episodes in 1 year post-transplant recipients of deceased donor and living donor grafts was 8% and 7%, respectively.[36] However, there remains a significant difference in 5- and 10-year death censored allograft survival rate between living and deceased donor kidney transplant (10% vs 15% and 20 vs 30%, respectively, in 2016). Given that the majority of graft failures after 5 years are related to antibody-mediated rejection,[37] it is possible that deceased donor grafts are more prone to chronic antibody-mediated rejection, but further larger scale studies are needed to confirm this. The Kidney Donor Profile Index (KDPI) system was introduced in 2009 to classify the risk of allograft failure based on donor profile.[38] For example, a KDPI of 80% indicates that an allograft from such a donor has a risk of graft failure of more than 80% of all kidney donors recovered in the previous year. A high KDPI score is associated with increased acute rejection.[39]

Previous sensitizing events and solid phase immunoassays
Prior sensitizing events should be carefully reviewed. The Sensitization in Transplantation working group has defined HLA sensitizing events as pregnancies, transfusions, previous transplant, and implants.[26] The Luminex solid phase immunoassay (Luminex, Austin, TX) is one of the most convenient and sensitive methods to check for circulating preformed antibodies before and after transplantation.[40,41] Owing to option of reporting so-called unacceptable antigens, it offers an efficient way of ruling out incompatible donors through a virtual crossmatch.[42] However, clinicians should be aware that there are many factors that go into determining what constitutes an unacceptable antigen.[43,44] The onus is on the individual center to determine the list of unacceptable antigens and the center may strategically set a different mean fluorescence intensity cutoff for positivity to support patients. Furthermore, technical variation between solid phase assays needs to be taken into account, as summarized in a recent review article.[45] Finally, the solid phase assay should not be used as a single tool for decision making, and it needs to be followed up with a functional assay such as cytotoxicity crossmatching as discussed elsewhere in this article.

HLA typing
HLA type identified during pretransplant evaluation helps find the best matching allograft. Traditionally, HLA-A, -B (class I) and HLA-DR (class II) were considered for determining a mismatch. The number of HLA mismatches shows a linear correlation with the incidence of acute rejection.[46,47] A couple of outcome studies using European

transplant databases have suggested that class II mismatches are more important than a class I mismatch,[48,49] especially showing the link between HLA-DR mismatch and antibody-mediated rejection. In recent years, HLA-DQ has been under the spotlight.[50] A series of reports showed an association with de novo anti-DQ antibody with increased acute rejection rate.[51,52] Nowadays, HLA can be characterized at the level of an eplet, the functional portion of epitope. The transplant community is actively working to refine the algorithms for immune risk assessment to incorporate eplet mismatches,[53] which may soon change the paradigm for approaching pretransplant evaluation.

Induction therapy

By reviewing the information collected as outlined, clinicians can obtain a general idea of which induction therapy to provide. There are 2 main categories of induction therapy: lymphodepleting agents (eg, antithymocyte globulin or anti-CD52 antibody) and immunomodulatory agents (eg, anti–IL-2R antibody). Studies have demonstrated the superiority of antithymocyte globulin in preventing acute rejection among high risk patients although this did not translate into improved 1-year allograft survival.[12] In addition, there was a higher incidence of infection with antithymocyte globulin.[12,13,54] Therefore, clinicians should identify lower risk patients—old, non-black, living donor, low panel reactive antibody, and no sensitization events—and provide anti–IL-2R antibody as an induction therapy to avoid exaggerated immunosuppression. In contrast, young, African American, deceased donor transplant recipients with prior sensitization events should be considered for antithymoglobulin antibody induction. There are no specific tools to guide therapy for patients who are at intermediate risk, and clinicians need to titrate the intensity of induction therapy and maintenance therapy to avoid overimmunosuppression or underimmunosuppression. Finally, the question arises if there are certain individuals who may not require induction therapy at all. The ratio of patients who do not receive any type of induction therapy has decreased to near 10% by 2017.[2] A study done with the patients on triple therapy for maintenance showed that low-risk recipients without induction therapy did as well as a group who received anti–IL-2R antibody, a standard choice for low-risk patients.[55] This finding highlights the need for further clinical trials to guide the precise use of induction therapy.

Special Considerations in Highly Sensitized Patients

The number of transplants in highly sensitized patients has increased over the past 5 years,[2] driven by changes in the allocation system that advocates for these patients.[56] The management of highly sensitized patients is a complex topic and the details are outside the scope of this article. However, we briefly discuss the current approach to highly sensitized patients, where availability of a potential living donor is crucial. If a living donor is available and compatible, the patient can proceed with a transplant; in cases with a concern for incompatible HLA, the team can seek a paired donor exchange. If a patient is offered a deceased donor allograft, most transplant centers in the United States activate a desensitization protocol to avoid hyperacute rejection. The protocol typically involves multiple rounds of intravenous immunoglobulin with plasmapheresis and, depending on the center, it includes rituximab or bortezomib to further suppress B cells and plasma cells. Once a patient has undergone a desensitization protocol, serum should be retested for the effective removal of antibodies. There are multiple ongoing clinical trials to find effective treatment approaches for sensitized patients and it will require a multi-institutional effort to recruit patients and follow their outcomes.[26,57]

Perioperative Assessment

Crossmatching

In the case of a deceased donor transplant, only virtual crossmatching is available until the donor blood sample becomes available. Once the deceased donor sample has arrived at the transplant center, or if a patient has a known living donor, functional capacity of preformed donor-specific antibodies can be performed as a final check point. CDC crossmatch (CDC-XM), one of the oldest tests invented for transplant compatibility,[58] remains a critical step in assessment. Donor B and T lymphocytes are incubated separately with recipient serum, and the presence of anti-HLA antibodies in the recipient serum is determined using CDC. Transplantation is aborted when T-cell CDC-XM shows a positive result. This result indicates that the recipient serum has strong reactivity against HLA class I antigens, which are expressed on all nucleated allograft cells. In contrast, if only the B-cell CDC-XM result is positive, this may be due to a low level of HLA class I antibody selectively targeting B cells or the presence of antibodies against HLA class II, and clinicians will weigh the risk and benefit of proceeding with the transplant.[59] It is also important to determine if the positivity is due to IgG antibody rather than IgM, and this can be tested by adding dithiothreitol to selectively inactivate IgM in the assay. A negative CDC-XM result should not completely obliviate the consideration of immunologic risks in further management decisions. There could be situations where the preformed donor-specific antibody titer is too low to fix complement or the antibody does not effectively bind complement. Although CDC-XM picks up the main pathogenic complement-fixing antibodies such as IgM, IgG1, and IgG3, the presence of other antibody isotypes can also contribute to rejection. This is where more sensitive assays, such as flow cytometry crossmatching, which detects donor-specific antibodies can be useful.[59] Positive flow cytometry crossmatching does increase the likelihood of antibody-mediated rejection[60] and should be taken into account for the long-term management of immunosuppressants.

Cold ischemia time

Recipients with an allograft that had a cold ischemia time of more than 24 hours were at an increased risk of acute rejection compared with those with a cold ischemia time of less than 12 hours (relative risk, 1.13). This effect was especially pronounced in patients who underwent repeat transplantation (relative risk, 1.66).[61]

One of the challenges in the new kidney allocation system is related to cold ischemia time. The high organ discard rate[62] is in part related to increased organ harvests from donors with a high kidney donor prolife index (KDPI), also known as a marginal kidney. These marginal kidneys are then shared at the regional level, which makes the matching process longer, and by the time of transplant, centers are worried about the association between long cold ischemia time and allograft outcome.[63] Along with revising the allocation system, technological improvements in organ preservation and perfusion techniques may be able to salvage more than 1000 kidneys per year.[62,64]

Warm ischemia time and anastomosis time

There are limited studies that have specifically investigated the association between warm ischemia time and the risk of acute rejection. Heylan and colleagues[65] conducted a single-center study in Belgium and concluded that, in patients who received kidney from a brain dead donor, there was no association with acute rejection in the first 3 months after transplantation and warm ischemia time. Now the technologies have improved and the interest has shifted to understanding the differences in the outcome of allograft survival between the traditional static cold storage preserved organs versus machine-perfused organs as well the use of a normothermic or hypothermic perfusion. More studies are required to understand the risk for immune response in the context of particular modes of organ preservation and guide the management strategies.

Delayed graft function

The rate of recovery of kidney function after transplantation is predictive of rejection, and is clinically classified into immediate (<1 day), slow (<5 days), and delayed (>7 days) recovery of graft function. A systematic metanalysis in 2009 showed a 38% increased risk of acute rejection within the first year in patients who suffered from delayed graft function.[66] A similar trend was reported again in 2016, when Gill and colleagues[67] looked into the long-term impact of delayed graft function. In this study, the group looked into data from the Scientific Registry of Transplant Recipients and analyzed data on patients where 2 group of patients received kidneys from the same deceased donor and only 1 transplant developed delayed graft function. This study revealed a 5-fold higher risk of acute rejection within 1 year for patients who suffered delayed graft function. In addition, patients who experience slow graft function are at higher risk of acute rejection within the first 6 months (40%) when compared with patients with immediate graft function (30%), but lower than patients who experienced delayed graft function (47%).[68]

Initial Response to the Immunosuppression Regimen

During postoperative care, patients are introduced to a number of new medications,[69] including immunosuppressants and infection prophylaxis. Clinicians should pay close attention if patients are experiencing any side effects. Not only can certain side effects be lethal, but unrecognized side effects can also lead to noncompliance and rejection episodes.[59,70]

The standard regimen in contemporary practice includes tacrolimus, mycophenolate, and prednisone. Mycophenolate, despite the development of an enteric-coated formula, remains a major cause of diarrhea after transplantation.[71] Diarrhea can significantly increase the circulating level of tacrolimus,[72] which leads to allograft injury[73] and overimmunosuppression. In contrast, the resolution of diarrhea can decrease serum tacrolimus level and, if this goes unnoticed, the patient may develop acute rejection. In addition, many antibiotics, antifungals, antiepileptics, or antihypertensive medications can either increase or decrease CNI levels.[74] If a patient who received an allograft with severe vascular disease shows sensitive vasoconstriction to CNI and the estimated glomerular filtration rate contraindicates the use of a mammalian target of rapamycin inhibitor, conversion to CTLA4-Ig can be considered.[75] However, premature conversion has been associated with a higher incidence or rejection[76]; therefore, clinicians should weigh the risk and benefit of the timing of conversion to CTLA4-Ig therapy.

Selective Tests to Guide Maintenance Therapy

There are a few tests for the post-transplant monitoring of cellular immunity to guide clinicians in managing maintenance immunosuppressants. Examples include the enzyme-linked immunosorbent spot for interferon-gamma,[77] a highly sensitive enzyme linked immunosorbent assay-like test used to infer the frequency of donor memory T-cell activity, which uses T-cell–depleted donor or third-party stimulator cells with donor HLA as an antigen. The Immuknow assay,[78,79] which measures the release of adenosine triphosphate by $CD4^+$ T cells upon Phytohemagglutinin mitogen treatment, provides a global measure of $CD4^+$ T-cell activation in the setting of alloimmune response. Each test has its own strengths and weaknesses but center-to-center variation and process standardization have prevented these tests from being more widely adopted across the country.[80–82] For in-depth information on biomarkers in transplantation, please refer to our recent review in *Clinics in Laboratory Medicine*.[83]

SUMMARY

The first human kidney transplantation in 1954 was performed between identical twins; nowadays, ABO blood group-incompatible organs are being transplanted successfully. The society endeavors to discover strategies of overcoming immunologic hurdles and expand eligible transplant candidates; in the near future, we may be witnessing xenotransplantation, which will significantly relieve the burden of the current organ shortage. In contrast, we ought to acknowledge the unmet needs for advancing the current immunologic risk assessment tools. Although the evaluation process described in this review provides a descriptive idea of immunologic risk, critical decisions such as listing transplant candidates and their unacceptable antigens, proceeding toward surgery with a high-risk organ donor, as well as the choice of immunosuppression is largely dictated by the intuition and experience of gathered by physicians at an individual center. Finally, as graft survival time increases with less acute rejection that is mainly T-cell driven,[84] antibody-mediated rejection has surfaced as a major threat against the long-term outcome of allografts.[37] This finding highlights the critical need for characterizing the immunologic risk of long-term B-cell–driven immunity.[85]

State-of-the-art biomarkers and targeted therapeutics are on the horizon.[83,86]

ACKNOWLEDGMENTS

Funding support was provided by NIH grants to author Dr.Choi T32DK007527; Dr. Chandraker has nothing to reveal. Authors report no conflict of interest.

REFERENCES

1. United States Renal Data System. 2018 USRDS annual data report: Epidemiology of kidney disease in the United States. National Institutes of Health, National Institute of Diabetes and Digestive and Kidney Diseases, Bethesda, MD, 2018. Available at: https://www.usrds.org/2018/download/Acknowledgments_18.pdf.
2. Hart A, Smith JM, Skeans MA, et al. OPTN/SRTR 2017 annual data report: kidney. Am J Transplant 2019. https://doi.org/10.1111/ajt.15274.
3. President Trump announces administration's bold vision for transforming kidney care. No title. National Kidney Foundation. 2019. Available at: https://www.kidney.org/news/president-trump-announces-administration's-bold-vision-transforming-kidney-care. Accessed August 10, 2019.
4. Sypek M, Kausman J, Holt S, et al. HLA epitope matching in kidney transplantation: an overview for the general nephrologist. Am J Kidney Dis 2018. https://doi.org/10.1053/j.ajkd.2017.09.021.
5. Kalluri HV. Current state of renal transplant immunosuppression: present and future. World J Transplant 2012. https://doi.org/10.5500/wjt.v2.i4.51.
6. Axelrod DA, Naik AS, Schnitzler MA, et al. National variation in use of immunosuppression for kidney transplantation: a call for evidence-based regimen selection. Am J Transplant 2016. https://doi.org/10.1111/ajt.13758.

7. Meier-Kriesche HU, Li S, Gruessner RWG, et al. Immunosuppression: evolution in practice and trends, 1994-2004. Am J Transplant 2006. https://doi.org/10.1111/j.1600-6143.2006.01270.x.

8. Gjertson D. Impact of delayed graft function and acute rejection on graft survival. Transplant Proc 2002. https://doi.org/10.1016/s0041-1345(02)03167-6.

9. Zand MS. Immunosuppression and immune monitoring after renal transplantation. Semin Dial 2005. https://doi.org/10.1111/j.1525-139X.2005.00098.x.

10. South AM, Grimm PC. Transplant immuno-diagnostics: crossmatch and antigen detection. Pediatr Nephrol 2016. https://doi.org/10.1007/s00467-015-3145-z.

11. Hardinger KL, Brennan DC, Klein CL. Selection of induction therapy in kidney transplantation. Transpl Int 2013. https://doi.org/10.1111/tri.12043.

12. Brennan DC, Daller JA, Lake KD, et al. Rabbit antithymocyte globulin versus basiliximab in renal transplantation. N Engl J Med 2006. https://doi.org/10.1056/nejmoa060068.

13. Lebranchu Y, Bridoux F, Büchler M, et al. Immunoprophylaxis with basiliximab compared with antithymocyte globulin in renal transplant patients receiving MMF-containing triple therapy. Am J Transplant 2002. https://doi.org/10.1034/j.1600-6143.2002.020109.x.

14. Mourad G, Rostaing L, Legendre C, et al. Sequential protocols using basiliximab versus anti-thymocyte globulins in renal-transplant patients receiving mycophenolate mofetil and steroids. Transplantation 2004. https://doi.org/10.1097/01.TP.0000129812.68794.CC.

15. Bataille S, Moal V, Gaudart J, et al. Cytomegalovirus risk factors in renal transplantation with modern immunosuppression. Transpl Infect Dis 2010. https://doi.org/10.1111/j.1399-3062.2010.00533.x.

16. Martins PNA, Tullius SG, Markmann JF. Immunosenescence and immune response in organ transplantation. Int Rev Immunol 2014. https://doi.org/10.3109/08830185.2013.829469.

17. Benavides CA, Pollard VB, Mauiyyedi S, et al. BK virus-associated nephropathy in sirolimus-treated renal transplant patients: incidence, course, and clinical outcomes. Transplantation 2007. https://doi.org/10.1097/01.tp.0000268524.27506.39.

18. Prince O, Savic S, Dickenmann M, et al. Risk factors for polyoma virus nephropathy. Nephrol Dial Transplant 2009. https://doi.org/10.1093/ndt/gfn671.

19. Dadhania D, Snopkowski C, Ding R, et al. Epidemiology of BK virus in renal allograft recipients: independent risk factors for bk virus replication. Transplantation 2008. https://doi.org/10.1097/TP.0b013e31817c6447.

20. Cherikh WS, Kauffman HM, McBride MA, et al. Association of the type of induction immunosuppression with posttransplant lymphoproliferative disorder, graft survival, and patient survival after primary kidney transplantation. Transplantation 2003. https://doi.org/10.1097/01.TP.0000100826.58738.2B.

21. Caillard S, Dharnidharka V, Agodoa L, et al. Posttransplant lymphoproliferative disorders after renal transplantation in the United States in era of modern immunosuppression. Transplantation 2005. https://doi.org/10.1097/01.tp.0000179639.98338.39.

22. Bustami RT, Ojo AO, Wolfe RA, et al. Immunosuppression and the risk of posttransplant malignancy among cadaveric first kidney transplant recipients. Am J Transplant 2004. https://doi.org/10.1046/j.1600-6135.2003.00274.x.

23. Luppi M, Barozzi P, Torelli G. Skin cancers after organ transplantation. N Engl J Med 2003;349(6):612–4 [author reply: 612–4].

24. Abramowicz D, Manas D, Lao M, et al. Cyclosporine withdrawal from a mycophenolate mofetil-containing immunosuppressive regimen in stable kidney transplant

recipients: a randomized, controlled study. Transplantation 2002. https://doi.org/10.1097/00007890-200212270-00015.

25. Kasiske BL, Heim-Duthoy K, Ma JZ. Elective cyclosporine withdrawal after renal transplantation: a meta-analysis. JAMA 1993. https://doi.org/10.1001/jama.1993.03500030093040.

26. Tambur AR, Campbell P, Claas FH, et al. Sensitization in transplantation: assessment of risk (STAR) 2017 working group meeting report. Am J Transplant 2018. https://doi.org/10.1111/ajt.14752.

27. Colvin MM, Smith CA, Tullius SG, et al. Aging and the immune response to organ transplantation. J Clin Invest 2017. https://doi.org/10.1172/JCI90601.

28. Zeier M, Döhler B, Opelz G, et al. The effect of donor gender on graft survival. J Am Soc Nephrol 2002. https://doi.org/10.1097/01.ASN.0000030078.74889.69.

29. Müller V, Szabó A, Viklicky O, et al. Sex hormones and gender-related differences: their influence on chronic renal allograft rejection. Kidney Int 1999. https://doi.org/10.1046/j.1523-1755.1999.00441.x.

30. Williams WW, Delmonico FL. The end of racial disparities in kidney transplantation? Not so fast! J Am Soc Nephrol 2016;27(8):2224–6. https://doi.org/10.1681/ASN.2016010005.

31. Gralla J, Le CN, Cooper JE, et al. The risk of acute rejection and the influence of induction agents in lower-risk African American kidney transplant recipients receiving modern immunosuppression. Clin Transplant 2014. https://doi.org/10.1111/ctr.12311.

32. Taber DJ, Douglass K, Srinivas T, et al. Significant racial differences in the key factors associated with early graft loss in kidney transplant recipients. Am J Nephrol 2014. https://doi.org/10.1159/000363393.

33. Taber DJ, Egede LE, Baliga PK. Outcome disparities between African Americans and Caucasians in contemporary kidney transplant recipients. Am J Surg 2017. https://doi.org/10.1016/j.amjsurg.2016.11.024.

34. Gore JL, Pham PT, Danovitch GM, et al. Obesity and outcome following renal transplantation. Am J Transplant 2006. https://doi.org/10.1111/j.1600-6143.2005.01198.x.

35. Sood A, Hakim DN, Hakim NS. Consequences of recipient obesity on postoperative outcomes in a renal transplant: a systematic review and meta-analysis. Exp Clin Transplant 2016. https://doi.org/10.6002/ect.2015.0295.

36. Kim WR, Lake JR, Smith JM, et al. OPTN/SRTR 2016 annual data report: kidney. Am J Transplant 2018. https://doi.org/10.1111/ajt.14558.

37. Sellarés J, De Freitas DG, Mengel M, et al. Understanding the causes of kidney transplant failure: the dominant role of antibody-mediated rejection and nonadherence. Am J Transplant 2012. https://doi.org/10.1111/j.1600-6143.2011.03840.x.

38. Rao PS, Schaubel DE, Guidinger MK, et al. A comprehensive risk quantification score for deceased donor kidneys: the kidney donor risk index. Transplantation 2009. https://doi.org/10.1097/TP.0b013e3181ac620b.

39. Keith D, Vranic G, Nishio Lucar A. Recipient Age and KDPI Are Potent Predictors of Early Acute Rejection in the Modern Era of Deceased Donor Kidney Transplantation. Am J Transplant 2016;16(suppl 3).

40. Lachmann N, Todorova K, Schulze H, et al. Luminex® and its applications for solid organ transplantation, hematopoietic stem cell transplantation, and transfusion. Transfus Med Hemother 2013. https://doi.org/10.1159/000351459.

41. Bettinotti MP, Zachary AA, Leffell MS. Clinically relevant interpretation of solid phase assays for HLA antibody. Curr Opin Organ Transplant 2016. https://doi.org/10.1097/MOT.0000000000000326.

42. Amico P, Hönger G, Steiger J, et al. Utility of the virtual crossmatch in solid organ transplantation. Curr Opin Organ Transplant 2009. https://doi.org/10.1097/MOT.0b013e328331c169.

43. Baxter-Lowe LA, Cecka M, Kamoun M, et al. Center-defined unacceptable HLA antigens facilitate transplants for sensitized patients in a multi-center kidney exchange program. Am J Transplant 2014. https://doi.org/10.1111/ajt.12734.

44. Zachary AA, Montgomery RA, Leffell MS. Defining unacceptable HLA antigens. Curr Opin Organ Transplant 2008. https://doi.org/10.1097/MOT.0b013e3283071450.

45. Konvalinka A, Tinckam K. Utility of HLA antibody testing in kidney transplantation. J Am Soc Nephrol 2015. https://doi.org/10.1681/asn.2014080837.

46. Shin S, Kim YH, Choi BH, et al. Long-term impact of human leukocyte antigen mismatches combined with expanded criteria donor on allograft outcomes in deceased donor kidney transplantation. Clin Transplant 2015. https://doi.org/10.1111/ctr.12487.

47. Cole EH, Johnston O, Rose CL, et al. Impact of acute rejection and new-onset diabetes on long-term transplant graft and patient survival. Clin J Am Soc Nephrol 2008. https://doi.org/10.2215/CJN.04681107.

48. Doxiadis IIN, De Fijter JW, Mallat MJK, et al. Simpler and equitable allocation of kidneys from postmortem donors primarily based on full HLA-DR compatibility. Transplantation 2007. https://doi.org/10.1097/01.tp.0000261108.27421.bc.

49. Gilks WR, Bradley BA, Gore SM, et al. Substantial benefits of tissue matching in renal transplantation. Transplantation 2006. https://doi.org/10.1097/00007890-198705000-00013.

50. Leeaphorn N, Pena JRA, Thamcharoen N, et al. HLA-DQ mismatching and kidney transplant outcomes. Clin J Am Soc Nephrol 2018. https://doi.org/10.2215/CJN.10860917.

51. Freitas MCS, Rebellato LM, Ozawa M, et al. The role of immunoglobulin-G subclasses and C1q in de novo HLA-DQ donor-specific antibody kidney transplantation outcomes. Transplantation 2013. https://doi.org/10.1097/TP.0b013e3182888db6.

52. Willicombe M, Brookes P, Sergeant R, et al. De novo DQ donor-specific antibodies are associated with a significant risk of antibody-mediated rejection and transplant glomerulopathy. Transplantation 2012. https://doi.org/10.1097/TP.0b013e3182543950.

53. Duquesnoy RJ. HLAMatchmaker: a molecularly based algorithm for histocompatibility determination. I. Description of the algorithm. Hum Immunol 2002. https://doi.org/10.1016/S0198-8859(02)00382-8.

54. Dharnidharka VR, Cherikh WS, Abbott KC. An OPTN analysis of national registry data on treatment of BK virus allograft nephropathy in the United States. Transplantation 2009. https://doi.org/10.1097/TP.0b013e31819cc383.

55. Tanriover B, Zhang S, MacConmara M, et al. Induction therapies in live donor kidney transplantation on tacrolimus and mycophenolate with or without steroid maintenance. Clin J Am Soc Nephrol 2015. https://doi.org/10.2215/CJN.08710814.

56. Formica RN. Allocating deceased donor kidneys to sensitized candidates. Clin J Am Soc Nephrol 2016. https://doi.org/10.2215/cjn.13641215.

57. Sethi S, Choi J, Toyoda M, et al. Desensitization: overcoming the immunologic Barriers to transplantation. J Immunol Res 2017. https://doi.org/10.1155/2017/6804678.

58. Patel R, Terasaki PI. Significance of the positive crossmatch test in kidney transplantation. N Engl J Med 2010. https://doi.org/10.1056/nejm196904032801401.

59. Mulley WR, Kanellis J. Understanding crossmatch testing in organ transplantation: a case-based guide for the general nephrologist. Nephrology 2011. https://doi.org/10.1111/j.1440-1797.2010.01414.x.

60. Karpinski M, Rush D, Jeffery J, et al. Flow cytometric crossmatching in primary renal transplant recipients with a negative anti-human globulin enhanced cytotoxicity crossmatch. J Am Soc Nephrol 2001;12(12):2807–14.

61. Postalcioglu M, Kaze AD, Byun BC, et al. Association of cold ischemia time with acute renal transplant rejection. Transplantation 2018. https://doi.org/10.1097/TP.0000000000002106.

62. Stewart DE, Klassen DK. Early experience with the new kidney allocation system: a perspective from UNOS. Clin J Am Soc Nephrol 2017. https://doi.org/10.2215/CJN.06380617.

63. Sampaio MS, Chopra B, Tang A, et al. Impact of cold ischemia time on the outcomes of kidneys with Kidney Donor Profile Index ≥85%: mate kidney analysis - a retrospective study. Transpl Int 2018. https://doi.org/10.1111/tri.13121.

64. Hameed AM, Pleass HC, Wong G, et al. Maximizing kidneys for transplantation using machine perfusion: from the past to the future: a comprehensive systematic review and meta-analysis. Medicine (Baltimore) 2016. https://doi.org/10.1097/MD.0000000000005083.

65. Heylen L, Pirenne J, Samuel U, et al. The impact of anastomosis time during kidney transplantation on graft loss: A eurotransplant cohort study. Am J Transplant 2017;17(3):724–32. https://doi.org/10.1111/ajt.14031.

66. Yarlagadda SG, Coca SG, Formica RN, et al. Association between delayed graft function and allograft and patient survival: a systematic review and meta-analysis. Nephrol Dial Transplant 2009. https://doi.org/10.1093/ndt/gfn667.

67. Gill J, Dong J, Rose C, et al. The risk of allograft failure and the survival benefit of kidney transplantation are complicated by delayed graft function. Kidney Int 2016. https://doi.org/10.1016/j.kint.2016.01.028.

68. Humar A, Johnson EM, Payne WD, et al. Effect of initial slow graft function on renal allograft rejection and survival. Clin Transplant 1997;11(6):623–7. Available at: http://www.ncbi.nlm.nih.gov/pubmed/9408697.

69. Hardinger KL, Hutcherson T, Preston D, et al. Influence of pill burden and drug cost on renal function after transplantation. Pharmacotherapy 2012. https://doi.org/10.1002/j.1875-9114.2012.01032.x.

70. Rianthavorn P, Ettenger RB, Malekzadeh M, et al. Noncompliance with immunosuppressive medications in pediatric and adolescent patients receiving solid-organ transplants. Transplantation 2004. https://doi.org/10.1097/01.TP.0000110410.11524.7B.

71. Shin HS, Chandraker A. Causes and management of postrenal transplant diarrhea: an underappreciated cause of transplant-associated morbidity. Curr Opin Nephrol Hypertens 2017. https://doi.org/10.1097/MNH.0000000000000368.

72. Sato K, Amada N, Sato T, et al. Severe elevations of FK506 blood concentration due to diarrhea in renal transplant recipients. Clin Transplant 2004. https://doi.org/10.1111/j.1399-0012.2004.00232.x.

73. Naesens M, Kuypers DRJ, Sarwal M. Calcineurin inhibitor nephrotoxicity. Clin J Am Soc Nephrol 2009. https://doi.org/10.2215/CJN.04800908.

74. Van Gelder T. Drug interactions with tacrolimus. Drug Saf 2002. https://doi.org/10.2165/00002018-200225100-00003.

75. Pérez-Sáez MJ, Yu B, Uffing A, et al. Conversion from tacrolimus to belatacept improves renal function in kidney transplant patients with chronic vascular lesions in allograft biopsy. Clin Kidney J 2018. https://doi.org/10.1093/ckj/sfy115.

76. Wojciechowski D, Vincenti F. Belatacept for prevention of acute rejection in adult patients who have had a kidney transplant: an update. Biologics 2012. https://doi.org/10.2147/BTT.S23561.

77. Hricik DE, Rodriguez V, Riley J, et al. Enzyme linked immunosorbent spot (ELISPOT) assay for interferon-gamma independently predicts renal function in kidney transplant recipients. Am J Transplant 2003. https://doi.org/10.1034/j.1600-6143.2003.00132.x.

78. Sottong PR, Rosebrock JA, Britz JA, et al. Measurement of T-lymphocyte responses in whole-blood cultures using newly synthesized DNA and ATP. Clin Diagn Lab Immunol 2002. https://doi.org/10.1128/cdli.7.2.307-311.2000.

79. Merrill JP, Murray JE, Harrison JH, et al. Successful homotransplantation of the human kidney between identical twins. J Am Med Assoc 1956. https://doi.org/10.1001/jama.1956.02960390027008.

80. Huskey J, Gralla J, Wiseman AC. Single time point immune function assay (Immu-Know™) testing does not aid in the prediction of future opportunistic infections or acute rejection. Clin J Am Soc Nephrol 2011. https://doi.org/10.2215/CJN.04210510.

81. Ashoor I, Najafian N, Korin Y, et al. Standardization and cross validation of alloreactive IFNγ ELISPOT assays within the clinical trials in organ transplantation consortium. Am J Transplant 2013. https://doi.org/10.1111/ajt.12286.

82. Wang Z, Liu X, Lu P, et al. Performance of the ImmuKnow assay in differentiating infection and acute rejection after kidney transplantation: a meta-analysis. Transplant Proc 2014. https://doi.org/10.1016/j.transproceed.2014.09.109.

83. Choi J, Bano A, Azzi J. Biomarkers in solid organ transplantation. Clin Lab Med 2019. https://doi.org/10.1016/j.cll.2018.11.003.

84. Halloran PF, Chang J, Famulski K, et al. Disappearance of T cell-mediated rejection despite continued antibody-mediated rejection in late kidney transplant recipients. J Am Soc Nephrol 2014. https://doi.org/10.1681/asn.2014060588.

85. Chong AS, Rothstein DM, Safa K, et al. Outstanding questions in transplantation: B cells, alloantibodies, and humoral rejection. Am J Transplant 2019. https://doi.org/10.1111/ajt.15323.

86. Stegall MD, Morris RE, Alloway RR, et al. Developing new immunosuppression for the next generation of transplant recipients: the path forward. Am J Transplant 2016. https://doi.org/10.1111/ajt.13582.

Laboratory Testing in the Context of Biologics and Cellular Therapies

Hugues Allard-Chamard, MD, PhD, FRCPC[a,b,c,d,*]

KEYWORDS

- Biological therapies • Monoclonal antibodies • Antidrug antibody • CAR T cells
- T-cell–mediated adverse drug reaction

KEY POINTS

- Antidrug antibodies can be divided into 2 categories: neutralizing antibodies (NABs) and binding antibodies; both may affect therapeutic performance.
- According to the Food and Drug Administration, the presence of NABs should be preferably evaluated using cell-based neutralization assays.
- The immunogenicity of a drug depends on the drug itself but also on its route of administration, the excipients, and its specific interactions with the immune system.
- Cytokine release syndrome and chimeric antigen receptor (CAR)-related encephalopathy syndrome are frequent complications of CAR T-cell therapy leading to significant comorbidities; a very high index of suspicion is necessary.
- Persistence of CAR T cells should be monitored by following the frequency of their targets as a surrogate marker.

INTRODUCTION

Therapeutic monoclonal antibodies (mabs) or biologics bearing an engineered component of an antibody such as the Fc domain are among the most common form of biological therapies in use today. There has been an explosion in the number of therapeutic monoclonal antibodies (mab)[1] used for the treatment of immune-mediated as well as

Disclosure Statement: Dr Hugues Allard-Chamard funding: Fellowship grant from the Faculté de médecine et des sciences de la santé de Sherbrooke.
[a] Ragon Institute of MGH, MIT and Harvard, Cambridge, MA, USA; [b] Division of Rheumatology, Faculty of Medicine and Health Sciences, Université de Sherbrooke, Sherbrooke, Québec, Canada; [c] Centre de Recherche Clinique du Centre Hospitalier Universitaire de Sherbrooke, Sherbrooke, Québec, Canada; [d] Division of Rheumatology, Centre intégré universitaire de santé et de service sociaux de l'Estrie – Centre hospitalier universitaire de Sherbrooke (CIUSSS de l'Estrie-CHUS), 3001, 12th Avenue North, Room 3853, Sherbrooke, Québec J1H 5N4, Canada
* Division of Rheumatology, Centre intégré universitaire de santé et de service sociaux de l'Estrie – Centre hospitalier universitaire de Sherbrooke (CIUSSS de l'Estrie-CHUS), 3001, 12th Avenue North, Room 3857, Sherbrooke, Québec J1H 5N4, Canada.
E-mail address: hugues.allard-chamard@USherbrooke.ca

Clin Lab Med 39 (2019) 657–668
https://doi.org/10.1016/j.cll.2019.07.011
0272-2712/19/© 2019 Elsevier Inc. All rights reserved.

labmed.theclinics.com

other diseases, such as migraine,[2] osteoporosis,[3] atherosclerosis,[4] and cancer.[5] Moreover, with the emergence of the chimeric antigen receptor (CAR) technology, which is used to redirect the antigenic specificity of T cells, immune cells themselves are being engineered into therapeutics, especially in oncology. Cytotoxic host T cells are expanded and transduced ex vivo with a CAR against a tumor antigen and reinfused into the host. Patients with documented sustained antitumor responses have been observed due to the generation of long-lived immune memory. The first CAR T cells successfully used in the clinic were directed against CD19, a protein highly expressed on B-cell malignancies.[6,7] CAR technology is set to explode and enter various fields of medicine, as it can be rationally designed against almost any protein, lipid, or carbohydrate target, and used to redirect the specificity of any type of immune response.

In the following chapter, the authors review the strategies used and challenges encountered in the design of assays for monitoring biological therapies and their side effects, in a clinical setting. Emphasis will be put on antidrug antibodies (ADA) detection, as it represents an active area of research with emerging scientific principles to guide assay design. Emerging guidelines for the development of assays to accurately measure ADAs are also discussed.

Antidrug Antibodies Against Biologics

Immunogenicity, or the capacity of an immunogen to elicit an immune response, spans from the activation of the innate immune system to the triggering of adaptive immune system, leading to highly specific immunity and the formation of immune memory. ADA responses likely span the entire gamut. It remains unclear why only some individuals mount a humoral response against a drug, while others do not. Sometimes, uncoupling the observed immune response against biological drugs into desired pharmacologic effects and undesired adverse effects can be a challenge. For instance, injection site reaction, cytokine storm, hypersensitivity reaction, generation of an antibody that cross-reacts with an endogenous protein, and the generation of ADA decreasing the therapeutic effect of a drug are clear examples of deleterious interactions of the drug with the immune system. Close to 1% of patients treated with biotherapies, mainly mabs, develop some form of measurable drug-induced immunogenicity.[8] However, an interaction with the immune system is not always detrimental. Many therapeutic mabs rely heavily on a strong and targeted interaction with the immune system to be fully effective. These interactions can take place in the following forms: antibody-dependent cellular cytotoxicity (ADCC), antibody-dependent phagocytosis, redirected killing using bispecific antibody cross-linking T cells and their target, complement-dependent cytotoxicity, and antibody-mediated opsonization or neutralization followed by clearance by the reticuloendothelial system.[9] Three therapeutic effects of mabs are thought to be largely independent of the immune system's activity: (1) disruption of a targeted ligand-receptor complex secondary to mab binding; (2) receptor downregulation due to synergistic interplay between internalization and degradation, triggered by the mab-mediated receptor activation; and (3) targeted drug delivery as in the case of antibody-drug conjugates.[10]

Some clinically measurable interactions of drugs with the immune system, such as allergic responses or infusion reactions, are thought to be idiosyncratic. But the generation of ADAs, in some clinical contexts or in association with particular human leukocyte antigen (HLA) alleles, has awakened the interest of the scientific community, as they can be monitored and used as a potential biomarker to predict the loss of efficacy during treatment and the emergence of side effects through the formation of immune complexes and cytokine release.[11] An understanding of the mechanisms underlying the development of ADAs has also opened the door to the design of potentially less antigenic drugs with the successive introduction of partially, and then fully, humanized mabs or mabs chemically modified by pegylation, or other modifications, aimed at both decreased immunogenicity and enhanced half-life. In 2010, in an attempt to specify the foundational principles and guidelines for testing the immunogenicity of biological drugs, an international conference was organized by the International Association for Biologicals, the Paul-Ehrlich-Institute (Federal Institute for Vaccines and Biologicals, Germany), and the International Federation of Pharmaceutical Manufacturers & Associations. This conference was followed by the publication of a guideline on immunogenicity assessment for biotechnology-derived therapeutic proteins.[8] In 2019, the Food and Drug Administration (FDA) released their own guidelines for the industry on Immunogenicity Testing of Therapeutic Protein Products, with specific guidance on the development and validation of assays for ADA detection.[12]

Types of antidrug antibodies

Based on Ehrlich's famous maxim *"corpora non agunt nisi fixata"* ("drugs will not act unless they are bound"), 2 main subsets of ADAs can be identified. The first group of ADAs is distinguished by their ability to bind a biological drug without significantly affecting the ability of the biological to interact with its target. Therapeutics that do not rely on the immune system to carry out their effect can usually still be functional despite being bound by this subset of ADAs. Such ADAs are called nonneutralizing or binding antibodies (BABs). BABs usually have a minor impact on the ability of the drug to find its target.[13] However, BABs can change the half-life of their drug targets or alter drug functions that are not strictly dependent on the physical effect of binding to their targets, such as activating the complement cascade. ADAs that increase the half-life of the drug are called sustaining ADAs, whereas ADAs that shorten the half life of the drug are called clearing ADAs.[14] More critically, it is important to identify patients at risk of developing the second type of ADAs that block the drug-target interaction: the neutralizing antibodies (NABs). NABs are able to prevent the drug from binding and interacting with its target, thus preventing the drug from acting. NABs either directly block the interaction between the biological therapeutic and its target or induce a change in the drug conformation, preventing the formation of a suitable binding interface between the drug and its target.

ADAs are implicated in a plethora of acute and delayed side effects. For instance, they are incriminated in immunoglobulin E (IgE)-mediated allergic anaphylactic reaction as well as non–IgE-mediated infusion reaction (anaphylactoid). They also can induce the formation of immune complexes, leading to serum sickness.[15] Although antidrug IgE antibodies and antibodies contributing to serum sickness are technically ADAs, we do not discuss these in depth in this article. We instead focus on the pharmacokinetic and pharmacodynamic effects of ADAs that result from their propensity to bind and neutralize a drug target and eliminate it from the circulation.

More importantly, there is a need to determine which ADAs have a clinical impact and require a change in the therapeutic strategy. NABs have been shown, in several instances, to muffle or abolish the therapeutic effect of a mab, but paradoxically, they may be transiently found in blood with a minimal functional impact. For instance, 9% of patients treated with natalizumab develop ADAs during the first 6 months of treatment, but only 6%, or two-thirds, remain positive in the long term.[16] Interestingly, the patients who remained positive had higher ADA titers. Biomarkers predicting the risk of developing persistent ADAs are still lacking for most biological therapies. This highlights both the risks of using poorly understood biomarkers and the fact that ADAs are clinically pertinent only if they remain in the blood over an extended period of time. In this specific study, if treatment had been discontinued based on

ADAs detected within the first 6 months of therapy, 3% of patients would have inappropriately terminated a potentially functional drug.[16] These gaps in our knowledge of ADAs should provide the impetus to better characterize and validate the use of ADAs.

Better characterization of ADAs has led to the paradigm of primary and secondary failure of therapeutic mabs. For example, in an attempt to treat a patient suffering from rheumatoid arthritis or Crohn disease with a biological therapy, the lack of any clinical improvement within the first few months may indicate either that the chosen mechanism of action is ineffective in the particular patient (primary failure) or that the drug failed to reach an adequate serum level (secondary failure). Anti-tumor necrosis factor (TNF) drugs only work in a ~30% of patients naive to biotherapies.[17,18] The need for distinguishing primary or secondary failure may also arise in a delayed context. For instance, a patient started on biotherapy may exhibit sustained remission for 5 years, but the disease may subsequently flare despite good compliance. In this delayed context, either the rheumatoid arthritis itself may have evolved into a more resistant phenotype (primary failure) or the drug may have induced neutralizing ADAs (secondary failure). Being able to distinguish between these 2 scenarios in the clinic would be of tremendous help. As the disease evolves, it might become resistant to a certain class of drugs, and clinicians could identify a different therapeutic regimen reliant on a distinct mechanism of action. Instead, if the loss in efficacy is solely due to the development of ADAs targeting the drug, another drug using the same mechanism of action could be administered, preserving other lines of treatment for future use.[19]

NABs have an even more dramatic impact when their level exceeds the capacity to neutralize the therapeutic agent. For instance, patients treated with recombinant erythropoietin who developed pure red cell aplasia (PRCA) were shown to have generated NABs reactive to both endogenous and recombinant erythropoietin.[20] Also, some patients with nonsevere forms of inherited hemophilia A or B, typically treated by supplementation of the missing factor only when severe bleeding was reported or before high bleeding risk surgery, can develop severe hemophilia due to the development of ADAs targeting the supplemented factor as well as the endogenous coagulation factor. The ability to rapidly identify such cases would be a game changer in the management of these devastating side effects. To avoid cross-neutralization by such NABs, engineered factors bearing minimal homology with their endogenous human counterparts are being developed.[21]

Factors triggering immunogenicity

The exact mechanisms of immunogenicity are not fully known and are probably heterogeneous, influenced by a complex interplay among various drug, host, and environmental factors. It is indeed widely accepted that both injection of foreign proteins or repeated injection of fully humanized proteins can eventually overcome the mechanisms of immune tolerance to self-antigens, hence triggering the activation of the adaptive immune system and the generation of a possibly autoreactive humoral response.[22] It is remarkable that drugs such as checkpoint inhibitors can by their very own nature be designed to trigger immunity. The factors intrinsic to a biological drug that may promote its immunogenicity can be divided into 3 categories: (1) the route of administration; (2) the bioactive compound; and (3) the excipient.

There is a growing body of evidence supporting the notion that the route of administration of a drug modulates its immunogenicity. Orally administered drugs are transported through the tolerogenic milieu present in the gut and may be less likely to induce an immune response. Similarly, intravenous infusions are also mildly immunogenic. The oral route is not suitable for most biological drugs, as they would be denatured or poorly absorbed through the gut. Although, subcutaneous administration of a drug is most likely to trigger immune activation, it is frequently used for the delivery of biological drugs due to reduced costs and the need for minimal infrastructure compared with intravenous administration. Albeit hard to distinguish in the clinic, epidermal delivery using skin patches seems to be more immunogenic than hypodermic or intramuscular injection.[23,24]

The structure of the bioactive compound clearly determines the potential for immunogenicity. Therapeutic antibodies or proteins that are fully humanized are less likely to trigger immune activation than their nonhumanized counterparts. As stated by the Committee for Medicinal Products for Human Use in their guideline on immunogenicity assessment of biotechnology-derived therapeutic proteins, increased vigilance is warranted when dealing with fusion proteins or partially humanized proteins. There are increasing reports of cases where the foreign moiety triggered the development of reactivity to the self portion of the therapeutic protein by epitope spreading and thus leading to autoimmunity. In that regard, fully humanized proteins are usually safer to use, although even they can harbor immunogenic posttranslational modifications, such as glycosylation, or bear a structural homology with an endogenous protein, against which the immune system may be triggered to react. Biological therapeutics are frequently modified to improve pharmacodynamic profiles, for example, mutant growth factors engineered to exhibit an higher affinity for their receptors.[25] These changes could be in the protein sequence itself, creating a neoantigen, or could be in the form of chemical modifications grafted onto the protein, such as pegylation or glycosylation that can change its affinity for various immune cells, sometimes at the risk of triggering an ADA response.[14] The FDA in its 2019 guideline for industry on developing and validating assays for ADA detection advocated for the development of assays specific for the non-Fc region of therapeutic mabs rather than the intact antibody to avoid false-positive signals from endogenous rheumatoid factor.[12]

Excipients are chosen to maximize the stability of a drug. Selection of an excipient is of paramount importance as it could also act as an adjuvant. An ideal excipient should minimize protein aggregation and not form stable complexes with the drug. However, excipients are far from perfect, and although they may promote the stability of the compound, they can also adversely affect the immunogenicity of a drug by creating immunogenic drug aggregates or drug-excipient complexes, resulting in either new epitopes or multivalent epitopes recognizable by the immune system. In the case of biological therapeutics, critical concerns arise from the possibility of contaminating side products (DNA, RNA, lipids, or proteins) from the cellular factory used in drug manufacture entering the final drug formulation. If the removal of these contaminating side products is incomplete, their adjuvant effects can promote immune activation. This is especially true of recombinant proteins expressed in bacteria or yeast. Moreover, experience has proved that even seemingly small changes during manufacturing and handling can have a dramatic effect on drug immunogenicity. For instance, organic compounds leaching from uncoated rubber stoppers in syringes were responsible for increasing the immunogenicity of an erythropoietin formulation, ultimately leading to PRCA through NABs cross-reacting to endogenous erythropoietin.[26]

Host factors are undeniably crucial in ADA development. Conceivably, in patients with a hyperactive immune system that is able to only partially discriminate self from nonself, there may be an amplified risk of immunogenicity toward therapeutics. Repeated exposure to a protein drug, even when fully humanized, can lead to immune activation. It is also important to consider the background of the patient in terms of immunosuppressive therapies. For instance, methotrexate is able to increase the lifespan of anti-TNF mab in patients with rheumatoid arthritis by decreasing the generation of ADAs.[27,28] The protective effect observed with methotrexate is not described with other immunosuppressive drugs. Age can also be an important factor. There are data suggesting that immunosenescence is associated with an increased propensity toward immune tolerance. Central tolerance mechanisms slowly fade with thymic involution and the maintenance of tolerance is delegated to peripheral lymphocytes such as regulatory T cells.[29] Moreover, the ratio of memory to naive lymphocytes increases with age, as progressive immunization occurs through accumulated environmental exposures creates a larger pool of memory lymphocytes with the potential to cross-react with a therapeutic agent. In addition, genetics plays a vital role in the development of ADAs. It is well known that different HLA alleles present distinct peptides from a proteinaceous antigen and that single nucleotide polymorphisms (SNP) in key immune genes can modulate the intensity of immune responses. For instance, SNPs in genes such as HLA-DR, ERAP, or interleukin 10 (IL-10) are associated with the development of specific patterns of autoimmunity. Moreover, a polymorphism in IL-10 has been associated with a ~4.5x increased risk of developing ADAs against adalimumab in patients with rheumatoid arthritis.[30] The adaptive immune system can occasionally induce cross-reacting responses to structurally similar antigens. The historic exposure of a patient to other biological drugs is therefore a key component of the assessment of immunogenicity. For instance, the use of a biosimilar is probably not appropriate in presence of ADAs targeting the original drug, as ADAs are likely to have high level of cross-reactivity against biosimilars. If a replacement drug is offered to a patient lacking an endogenous protein, such as in the case of hemophilia related to factor VIII deficiency, ADAs can develop following recombinant factor VIII therapy, as the host sees it as a foreign protein. Moreover, once an ADA develops against recombinant factor VIII, it is likely to cross-react with other recombinant factor VIII formulations on the market. Currently, treatment of hemophilia in presence of ADAs to coagulation factors is empirically managed. Evaluating the epitope specificity of ADAs in these contexts could give physicians a new handle to address such clinical challenges.

Testing for antidrug antibodies

Screening for ADAs can be performed using a plethora of immunoassays, such as enzyme-linked immunosorbent assay, fluoroenzyme immunoassay, radioimmunoprecipitation assay, chemiluminescent immunoassay, electrochemiluminescence, dissociation enhanced lanthanide fluoroimmunoassay, and surface plasmon resonance. ADA screening should allow the determination of the presence of a "binding" antibody, regardless of its isotype. It should be aimed at providing an ADA titer and a quantification of its neutralizing capacity. Further characterization, depending on the clinical need, could include determination of the isotype if an IgE-mediated allergic reaction is suspected or epitope mapping if cross-reactivity to an endogenous protein is suspected such as in the case of NABs targeting endogenous factor VIII.

Nonetheless, definitive demonstration of the presence of NABs requires a confirmatory test showing functional impairment of the drug's action. Monitoring ADAs in terms of the biological function can be challenging because the function of biologics depends on complex interactions that either block or activate their targets, depending on the clinical context. A typical example of a complex drug-target interaction in which investigating adverse immune interferences must be tailored with an a priori knowledge of the pathway are the therapeutics that target immune checkpoints. CTLA4 is an interesting conceptual case, a Janus incarnate in its duality. The therapeutic potential of targeting CTLA4 can be achieved both by blocking or enhancing its functionality. Ipilimumab binds to and blocks CTLA4 on T regulatory cells. It is used to interfere with the suppressive effect of CTLA4 on T regulatory cells and promote T-cell dependent elimination of the tumor cells.[31] On the other hand, abatacept, a fusion protein coupling the CTLA4 protein to the Fc of an immunoglobulin, is used to dampen inappropriate immune activation in autoimmune diseases, such as rheumatoid arthritis and polyarticular juvenile idiopathic arthritis.[32] Abatacept thus directly acts on effector T cells bypassing T regulatory cells. In this context, developing immunoassays to reliably detect the activity of the CTLA4 pathway in the presence of the drug and a possible ADA is not as straightforward. It is imperative for bioassays to detect that the development of antibodies interacting with drugs targeting the CTLA4/CD80-86 axis are also able to assess the functional impact of such interactions. However, there is no simple surrogate plasma biomarker that directly corresponds to the activity of the CTLA4/CD80-86 axis. ADA assays need to be designed to look beyond just the simple physical interaction between the therapeutic and the ADA and analyze alterations in the pharmacokinetic and pharmacodynamic parameters or include assessment of relevant surrogate biomarkers that inform the presence of functionally significant ADAs. A simplistic quantification of the drug target or the plasma level of the drug itself based on a competitive binding assay may not provide a complete picture of the impact of ADAs on secondary functions of the drug such as its propensity to activate, complement, and kill the target cell or recruit innate immune cells. Moreover, abatacept and ipilimumab do not exert their effect through the same "secondary" feature of their Fc.

The presence of NABs can be assessed using both cell-based assays, such as proliferation assays, gene reporter assays, gene expression measurements, ADCC, and complement-dependent cytotoxicity, and other acellular assays, such as competitive ligand binding. In its current guideline on Immunogenicity Testing of Therapeutic Protein Products, the FDA favors the use of neutralizing cell-based assays, which are thought to more closely reflect physiologic systems. If such assays cannot be performed, ligand-binding competition assays are considered a suitable alternative.[12,19,33] However, when designing ligand-binding assays, it is important to keep in mind that many immunoassays are susceptible to epitope masking or matrix effect, leading to a potential for false negatives. The matrix effect is a poorly characterized phenomenon by which components added with the analyte, usually carbohydrates, proteins, and phospholipids, from the serum, interfere with the ability of the antibody to bind its target. Moreover, the choice of a blocking reagent in an immunoassay can interfere with the ADA testing as both bovine serum albumin and milk-based blocking buffers contain nonhuman glycans that are found on therapeutics produced in nonhuman cells.

If the signaling pathway targeted by a drug is known, a common strategy is to design a reporter cell line to directly evaluate the presence of ADAs in the serum (**Fig. 1**). Owing to the widespread use of anti-TNF drugs in the clinic, reporter cell lines are available to evaluate the presence of ADAs against these drugs. Anti-TNF mabs and decoy receptors are among the most widely used biologics in rheumatology, dermatology, as well as gastroenterology. The knowledge that their efficacy can be impaired by the development of ADAs has triggered intense investigation into understanding the implications of developing ADAs, how they affect response to treatment, and how they can be best monitored. A genetically modified K562 erythroleukemic cell line that constitutively expresses a Renilla luciferase, and an inducible firefly luciferase responsive to TNF signaling under a NFκB promoter, has been developed to assay for the presence of anti-TNF ADAs. These cells are cultured with a fixed amount of TNF-α in the presence of increasing concentrations of both test and control serum to assess ADA activity. Unopposed TNF-α triggers the activation of nuclear factor-kappa B and its migration to the nucleus, where it induces the expression of the firefly luciferase reporter gene.

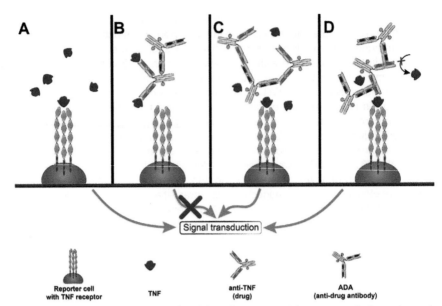

Fig. 1. ADAs are best assayed using a cell-based system, as it better recapitulates the under-lying biology of drug action and the complex interplay between the drug, the ADA, and the receptor-ligand dyad. Here, cell-based assays for ADAs against anti-TNF mabs are illustrated as an example. In the absence of any anti-TNF in the blood, soluble TNF is free to interact with its receptor and induce signal transduction leading to activation of the reporter gene. In the presence of test serum, the following scenarios may be encountered. (*A*) The serum assayed contains no ADAs and active anti-TNF can neutralize its ligand and prevent signal transduction. (*B*) Nonneutralizing BABs and the therapeutic are present; BABs are un-able to interfere with the ability of anti-TNF to prevent signal transduction. NABs, which impinge on the ability of a therapeutic to bind its target, are present; TNF signal will be transduced in this assay. Therapeutic hindrance from NABs can be the result of (*C*) occlusion of the binding site of the drug or (*D*) binding of the NAB close to the interface between the drug and its target, inducing a conformational change that reduces the affinity of the drug for its target.

The use of reporter cell lines ensures reproducibility, and because the transcriptional response to TNF is very fast, this test can be performed in less than 4 hours.[34]

Testing for adverse T-cell responses Biological drugs are generally composed of a pro-teinaceous core, and peptides derived from the drugs can therefore be displayed by major histocompatibility complex I (MHC-I) or MHC-II and recognized by CD8+ and CD4+ T cells respectively. Drug-induced activation of T cells can sometimes induce an exuberant cytokine release or direct cytotoxicity and result in a T-cell–mediated adverse drug reaction (TADR). TADRs can be just as dramatic as neutralizing ADAs and result in irreversible end organ damage. The most severe TADRs encompass the drug rash with eosinophilia and systemic symptoms syndrome or the Stevens-Johnson syndrome (SJS)/toxic epidermal necrolysis (TEN) spectrum. Activated T cells can also lead to profound drug-induced liver injury causing acute liver failure and eventually cirrhosis. TADRs can develop days to weeks after drug exposure. Currently, there are no biomarkers that can preemptively determine the risk for TADR and guide clinical decision, but some HLA alleles linked to autoimmunity are associated with the risk of TADR.

A TADR is generally approached as a clinical diagnosis and managed by avoidance of the presumed triggering drug. However, if an immunologic confirmation is desired, as in the case of multiple concomitant putative drug triggers or in the case of a drug that has no easy substitute, evaluation of TARDs is performed using standard functional assays. Commonly, peripheral blood mononuclear cells from patients with suspected TADRs are isolated and incubated with the putative triggering drug. The proliferation response of T cells is then evaluated in culture using assays based on either fluorescent (carboxyfluorescein succinimidyl ester, Ki-67) or radioactive (3H-thymidine incorporation) tracers. The ratio of the proportion of proliferating cells in the presence or absence of the drug is used to calculate a stimulation index that indicates T-cell responsiveness.[35] Once a TADR is confirmed, further characterization can be performed. TADR are sometimes referred to as delayed-type hypersensitivity (DTH), as they develop days to weeks after drug exposure and are divided into 4 categories (a to d) based on the predominantly expanded T-cell subset and cytokines produced. In type IVa DTH, immunity is skewed toward T helper 1 (Th1) and interferon gamma (IFN-γ) production. In type IVb DTH, immunity leans toward a Th2 phenotype with enhanced production of IL-4, IL-5, and IL-13. Type IVc DTH is characterized by activation of CD8+ T cells and an increased expression of granzyme B, perforin, and Fas ligand in tissues. SJS/TEN syndrome falls into this category of TADR. Type IVd DTH is marked by T-cell–driven neutrophilic infiltration that is sustained by T-cell–derived CXCL8 and GM-CSF. Assaying various types of DTH is performed using a combination of flow cytometry and ELISPOT.[36]

Monitoring Chimeric Antigen Receptor T-Cell Therapeutics

The advent of tisagenlecleucel, a CAR T-cell immunotherapy directed at CD19 + cells, in clinical practice, was the latest milestone in cancer immunotherapy. CAR T-cell immunotherapy has unparalleled therapeutic potential as highlighted by the American Society of Clinical Oncology, naming them the "advance of the year" in 2018.[37] CAR T cells are highly customizable, as the transgenic receptor could, in theory, target any class of chemical and eliminate the need for continued dosing. CAR T cells are being developed as candidate therapeutics in many fields but several questions remain to be answered. How should one monitor the administered CAR T cells themselves? How does one deal with therapeutics that cannot be removed once they are administered? The literature is currently at its inception; however, important messages are emerging on how CAR T-cell–mediated side effects should be monitored and how technological improvement in CAR T-cell design, such as in-built inducible suicide switches, may lead to better tolerability.

Despite being extremely efficient in clinical settings where other therapeutics have failed to provide sustained benefits, patients treated with CAR T cells still remain vulnerable to relapse. Approximately 30% to 50% of patients with acute lymphoblastic leukemia remain disease free at 5 years.[38] Moreover, cytokine release syndrome (CRS) and CAR-related encephalopathy syndrome are frequently encountered complications and can be challenging diagnoses to make, as they can mimic sepsis, hemophagocytic lymphohistiocytosis, and tumor lysis syndrome. To overcome the clinical difficulties in diagnosing CRS, cytokine screening is performed to find biomarkers that can inform clinical judgment in the presence of compatible manifestations. The core hallmark cytokines of CRS are IL-6, IL-10, and IFN-γ.[39] They are thought to be released after the CAR T cells engage with their targets, leading to the activation of bystander cells and endothelium activation. CRS is characterized by a systemic vasculopathy with endothelial activation and leakiness and complement activation, often resulting in disseminated intravascular coagulation. Peak serologic levels of IL-6, soluble IL-6 receptor, IFN-γ, and sgp130 were shown to correlate with CRS and are considered potentially helpful biomarkers for this condition. This panel of biomarkers may also help discriminate CRS from other related conditions such as sepsis, which are not strong inducers of IFN-γ.[39,40]

The evaluation of the long-term safety of CAR T cells is still lacking. In the meantime, the National Comprehensive Cancer Network (NCCN) CAR T-Cell Therapy Task Force recommends monitoring CAR T-cell persistence. Conventional flow cytometric measurement of circulating CD19 + lymphocytes is the preferred method for monitoring anti-CD19 CAR T cells. The absence of CD19 + lymphocytes is a good surrogate marker of residual CD19 CAR T-cell activity. This assessment should be performed at each follow-up visit. The recommendation does not include testing specifically for the presence of CAR T cells, although most patients in clinical trials typically undergo direct assessment of CAR T cells.[41] In addition to the standard care, the NCCN CAR T-Cell Therapy Task Force also recommends monitoring gamma-globulin levels, B- and T-cell reconstitution, as well as conventional immunoprophy-laxis and revaccination in keeping with the currently available guidelines for autologous transplantation.[41,42]

SUMMARY

The use of biological drugs, such as recombinant proteins, mab, and molecularly engineered cell-based therapies has raised new challenges in diagnostic immunology. The use of drugs that are either able to interact with the immune system or that depend on the interaction with immune cells for their action can trigger unpredictable immune responses. Indeed, unlike small molecule therapeutics, the interaction of biological drugs with the immune system is much stronger and often immunogenic. This immunogenicity of biologics can lead to the development of ADAs and a loss of drug efficacy, as well as other major side effects. It is thus critical to be able to monitor the impact of biologics on the immune system, as well as to understand the mechanisms underlying their antigenicity. A thorough understanding of these mechanisms could lead to better drugs with increased efficacy and tolerability.

REFERENCES

1. Kelley B. Industrialization of mAb production technology: the bioprocessing industry at a crossroads. MAbs 2009;1(5):443–52.

2. Garland SG, Smith SM, Gums JG. Erenumab: a first-in-class monoclonal antibody for migraine prevention. Ann Pharmacother 2019;53(9):933–9, 1060028019835166. [Epub ahead of print].

3. Rifkin WD. Denosumab in postmenopausal women with low bone mineral density. N Engl J Med 2006;354(22):2390–1 [author reply: 2390–1].

4. Wong ND, Rosenblit PD, Greenfield RS. Advances in dyslipidemia management for prevention of atherosclerosis: PCSK9 monoclonal antibody therapy and beyond. Cardiovasc Diagn Ther 2017;7(Suppl 1):S11–20.

5. Ayyar BV, Arora S, O'Kennedy R. Coming-of-age of antibodies in cancer therapeutics. Trends Pharmacol Sci 2016;37(12):1009–28.

6. Roberts ZJ, Better M, Bot A, et al. Axicabtagene ciloleucel, a first-in-class CAR T cell therapy for aggressive NHL. Leuk Lymphoma 2018;59(8):1785–96.

7. Wang Z, Wu Z, Liu Y, et al. New development in CAR-T cell therapy. J Hematol Oncol 2017;10(1):53.

8. Büttel IC, Chamberlain P, Chowers Y, et al. Taking immunogenicity assessment of therapeutic proteins to the next level. Biologicals 2011;39(2):100–9.
9. Suzuki M, Kato C, Kato A. Therapeutic antibodies: their mechanisms of action and the pathological findings they induce in toxicity studies. J Toxicol Pathol 2015;28(3):133–9.
10. Weiner GJ. Monoclonal antibody mechanisms of action in cancer. Immunologic research 2007;39(1–3):271–8.
11. Tovey MG, Legrand J, Lallemand C. Overcoming immunogenicity associated with the use of biopharmaceuticals. Expert Rev Clin Pharmacol 2011;4(5): 623–31.
12. Cder F. Immunogenicity testing of therapeutic protein products —developing and validating assays for anti-drug antibody detection guidance for industry. Rockville: Food and Drug Administration; 2019. p. 1–37.
13. Rup B, Pallardy M, Sikkema D, et al. Standardizing terms, definitions and concepts for describing and interpreting unwanted immunogenicity of biopharmaceuticals: recommendations of the Innovative Medicines Initiative ABIR-ISK consortium. Clin Exp Immunol 2015;181(3):385–400.
14. Medicines CFMPFHULE. Guideline on immunogenicity assessment of biotechnology-derived therapeutic proteins. London: European Medicines Agency; 2007.
15. Lichtenstein L, Ron Y, Kivity S, et al. Infliximab-related infusion reactions: systematic review. J Crohns Colitis 2015;9(9):806–15.
16. Deisenhammer F, Jank M, Lauren A, et al. Prediction of natalizumab anti-drug antibodies persistency. Mult Scler 2019;25(3):392–8.
17. Rubbert-Roth A, Finckh A. Treatment options in patients with rheumatoid arthritis failing initial TNF inhibitor therapy: a critical review. Arthritis Res Ther 2009; 11(Suppl 1):S1.
18. Ding NS, Hart A, De Cruz P. Systematic review: predicting and optimising response to anti-TNF therapy in Crohn's disease - algorithm for practical management. Aliment Pharmacol Ther 2016;43(1):30–51.
19. Kalden JR, Schulze-Koops H. Immunogenicity and loss of response to TNF inhibitors: implications for rheumatoid arthritis treatment. Nat Rev Rheumatol 2017; 13(12):707–18.
20. Casadevall N, Nataf J, Viron B, et al. Pure red-cell aplasia and antierythropoietin antibodies in patients treated with recombinant erythropoietin. N Engl J Med 2002;346(7):469–75.
21. Mannucci PM, Franchini M. Porcine recombinant factor VIII: an additional weapon to handle anti-factor VIII antibodies. Blood Transfus 2017;15(4):365–8.
22. Wadhwa M, Thorpe R. Unwanted immunogenicity: lessons learned and future challenges. Bioanalysis 2010;2(6):1073–84.
23. Hamuro L, Kijanka G, Kinderman F, et al. Perspectives on subcutaneous route of administration as an immunogenicity risk factor for therapeutic proteins. J Pharm Sci 2017;106(10):2946–54.
24. Brohem CA, Cardeal LBDS, Tiago M, et al. Artificial skin in perspective: concepts and applications. Pigment Cell Melanoma Res 2011;24(1):35–50.
25. Lahti JL, Lui BH, Beck SE, et al. Engineered epidermal growth factor mutants with faster binding on-rates correlate with enhanced receptor activation. FEBS Lett 2011;585(8):1135–9.
26. Boven K, Stryker S, Knight J, et al. The increased incidence of pure red cell aplasia with an Eprex formulation in uncoated rubber stopper syringes. Kidney Int 2005;67(6):2346–53.

27. Bitoun S, Nocturne G, Ly B, et al. Methotrexate and BAFF interaction prevents immunization against TNF inhibitors. Ann Rheum Dis 2018;77(10):1463–70.

28. Cronstein BN. Methotrexate BAFFles anti-drug antibodies. Nat Rev Rheumatol 2018;14(9):505–6.

29. Stacy S, Williams EL, Standifer NE, et al. Maintenance of immune tolerance to a neo-self acetylcholine receptor antigen with aging: implications for late-onset autoimmunity. J Immunol 2010;184(11):6067–75.

30. Bartelds GM, Wijbrandts CA, Nurmohamed MT, et al. Anti-adalimumab antibodies in rheumatoid arthritis patients are associated with interleukin-10 gene polymorphisms. Arthritis Rheum 2009;60(8):2541–2.

31. Camacho LH. CTLA-4 blockade with ipilimumab: biology, safety, efficacy, and future considerations. Cancer Med 2015;4(5):661–72.

32. Maxwell L, Singh JA. Abatacept for rheumatoid arthritis. Cochrane Database Syst Rev 2009;(4):CD007277.

33. Wu B, Chung S, Jiang X-R, et al. Strategies to determine assay format for the assessment of neutralizing antibody responses to biotherapeutics. AAPS J 2016;18(6):1335–50.

34. Lallemand C, Kavrochorianou N, Steenholdt C, et al. Reporter gene assay for the quantification of the activity and neutralizing antibody response to TNFα antagonists. J Immunol Methods 2011;373(1–2):229–39.

35. Thong BY, Mirakian R, Castells M, et al. A world allergy organization international survey on diagnostic procedures and therapies in drug allergy/hypersensitivity. World Allergy Organ J 2011;4(12):257–70.

36. Uzzaman A, Cho SH. Chapter 28: classification of hypersensitivity reactions. Allergy Asthma Proc 2012;33(Suppl 1):96–9.

37. Madden DL. From a patient advocate's perspective: does cancer immunotherapy represent a paradigm shift? Curr Oncol Rep 2018;20(1):8.

38. Forsberg MH, Das A, Saha K, et al. The potential of CAR T therapy for relapsed or refractory pediatric and young adult B-cell ALL. Ther Clin Risk Manag 2018;14:1573–84.

39. Shimabukuro-Vornhagen A, Gödel P, Subklewe M, et al. Cytokine release syndrome. J Immunother Cancer 2018;6(1):56.

40. Teachey DT, Lacey SF, Shaw PA, et al. Identification of predictive biomarkers for cytokine release syndrome after chimeric antigen receptor T-cell therapy for acute lymphoblastic leukemia. Cancer Discov 2016;6(6):664–79.

41. Ogba N, Arwood NM, Bartlett NL, et al. Chimeric antigen receptor T-cell therapy. J Natl Compr Canc Netw 2018;16(9):1092–106.

42. Palazzo M, Shah GL, Copelan O, et al. Revaccination after autologous hematopoietic stem cell transplantation is safe and effective in patients with multiple myeloma receiving lenalidomide maintenance. Biol Blood Marrow Transplant 2018;24(4):871–6.

Testing Immune-Related Adverse Events in Cancer Immunotherapy

Jocelyn R. Farmer, MD, PhD[a,b,]*

KEYWORDS

- Immune checkpoint inhibitor ● Immune-related adverse event ● CTLA-4 ● LRBA

KEY POINTS

- Immune checkpoint inhibitors are promising new therapeutics in advanced-stage cancers, which target signal 2 in T-cell activation (eg, anti-CTLA-4 and anti-PD-1/PD-L1).
- Immune checkpoint inhibitors can adversely cause severe autoimmune and hyperinflammatory diseases, known as immune-related adverse events (irAEs).
- Currently, there are no clinically available biomarkers to aid in the acute diagnosis of irAEs, and limited data to guide treatment selection for severe (grade ≥3) life-threatening toxicities.
- Patients with congenital T-cell hyperactivation syndromes, such as CTLA-4 deficiency may critically inform our ability to diagnosis and treat irAEs to checkpoint inhibitors.

INTRODUCTION

The promise of immune-targeted therapeutics in cancer has been fulfilled. Starting with the US Food and Drug Administration (FDA) approval of ipilimumab for the treatment of metastatic melanoma in 2011, immune "checkpoint inhibition" provides a rare promise for prolonged disease-free patient survival in severe and otherwise treatment-refractory forms of cancer. However, growing clinical use of checkpoint inhibitors has coincided with the observation of immune-related adverse events (irAEs). irAEs are caused by a break in host self-tolerance and can include both autoantibody production and prominent autoinflammatory lymphocytic trafficking to end-organs, both of which can be deadly in their most severe forms. Moreover, acute management of irAEs is often complicated by difficulty making a prompt clinical diagnosis given the concomitant risk for severe infectious and malignant complications in these patients.

Disclosure: This work was supported by the National Institutes of Health (T32-HL116275 to J.R.F.).
[a] Division of Rheumatology, Allergy and Immunology, Massachusetts General Hospital, COX 201, MGH, 55 Fruit Street, Boston, MA 02114, USA; [b] Ragon Institute of MGH, MIT and Harvard, Cambridge, MA, USA
* Division of Rheumatology, Allergy and Immunology, Massachusetts General Hospital, COX 201, MGH, 55 Fruit Street, Boston, MA 02114.
E-mail address: jrfarmer@partners.org

The overarching goal is to maximize anticancer benefit while minimizing irAE risk. However, we currently lack the clinical diagnostic tools with which to assess for pre-treatment irAE risk and facilitate acute irAE diagnosis. This article discusses our current immunologic understanding of irAEs, in addition to how patients with rare primary immune deficiencies, specifically patients with congenital cytotoxic T lymphocyte antigen-4 (CTLA-4) deficiency, can inform this understanding. In conclusion, the prospects of improving diagnostics for, and treatment of, checkpoint inhibitor-mediated irAEs, are discussed.

WHAT ARE IMMUNE CHECKPOINTS?

The activation of a T cell by an antigen-presenting cell occurs in the periphery through 3 major signals. Signal 1 is the activation of the T-cell receptor via recognition of its cognate peptide antigen as presented in the context of a major histocompatibility complex molecule. Signal 2 is co-stimulatory activation, classically through the binding of CD28 on the T-cell surface to CD80/86 on the antigen-presenting cell surface. Signal 3 is the cytokine milieu that dictates downstream T lineage differentiation. The co-stimulatory molecules that regulate signal 2 in T-cell activation are upregulated in the context of inflammation, including signaling downstream of innate immune receptors. Thus, signal 2 informs the T cell that the recognized antigen is being presented in the context of host inflammation and appropriately augments T-cell activation. To keep co-stimulation in check and protect against hyperinflammatory disease, the mammalian immune system has evolved mechanisms to inhibit signal 2 in T-cell activation that include the regulated expression of CTLA-4 and PD-1/PD-L1.

Cytotoxic T Lymphocyte Antigen-4

CTLA-4 is a homolog of CD28 that is expressed on the cell surface of activated and regulatory T cells. CTLA-4 functions as a negative T-cell regulator by specifically competing for and depleting CD80/86 on the surface of antigen-presenting cells, which in turn results in less co-stimulatory T-cell activation. The role of CTLA-4 in negatively regulating T-cell activation and maintaining T-cell tolerance in the periphery was first elucidated through genetically engineered mice. Germline knockout of CTLA-4 resulted in a dramatic phenotype of diffuse T-cell infiltration to and destruction of end-organs, resulting in lethality as early as 3 to 4 weeks of age.[1,2] A milder phenotype, albeit still lethal, was observed in the regulatory (FoxP3+) T cell-specific CTLA-4 knockout mouse.[3] Finally, the autoinflammatory phenotype was recapitulated on transfer of splenic T cells from CTLA-4 knockout mice to wild-type T-cell-depleted recipient animals.[4] Together, these data elucidated a critical role for CTLA-4 in maintaining T-cell host tolerance in the periphery.

Programmed Cell Death Protein 1/Programmed Cell Death-Ligand 1

The programmed cell death protein 1 (PD-1) receptor is induced in lymphocytes and monocytes following activation. The role of PD-1 in maintaining peripheral T-cell tolerance was similarly first elucidated through knockout studies in mice, whereby germline deletion of PD-1 led to a lupus-like phenotype with augmented T-cell proliferation.[5] Subsequently, the ligand for PD-1 (PD-L1) was identified. A member of the CD80 gene family, engagement of PD-L1 by its cognate PD-1 receptor was shown to negatively regulate T-cell receptor-mediated lymphoproliferation and cytokine secretion. The further demonstration that PD-L1 was expressed on end-organ tissues (eg, heart and lung) provided a potential mechanism for end-organ-specific control of T-cell autoreactivity in the periphery.[6]

HOW DOES CHECKPOINT INHIBITOR THERAPY WORK IN CANCER?
Targeting Cytotoxic T Lymphocyte Antigen-4

Based on the knockout mouse models, researchers theorized that CTLA-4 blockade could be used to augment T-cell effector numbers and function in the periphery, culminating in an antitumor benefit. CTLA-4 blockade was first trialed in murine cancer models and was observed to increase tumor-free survival in a subset of cancer types and combination regimens.[7] Specifically, CTLA-4 blockade was trialed as monotherapy as well as in combination with vaccines, chemotherapy, and radiation therapy as mechanisms to enhance tumor-specific antigen presentation. Based on the success of these murine studies, 2 human monoclonal antibodies targeting CTLA-4, ipilimumab and tremelimumab, were subsequently developed. Ipilimumab became the first FDA-approved CTLA-4 targeting biologic following a phase III study in metastatic melanoma, demonstrating that monotherapy could improve overall patient survival.[8] Both biologics are now FDA-approved for the treatment of advanced melanoma, and ipilimumab is also approved as a combination agent for a broad spectrum of malignancies (**Table 1**).

Targeting Programmed Cell Death Protein 1/Programmed Cell Death-Ligand 1

Insight that targeting PD-1/PD-L1 might be beneficial in cancer was initially driven by observational and *in vitro* studies. Specifically, PD-L1 was found to be significantly upregulated in tumors compared with normal host tissues.[9] Moreover, cancer cells transgenically overexpressing PD-L1 were rendered less susceptible to T cell receptor-mediated lysis by cytotoxic T cells *in vitro*.[10] These data led to the first phase I studies of humanized monoclonal antibodies targeting PD-1 and PD-L1 in advanced solid tumors,[11,12] and, subsequently, the first FDA-approved biologic, pembrolizumab, for the treatment of advanced-stage melanoma in 2014.[13,14] Currently, there are numerous PD-1 and PD-L1 inhibitors approved for use in cancer as monotherapy and also in combination with CTLA-4 blockade (see **Table 1**).

Table 1			
Approved immune checkpoint inhibitors in cancer			
Target	**Drug**	**FDA Approval**	**Indication**
CTLA-4	Ipilimumab	2011	Melanoma
CTLA-4	Tremelimumab	2015	Melanoma
PD-1	Nivolumab	2014	Melanoma, renal cell carcinoma, Hodgkin's lymphoma, squamous cell carcinoma, non-small cell lung cancer, ovarian cancer
PD-1	Pembrolizumab	2014	Melanoma, Merkel cell carcinoma, non-small cell lung cancer, progressive metastatic colorectal cancer
PD-1	Cemiplimab	2018	Squamous cell carcinoma
PD-L1	Atezolizumab	2016	Non-small-cell lung cancer, urothelial carcinoma
PD-L1	Durvalumab	2018	Non-small-cell lung cancer, urothelial carcinoma
PD-L1	Avelumab	2017	Merkel cell carcinoma, renal cell carcinoma, urothelial carcinoma
CTLA-4/PD-1	Ipilimumab/nivolumab	2018	Renal cell cancer, colorectal cancer

WHAT ARE THE IMMUNE-RELATED ADVERSE EVENTS TO CHECKPOINT INHIBITORS?

An irAE is the development of host autoinflammatory disease subsequent to the administration of an immune checkpoint inhibitor. irAEs may occur as early as days (eg, dermatitis) or as late as moths (eg, pneumonitis) following drug administration. A wide range of systemic and end-organ-specific complications have been described, including entities of autoantibody-predominant disease (eg, autoimmune cytopenias, vasculitis, and myasthenia gravis) as well as diseases predominated by lymphocytes trafficking to end-organs (eg, dermatitis, colitis, hepatitis, nephritis, arthritis, pneumonitis, and myocarditis, as well as a spectrum of neuropathies and endocrinopathies).[15] However, the role of autoantibodies and autoreactive immune cells in directly mediating host autoinflammatory disease pathogenesis in the context of checkpoint inhibitor therapy is currently unknown and an area of active research investigation.

irAE severity is graded 1 to 4, with grade 1 being subclinical or mild disease and grade 4 being acutely life-threatening.[16] The occurrence of irAEs does not seem to be fundamentally influenced by cancer type. An exception is the observation of dermatitis and vitiligo, specifically, following checkpoint inhibitor therapy in patients with underlying melanoma. The onset of vitiligo in this clinical context has been considered a cross-reactive yet still tumor-directed immune response, consistent with the observation that vitiligo significantly associates with improved melanoma outcomes.[17,18] In contrast, irAE risk correlates strongly with checkpoint inhibitor drug target. irAEs occur more commonly following CTLA-4 blockade (60%–85%) than PD-1 blockade (16%–37%) than PD-L1 blockade (12%–24%).[19] The use of dual inhibitor therapy, most often in advanced-stage melanoma, may exacerbate this risk even further.[19] Finally, some irAEs do demonstrate checkpoint inhibitor drug target specificity. For example, colitis and hypophysitis are more prevalent following CTLA-4 blockade, whereas pneumonitis and thyroiditis are more prevalent following anti-PD-1/PD-L1 therapy.[15]

HOW DO WE DIAGNOSE IMMUNE-RELATED ADVERSE EVENTS TO CHECKPOINT INHIBITORS?

The difficulty in irAE diagnosis stems from the broad range of clinical presentations that can occur following checkpoint inhibitor therapy (eg, skin manifestations ranging from dermatitis to bullous disease[20]) and the concomitant risk for severe infectious and malignant complications. Most often, irAEs are diagnosed by the clinical demonstration of end-organ disease (eg, transaminitis in the case of hepatitis) in the absence of confounding infectious causes or metastatic tumor involvement. Biopsy can be extremely helpful. In the case of irAEs, a dense lymphocytic infiltrate often predominates.[21] However, biopsy is not always feasible (eg, diagnosis of myocarditis in a clinically unstable patient) and is often limited by the patchy nature of the lymphocytic involvement adjacent to normal (early in toxicity) or necrotic (late in toxicity) host tissues.[22] At present, there are no clinically available biomarkers to further facilitate irAE diagnosis.

HOW DO WE TREAT IMMUNE-RELATED ADVERSE EVENTS TO CHECKPOINT INHIBITORS?

There are limited consensus guidelines available that inform the management of irAEs to checkpoint inhibitor therapy. In the case of low-grade toxicities, checkpoint inhibitor continuation or brief hiatus followed by re-challenge may be considered. In some instances, discontinuation alone may suffice to address the toxicity. In contrast, grade ≥2 toxicities generally warrant management with an immune-suppressive strategy. Steroids are frequently first-line therapy, with a range of dosing used (eg, methylprednisolone 0.5–4 mg/kg daily for grade 1–4 pneumonitis).[23] Steroid therapy is typically prolonged, with most practitioners tapering over several weeks.[23] Whereas steroids have shown benefit over a wide spectrum of irAEs, risks include prominent and broad immune suppression predisposing to infection, as well as the potential risk of blunting the anticancer immune response.[19] More targeted immune suppression has also been tried, most often as a second-line approach, with agent selection largely guided by end-organ-specific disease correlates. For example, tumor necrosis factor-alpha (TNF-α) inhibitors, which have known benefit in the management of inflammatory bowel disease, have been efficacious in the management of checkpoint inhibitor colitis.[24] In contrast, other irAEs have less standardized second-line treatment approaches, including checkpoint inhibitor pneumonitis and myocarditis, which can quickly deteriorate into life-threatening disease. Furthermore, multiple irAEs may co-occur in a single patient,[25,26] limiting the applicability of an end-organ-centric treatment approach. Thus, the need for a more mechanism-based understanding of checkpoint inhibitor toxicity to inform precision immune suppression that limits irAEs while maintaining antitumor benefit is greatly needed in the field.

WHAT CAN WE LEARN FROM PATIENTS WITH CONGENITAL LOSS OF CHECKPOINT INHIBITION?

Genetic polymorphisms in *CTLA4*, including coding and noncoding region variants, have been shown to correlate with increased risk for autoimmune disease in humans.[27–30] A further breakthrough occurred in 2014 with the description of CTLA-4 haploinsufficiency in humans as an autosomal dominant condition of primary immune dysregulation.[31,32] Specifically, patients with heterozygous loss-of-function *CTLA4* mutations demonstrate enhanced T-cell activation in the periphery with a marked shift away from naive T cells toward T effector memory cells in circulation. They also have marked pathologic lymphocyte trafficking to end-organs, which can include the lungs, liver, gastrointestinal lumen, kidneys, joints, endocrine organs, bone marrow, and brain.[33,34] Finally, these patients develop prominent autoantibody-mediated diseases, including a predominance of autoimmune cytopenias.[33,34] In 2015, an additional human condition of functional CTLA-4 deficiency was described in patients with autosomal recessive inheritance of LRBA deficiency, which results in aberrant and enhanced CTLA-4 trafficking and turnover.[35] Patients with congenital LRBA deficiency demonstrate a similar spectrum of T-cell hyperactivation in the peripheral blood as well as pathologic T-cell infiltrative disease in end-organs and enhanced susceptibility to autoantibody diseases.[36]

Although CTLA-4 and LRBA deficiencies are by definition rare primary immune disorders, these patients may have critical lessons to teach us about the pathogenesis of immune checkpoint toxicity.[37] First, the clinical spectra of disease are highly overlapping. Multiorgan lymphocyte-predominant inflammation can occur in both conditions, with a majority of T cells and B cells noted on histopathology.[31,38] Following CTLA-4 blockade, CD4+ T-cell infiltrates are particularly prominent.[39] The spectrum of affected organs is also similar and may include the skin, lungs, gastrointestinal lumen, liver, joints, hematologic, endocrine, and nervous systems. Rare exceptions include hypophysitis, which is best described following anti-CTLA-4 therapy and potentially mediated by high CTLA-4 expression mediating direct T-cell targeting of the pituitary gland in a subset of patients.[40] Congenital and iatrogenic loss of CTLA-4 also drives a largely convergent peripheral immune phenotype, characterized by decreased naive T cells and increased effector T cells in circulation. In patients with congenital CTLA-4 deficiency, further detailed immunophenotyping has elucidated aberrant B-cell maturation to the class-switched memory stage, defective humoral immunity (with a spectrum of selective antibody deficiency to overt hypogammaglobulinemia described), and an expansion of autoreactive CD21[lo] B cells in circulation.[32] More recently, a CD21[lo] B-cell expansion was similarly observed in patients with melanoma who received checkpoint inhibitor blockade (anti-CTLA-4, anti-PD-1, or combination therapy), detectable as early as the first cycle of therapy.[41] Moreover, ≥2-fold expansion in CD21[lo] B cells or plasmablasts in conjunction with B-cell lymphopenia was shown to predict the onset of grade ≥3 irAEs by a median of 3 weeks.[41] These data suggest that lessons learned from rare patients with congenital loss of CTLA-4 expression and/or function may critically inform our ability to understand and diagnose checkpoint inhibitor toxicity.

HOW MIGHT WE BE ABLE TO BETTER DIAGNOSE IMMUNE-RELATED ADVERSE EVENTS TO CHECKPOINT INHIBITORS?

At present, biomarker research has focused predominantly on predicting the subset of patients with cancer who will receive the most antitumor benefit from immune checkpoint inhibitor therapy.[42,43] Just as critical, however, will be early prediction and/or detection of the subset of patients with cancer who are at greatest risk for toxicity from immune checkpoint inhibition.

Genetics

Genetics play a significant role in determining host risk for autoimmune disease pathogenesis, underscored by the discovery, now 60 years previously, that distinct human leukocyte antigen (HLA) alleles, which encode for the major histocompatibility complex class I and II molecules involved in T-cell receptor antigen presentation, associated with risk for autoimmune disease pathogenesis in humans.[44] Not surprisingly, distinct HLA genotypes have more recently been associated both with antitumor benefit[45] and irAE risk[46] in patients receiving checkpoint inhibitor therapy. Moreover, HLA genotype specificity for end-organ disease has been shown, for example, carriers of HLA-DQB1*03:01 who are predisposed to checkpoint inhibitor colitis.[46] Beyond genetic variants that control signal 1 in T-cell activation, many more may ultimately control overall irAE risk. For example, increased rates of malignancy have been described in patients with congenital signal 2 hyperactivation, including CTLA-4 deficiency,[47] and a retrospective diagnosis of CTLA-4 haploinsufficiency was recently described in a patient receiving anti-CD25 therapy who developed wide-spread lymphoproliferative complications from the additional iatrogenic checkpoint inhibition.[48] These data suggest that we must consider the broad potential for genetic influences on T-cell activation, including coding gene variants (eg, HLA[46] and CTLA4[48]), noncoding gene variants (eg, CTLA4 3' UTR[30]), gene modifiers (eg, LRBA[35]), and epigenetic changes,[49] as potential contributors to irAE risk in the context of immune checkpoint inhibitor therapy. Finally, as there are limited data available looking at immune checkpoint inhibitor safety profiling in patients with preexisting autoimmunity,[50] prospective longitudinal studies are warranted to address more accurately irAE risk in this patient demographic moving forward. In patients with known personal and/or family history of autoimmunity, precision genotyping may prove to be a critical diagnostic tool for more accurately defining pretreatment irAE risk.

Immune Cell Profiling

There is currently great momentum toward identifying a unique immune cell phenotype in the peripheral blood that may aid in the prediction or acute diagnosis of checkpoint inhibitor-mediated irAEs. At baseline and acutely (1 month) postcheckpoint inhibitor therapy, higher absolute counts of lymphocytes (>2000 cells/μL) and eosinophils in circulation were associated with increased rates of grade $\geq$2 irAEs in patients with solid tumor receiving anti-PD-1 therapy.[51] In contrast, leukocytosis with a decreased relative lymphocyte count was shown to coincide with the onset of severe (grade $\geq$3) lung and gastrointestinal irAEs in patients with melanoma receiving anti-PD-1 therapy.[52] These latter data suggest a relative depletion of lymphocytes from the circulating pool coincident with irAE onset, potentially mediated by robust lymphocyte trafficking out of the blood and into end-organs. Finally, given the use of detailed B-cell and T-cell immunophenotyping previously demonstrated in congenital T-cell hyperactivation syndromes,[31–34] advanced lymphocyte profiling by surface marker levels and functional status are likely to benefit checkpoint inhibitor irAE diagnostics moving forward. Recently, a $\geq$2-fold expansion of either CD21^{lo} B cells or plasmablasts in conjunction with B-cell lymphopenia was demonstrated to predict the onset of grade $\geq$3 irAEs by a median of 3 weeks in patients with melanoma treated with anti-CTLA-4, anti-PD-1, or combination therapy.[41] Whether detailed T-cell immunophenotyping can further refine this diagnostic model is yet to be seen.

Cytokines/Chemokines

Cytokines and chemokines, as regulators of T-cell differentiation, activation, and trafficking, have been profiled in checkpoint inhibitor-treated patients with cancer. At present, much attention has centered on Th17 cell signaling. Interleukin-6 (IL-6), an inducer of Th17 and T follicular helper cell differentiation, was found to be increased posttreatment in patients who developed psoriasiform dermatitis following PD-1 inhibition using nivolumab.[53] IL-17, the major unique cytokine product of Th17 cells, was found to be increased at baseline in patients with melanoma treated with neoadjuvant ipilimumab who progressed to grade 3 checkpoint inhibitor-associated diarrhea and/or colitis.[54] Finally, sCD163 and CXCL5, markers of macrophage activation both upstream and downstream of Th17 cell differentiation and activation, were examined in patients with advanced-stage melanoma treated with the PD-1 inhibitor, nivolumab.[55] Higher absolute change rate of sCD163 at baseline compared with day 42 of treatment correlated with overall irAE risk. Together, these data suggest that Th17 skewing in association with increased macrophage activation may contribute to irAE pathogenesis. For checkpoint colitis, these data are consistent with the observation of Th1 and Th17 signaling profiles (interferon-γ [IFN-γ] and IL-17A messenger RNA, respectively) in gut lamina propria from patients with melanoma who developed ipilimumab-associated toxicity.[56] Whereas increased circulating IL-17 levels are also described in patients with inflammatory bowel disease,[57] a direct role for Th17 cells in the pathogenesis of checkpoint inhibitor colitis and/or the efficacy of Th17 cell targeting have yet to be demonstrated.

Autoantibodies

As the question of checkpoint inhibitor safety has arisen in patients with preexisting autoimmunity,[50] researchers also have screened pretreatment for the presence of autoantibodies. These data demonstrate some utility in predicting end-organ-specific toxicities, for example, baseline antithyroid and anti-islet cell autoantibodies correlating with posttreatment autoimmune thyroiditis[58,59] and type I diabetes,[60] respectively. However, in patients with advanced non-small cell lung cancer receiving anti-PD-1 monotherapy, baseline presence of circulating rheumatoid factor, antinuclear antibodies, antithyroglobulin antibodies, or antithyroid peroxidase antibodies was recently shown to correlate with both irAE risk and progression-free cancer survival.[58] These data suggest that pretreatment screening for the presence of autoantibodies is likely insufficient in isolation to diagnostically uncouple irAE risk from antitumor benefit, consistent with the finding that irAE occurrence in non-small cell lung cancer, specifically, correlates positively with progression-free patient survival.[61] However, unique autoantibodies may still have diagnostic use in this regard, for example, circulating rheumatoid factor was identified in 39% of all patients with advanced non-small cell lung cancer who developed irAEs.[58] Finally, the positive correlation between irAE occurrence and anti-PD-1 therapy response, as measured by overall response rate and time to next therapy or death, was shown to be limited to low-grade irAEs.[62] Therefore, the overarching goal is really to identify predictive biomarkers specific for the subset of patients who will progress to severe and life-threatening check point inhibitor toxicities.

Repertoire

The antitumor benefit derived from immune checkpoint inhibitor therapy has been shown to coincide with unique T-cell receptor repertoire parameters, including increased baseline diversity[63] as well as early diversification posttherapy.[64] In addition, broadening of the T-cell receptor repertoire as early as 2 weeks following anti-CTLA-4 therapy has been shown to predict the onset of irAEs.[64] Thus, whether T-cell repertoire alone can uncouple antitumor benefit from irAE risk remains unclear. To this end, a case series of significantly overlapping T-cell receptor clonotypes in tumor versus irAE lung tissue was recently presented.[65] The additional potential utility of B-cell receptor repertoire profiling is yet unknown. Finally, combination approaches that examine T-cell receptor sequences as well as antigen specificity in conjunction with overall T-cell phenotype and functional status may be warranted.[66]

Environmental Factors

There is growing evidence that environmental factors, such as acute infections and composition of the host commensal microbiota play important roles in global immune system function, including anticancer surveillance.[67] In patients with primary immune deficiency, onset of autoimmunity has been described in close temporal association (days to weeks) following live viral vaccinations and/or naturally acquired infections.[68] Whether acute and/or chronically active infections may precipitate the onset of irAEs in the context of checkpoint inhibitor therapy remains unclear. In addition, host gut microbiota have been analyzed, most prominently in the clinical context of ipilimumab-induced colitis.[69] An increase in baseline gut *Bacteroidetes* species was found to associate with decreased rates of colitis in 2 consecutive studies[70,71]; and, an increase in baseline gut *Firmicutes* species was found to associate with decreased rates of colitis in the latter study.[71] A mechanism of new-onset commensal pathogenicity driving enhanced immune activation has been proposed[19]; however, we currently lack a definitive understanding as to how alterations in host microbiota may directly mediate or not host autoinflammatory disease pathogenesis in the context of checkpoint inhibitor therapy.

HOW MIGHT WE BE ABLE TO BETTER TREAT IMMUNE-RELATED ADVERSE EVENTS TO CHECKPOINT INHIBITORS?

Steroids are proving effective in the management of low-grade irAEs, yet high-dose and prolonged steroid use in this patient demographic risks both secondary infections and loss of antitumor benefit from the broad immune suppression.[19] Moreover, a standardized second-line treatment approach across irAEs is lacking in the field, with particularly limited data available for the management of steroid-refractory grade ≥3 toxicities.[23]

Currently, clinicians are using end-organ disease mimetics (eg, inflammatory bowel disease in the case of checkpoint inhibitor colitis) to guide therapeutic intervention. Could we glean additional insights from patients who mirror the pathophysiology of these iatrogenic toxicities in terms of systemic T-cell hyperactivation? In a retrospective cohort of 22 CTLA-4-deficient patients with autoimmune cytopenias managed at the National Institutes of Health (NIH), CTLA-4-Ig replacement therapy (abatacept) was tried in 10 patients, given at a dose of 500 to 750 mg intravenously twice monthly.[72] Either complete or partial response, as measured by stabilization of cytopenias and/or improvement in end-organ lymphoproliferative disease (gastrointestinal or brain), was observed in all abatacept-treated participants. Furthermore, no significant adverse complications were appreciated over the retrospective follow-up period of 17 patient-years, including infusion reactions, infections, or malignancies. Clinical benefits of abatacept therapy, as measured by reduced rates of lymphoproliferation, immune dysregulation, and chronic diarrhea, specifically, also have been demonstrated in patients with LRBA deficiency.[35,73] Beyond CTLA-4-Ig, mammalian target of rapamycin inhibitors that block T-cell activation directly downstream of T-cell receptor recognition and co-stimulatory CD28 activation (eg, sirolimus and everolimus) have been tried in CTLA-4 deficiency for the primary indication of autoimmune cytopenias.[72] The benefit of sirolimus for the management of severe autoimmune enteropathy in a patient with LRBA deficiency over a 33-month follow-up period has also been described.[74] This patient was requiring total parenteral nutrition, was refractory to attempts at management using steroids and tacrolimus, on which therapy the patient developed hepatitis, and sirolimus intervention was observed to improve the clinical course of autoimmune enteropathy as well as ameliorate excess Th17 signaling (IL-17 production from CD4+ T cells) in this case.

Despite the growing evidence that targeting signal 2 in T-cell activation for congenital syndromes of CTLA-4 deficiency is effective in the management of autoinflammatory disease, it is yet to be determined whether this therapeutic approach will be effective and/or safe in patients with checkpoint inhibitor toxicity. Recently, single case reports of efficacy were documented for alemtuzumab, an anti-CD52 monoclonal antibody that targets mature lymphocytes, and abatacept, at a dose of 500 mg intravenously every 2 weeks for a total of 5 doses, in steroid-refractory cases of severe checkpoint inhibitor-mediated myocarditis.[75,76] A case report of abatacept efficacy also has been described in the clinical context of a myasthenia gravis flare after 2 doses of pembrolizumab, which necessitated noninvasive positive pressure ventilation support for diaphragmatic weakness.[77] The patient was unresponsive to plasma exchange, mycophenolate mofetil (at a dose of 500 mg twice daily), methylprednisolone (1 g daily), intravenous immunoglobulin (2 g/kg of body weight daily), and 4 weekly doses of rituximab (375 mg/m^2 of body surface area). The patient received abatacept (1 g every 2 weeks for a total of 2 doses) with subsequent wean from ventilator support at day 7 posttreatment, hospital discharge at day 21, and absence of muscle weakness at the 3-month follow-up. Together, these data suggest that targeting signal 2 in T-cell activation may be efficacious, including for antibody-predominant immune checkpoint toxicities. However, larger case series and, ideally, prospective studies that address infection risk and cancer-free survival, specifically, are warranted.

Beyond targeting signal 2 in T-cell activation, targeting cytokines such as TNF-α and, more recently, IL-6 using tocilizumab, a humanized monoclonal antibody against the IL-6 receptor, have shown benefit in the management of steroid-refractory checkpoint colitis,[24] and severe grade 3 to 4 checkpoint inhibitor toxicities,[78] respectively. TNF-α and IL-6 are pleiotropic cytokines with broad influences on innate and adaptive immune signaling; however, both convergently influence T-cell activation. Specifically, tocilizumab therapy has been shown to restore Th17 to T regulatory cell imbalances in patients with rheumatoid arthritis.[79,80] In addition, TNF-α inhibitors can modulate the production and activation of Th1, Th17, and T regulatory cells in patients with psoriasis.[81] The use of TNF-α inhibitors may be limited to gastrointestinal toxicities and there is the potential for paradoxic adverse events (eg, flares of psoriasis, inflammatory bowel disease, lung granulomas, and uveitis).[82,83] Here again, prospective studies addressing infection risk and cancer-free survival will be warranted, especially because a role for TNF-α in antitumor immunity has been described.[84] Conversely, anti-IL-6 therapy has shown use across a broad spectrum of irAEs, including pneumonitis, colitis, hepatitis, and even systemic inflammatory response syndrome.[78] Furthermore, IL-6 may suppress antitumor immunity,[85,86] making it a particularly attractive drug target in patients with advanced-stage malignancies. Finally, anti-IL-17, anti-IL-1, and/or anti-IL-12/23 have known use in the management of autoinflammatory diseases in humans, but with limited direct application to the management of checkpoint toxicities to date.[82]

Beyond intervening at the level of T-cell activation, attempts at stopping downstream T-cell trafficking to end-organs has shown efficacy the management of irAEs. Treatment with vedolizumab, an anti-integrin α4/β7 monoclonal antibody that predominantly blocks T-cell trafficking to the gastrointestinal lumen, recently achieved sustained clinical remission in 24 of 28 (86%) of patients retrospectively reviewed in a multicenter study as having steroid- and/or infliximab-refractory checkpoint inhibitor colitis with a favorable safety profile.[87] Finally, given the potential impact of microbiome on checkpoint inhibitor-mediated colitis, treatment with fecal transplant has been tried with the goal of reducing secondary immune recruitment to the tissue, with some demonstration of efficacy in otherwise treatment-refractory disease.[88] Although larger prospective studies are warranted, these approaches have the potential to maximize antitumor benefit by limiting irAE intervention to the affected end-organ.

CONCLUDING REMARKS

As discoveries in the area of checkpoint inhibitor toxicity will undoubtedly rely on a cross-discipline understanding of tumor biology, immunology—with a focus on mechanisms governing host T-cell tolerance—and end-organ-specific disease pathophysiology, this field can only advance in a significant way from cross-disciplinary clinical and research endeavors. The overarching goal is to develop superior diagnostic tools that will facilitate predictive modeling and early diagnostic screening of irAEs with the far-reaching potential benefit of improving the safety profile of immune checkpoint inhibitor therapy in cancer.

REFERENCES

1. Tivol EA, Borriello F, Schweitzer AN, et al. Loss of CTLA-4 leads to massive lymphoproliferation and fatal multiorgan tissue destruction, revealing a critical negative regulatory role of CTLA-4. Immunity 1995;3(5):541–7.
2. Waterhouse P, Penninger JM, Timms E, et al. Lymphoproliferative disorders with early lethality in mice deficient in CTLA-4. Science 1995;270(5238):985–8.
3. Wing K, Onishi Y, Prieto-Martin P, et al. CTLA-4 control over Foxp3+ regulatory T cell function. Science 2008;322(5899):271–5.
4. Klocke K, Sakaguchi S, Holmdahl R, et al. Induction of autoimmune disease by deletion of CTLA-4 in mice in adulthood. Proc Natl Acad Sci U S A 2016; 113(17):E2383–92.
5. Nishimura H, Nose M, Hiai H, et al. Development of lupus-like autoimmune diseases by disruption of the PD-1 gene encoding an ITIM motif-carrying immunoreceptor. Immunity 1999;11(2):141–51.
6. Freeman GJ, Long AJ, Iwai Y, et al. Engagement of the PD-1 immunoinhibitory receptor by a novel B7 family member leads to negative regulation of lymphocyte activation. J Exp Med 2000;192(7):1027–34.
7. Grosso JF, Jure-Kunkel MN. CTLA-4 blockade in tumor models: an overview of preclinical and translational research. Cancer Immun 2013;13:5.
8. Hodi FS, O'Day SJ, McDermott DF, et al. Improved survival with ipilimumab in patients with metastatic melanoma. N Engl J Med 2010;363(8):711–23.
9. Dong H, Strome SE, Salomao DR, et al. Tumor-associated B7-H1 promotes T-cell apoptosis: a potential mechanism of immune evasion. Nat Med 2002;8(8): 793–800.
10. Iwai Y, Ishida M, Tanaka Y, et al. Involvement of PD-L1 on tumor cells in the escape from host immune system and tumor immunotherapy by PD-L1 blockade. Proc Natl Acad Sci U S A 2002;99(19):12293–7.
11. Patnaik A, Kang SP, Rasco D, et al. Phase I study of pembrolizumab (MK-3475; anti-PD-1 monoclonal antibody) in patients with advanced solid tumors. Clin Cancer Res 2015;21(19):4286–93.
12. Brahmer JR, Tykodi SS, Chow LQ, et al. Safety and activity of anti-PD-L1 antibody in patients with advanced cancer. N Engl J Med 2012;366(26):2455–65.
13. Robert C, Ribas A, Wolchok JD, et al. Anti-programmed-death-receptor-1 treatment with pembrolizumab in ipilimumab-refractory advanced melanoma: a randomised dose-comparison cohort of a phase 1 trial. Lancet 2014;384(9948): 1109–17.
14. Hamid O, Robert C, Daud A, et al. Safety and tumor responses with lambrolizumab (anti-PD-1) in melanoma. N Engl J Med 2013;369(2):134–44.
15. Postow MA, Sidlow R, Hellmann MD. Immune-related adverse events associated with immune checkpoint blockade. N Engl J Med 2018;378(2):158–68.
16. Myers G. Immune-related adverse events of immune checkpoint inhibitors: a brief review. Curr Oncol 2018;25(5):342–7.
17. Hua C, Boussemart L, Mateus C, et al. Association of vitiligo with tumor response in patients with metastatic melanoma treated with pembrolizumab. JAMA Dermatol 2016;152(1):45–51.
18. Teulings HE, Limpens J, Jansen SN, et al. Vitiligo-like depigmentation in patients with stage III-IV melanoma receiving immunotherapy and its association with survival: a systematic review and meta-analysis. J Clin Oncol 2015;33(7):773–81.
19. Pauken KE, Dougan M, Rose NR, et al. Adverse events following cancer immunotherapy: obstacles and opportunities. Trends Immunol 2019;40(6):511–23.

20. Plachouri KM, Vryzaki E, Georgiou S. Cutaneous adverse events of immune checkpoint inhibitors: a summarized overview. Curr Drug Saf 2019;14(1):14–20.

21. Johncilla M, Misdraji J, Pratt DS, et al. Ipilimumab-associated hepatitis: clinico-pathologic characterization in a series of 11 cases. Am J Surg Pathol 2015; 39(8):1075–84.

22. Neilan TG, Rothenberg ML, Amiri-Kordestani L, et al. Myocarditis associated with immune checkpoint inhibitors: an expert consensus on data gaps and a call to action. Oncologist 2018;23(8):874–8.

23. Friedman CF, Proverbs-Singh TA, Postow MA. Treatment of the immune-related adverse effects of immune checkpoint inhibitors: a review. JAMA Oncol 2016; 2(10):1346–53.

24. Dougan M. Checkpoint blockade toxicity and immune homeostasis in the gastro-intestinal tract. Front Immunol 2017;8:1547.

25. Weber JS. Challenging cases: management of immune-related toxicity. Am Soc Clin Oncol Educ Book 2018;38:179–83.

26. Chen JH, Lee KY, Hu CJ, et al. Coexisting myasthenia gravis, myositis, and poly-neuropathy induced by ipilimumab and nivolumab in a patient with non-small-cell lung cancer: a case report and literature review. Medicine (Baltimore) 2017; 96(50):e9262.

27. Wang K, Zhu Q, Lu Y, et al. CTLA-4 +49 G/A polymorphism confers autoimmune disease risk: an updated meta-analysis. Genet Test Mol Biomarkers 2017;21(4): 222–7.

28. Chen Y, Chen S, Gu Y, et al. CTLA-4 +49 G/A, a functional T1D risk SNP, affects CTLA-4 level in Treg subsets and IA-2A positivity, but not beta-cell function. Sci Rep 2018;8(1):10074.

29. Ting WH, Chien MN, Lo FS, et al. Association of cytotoxic T-lymphocyte-associ-ated protein 4 (CTLA4) gene polymorphisms with autoimmune thyroid disease in children and adults: case-control study. PLoS One 2016;11(4):e0154394.

30. de Jong VM, Zaldumbide A, van der Slik AR, et al. Variation in the CTLA4 3' UTR has phenotypic consequences for autoreactive T cells and associates with ge-netic risk for type 1 diabetes. Genes Immun 2016;17(1):75–8.

31. Schubert D, Bode C, Kenefeck R, et al. Autosomal dominant immune dysregula-tion syndrome in humans with CTLA4 mutations. Nat Med 2014;20(12):1410–6.

32. Kuehn HS, Ouyang W, Lo B, et al. Immune dysregulation in human subjects with heterozygous germline mutations in CTLA4. Science 2014;345(6204):1623–7.

33. Schwab C, Gabrysch A, Olbrich P, et al. Phenotype, penetrance, and treatment of 133 cytotoxic T-lymphocyte antigen 4-insufficient subjects. J Allergy Clin Immunol 2018;142(6):1932–46.

34. Verma N, Burns SO, Walker LSK, et al. Immune deficiency and autoimmunity in patients with CTLA-4 (CD152) mutations. Clin Exp Immunol 2017;190(1):1–7.

35. Lo B, Zhang K, Lu W, et al. Autoimmune disease. Patients with LRBA deficiency show CTLA4 loss and immune dysregulation responsive to abatacept therapy. Science 2015;349(6246):436–40.

36. Alkhairy OK, Abolhassani H, Rezaei N, et al. Spectrum of phenotypes associated with mutations in LRBA. J Clin Immunol 2016;36(1):33–45.

37. Bakacs T, Mehrishi JN. Anti-CTLA-4 therapy may have mechanisms similar to those occurring in inherited human CTLA4 haploinsufficiency. Immunobiology 2015;220(5):624–5.

38. Moreira A, Loquai C, Pfohler C, et al. Myositis and neuromuscular side-effects induced by immune checkpoint inhibitors. Eur J Cancer 2019;106:12–23.

39. Coutzac C, Adam J, Soularue E, et al. Colon immune-related adverse events: anti-CTLA-4 and anti-PD-1 blockade induce distinct immunopathological entities. J Crohns Colitis 2017;11(10):1238–46.

40. Caturegli P, Di Dalmazi G, Lombardi M, et al. Hypophysitis secondary to cytotoxic T-lymphocyte-associated protein 4 blockade: insights into pathogenesis from an autopsy series. Am J Pathol 2016;186(12):3225–35.

41. Das R, Bar N, Ferreira M, et al. Early B cell changes predict autoimmunity following combination immune checkpoint blockade. J Clin Invest 2018;128(2):715–20.

42. Nakamura Y. Biomarkers for immune checkpoint inhibitor-mediated tumor response and adverse events. Front Med (Lausanne) 2019;6:119.

43. Anderson R, Rapoport BL. Immune dysregulation in cancer patients undergoing immune checkpoint inhibitor treatment and potential predictive strategies for future clinical practice. Front Oncol 2018;8:80.

44. Bodis G, Toth V, Schwarting A. Role of human leukocyte antigens (HLA) in autoimmune diseases. Methods Mol Biol 2018;1802:11–29.

45. Chowell D, Morris LGT, Grigg CM, et al. Patient HLA class I genotype influences cancer response to checkpoint blockade immunotherapy. Science 2018;359(6375):582–7.

46. Hasan Ali O, Berner F, Bomze D, et al. Human leukocyte antigen variation is associated with adverse events of checkpoint inhibitors. Eur J Cancer 2019;107:8–14.

47. Egg D, Schwab C, Gabrysch A, et al. Increased risk for malignancies in 131 affected CTLA4 mutation carriers. Front Immunol 2018;9:2012.

48. Watson LR, Slade CA, Ojaimi S, et al. Pitfalls of immunotherapy: lessons from a patient with CTLA-4 haploinsufficiency. Allergy Asthma Clin Immunol 2018;14:65.

49. Coit P, Dozmorov MG, Merrill JT, et al. Epigenetic reprogramming in naive CD4+ T cells favoring T cell activation and non-Th1 effector T cell immune response as an early event in lupus flares. Arthritis Rheumatol 2016;68(9):2200–9.

50. Abdel-Wahab N, Shah M, Lopez-Olivo MA, et al. Use of immune checkpoint inhibitors in the treatment of patients with cancer and preexisting autoimmune disease: a systematic review. Ann Intern Med 2018;168(2):121–30.

51. Diehl A, Yarchoan M, Hopkins A, et al. Relationships between lymphocyte counts and treatment-related toxicities and clinical responses in patients with solid tumors treated with PD-1 checkpoint inhibitors. Oncotarget 2017;8(69):114268–80.

52. Fujisawa Y, Yoshino K, Otsuka A, et al. Fluctuations in routine blood count might signal severe immune-related adverse events in melanoma patients treated with nivolumab. J Dermatol Sci 2017;88(2):225–31.

53. Tanaka R, Okiyama N, Okune M, et al. Serum level of interleukin-6 is increased in nivolumab-associated psoriasiform dermatitis and tumor necrosis factor-alpha is a biomarker of nivolumab recativity. J Dermatol Sci 2017;86(1):71–3.

54. Tarhini AA, Zahoor H, Lin Y, et al. Baseline circulating IL-17 predicts toxicity while TGF-beta1 and IL-10 are prognostic of relapse in ipilimumab neoadjuvant therapy of melanoma. J Immunother Cancer 2015;3:39.

55. Fujimura T, Sato Y, Tanita K, et al. Serum levels of soluble CD163 and CXCL5 may be predictive markers for immune-related adverse events in patients with advanced melanoma treated with nivolumab: a pilot study. Oncotarget 2018;9(21):15542–51.

56. Bamias G, Delladetsima I, Perdiki M, et al. Immunological characteristics of colitis associated with anti-CTLA-4 antibody therapy. Cancer Invest 2017;35(7):443–55.

57. Abraham C, Cho J. Interleukin-23/Th17 pathways and inflammatory bowel disease. Inflamm Bowel Dis 2009;15(7):1090–100.

58. Toi Y, Sugawara S, Sugisaka J, et al. Profiling preexisting antibodies in patients treated with anti-PD-1 therapy for advanced non-small cell lung cancer. JAMA Oncol 2018. https://doi.org/10.1001/jamaoncol.2018.5860.

59. Kimbara S, Fujiwara Y, Iwama S, et al. Association of antithyroglobulin antibodies with the development of thyroid dysfunction induced by nivolumab. Cancer Sci 2018;109(11):3583–90.

60. Stamatouli AM, Quandt Z, Perdigoto AL, et al. Collateral damage: insulin-dependent diabetes induced with checkpoint inhibitors. Diabetes 2018;67(8): 1471–80.

61. Toi Y, Sugawara S, Kawashima Y, et al. Association of immune-related adverse events with clinical benefit in patients with advanced non-small-cell lung cancer treated with nivolumab. Oncologist 2018;23(11):1358–65.

62. Judd J, Zibelman M, Handorf E, et al. Immune-related adverse events as a biomarker in non-melanoma patients treated with programmed cell death 1 inhibitors. Oncologist 2017;22(10):1232–7.

63. Postow MA, Manuel M, Wong P, et al. Peripheral T cell receptor diversity is associated with clinical outcomes following ipilimumab treatment in metastatic melanoma. J Immunother Cancer 2015;3:23.

64. Oh DY, Cham J, Zhang L, et al. Immune toxicities elicted by CTLA-4 blockade in cancer patients are associated with early diversification of the T-cell repertoire. Cancer Res 2017;77(6):1322–30.

65. Laubli H, Koelzer VH, Matter MS, et al. The T cell repertoire in tumors overlaps with pulmonary inflammatory lesions in patients treated with checkpoint inhibitors. Oncoimmunology 2018;7(2):e1386362.

66. Jiang N, Schonnesen AA, Ma KY. Ushering in integrated T cell repertoire profiling in cancer. Trends Cancer 2019;5(2):85–94.

67. Routy B, Gopalakrishnan V, Daillere R, et al. The gut microbiota influences anticancer immunosurveillance and general health. Nat Rev Clin Oncol 2018;15(6): 382–96.

68. Farmer JR, Foldvari Z, Ujhazi B, et al. Outcomes and treatment strategies for autoimmunity and hyperinflammation in patients with RAG deficiency. J Allergy Clin Immunol Pract 2019;7(6):1970–85.e4.

69. Som A, Mandaliya R, Alsaadi D, et al. Immune checkpoint inhibitor-induced colitis: a comprehensive review. World J Clin Cases 2019;7(4):405–18.

70. Dubin K, Callahan MK, Ren B, et al. Intestinal microbiome analyses identify melanoma patients at risk for checkpoint-blockade-induced colitis. Nat Commun 2016;7:10391.

71. Chaput N, Lepage P, Coutzac C, et al. Baseline gut microbiota predicts clinical response and colitis in metastatic melanoma patients treated with ipilimumab. Ann Oncol 2017;28(6):1368–79.

72. Gulbu Uzel DK, Su H, Rump A, et al. Management of cytopenias in CTLA4 haploinsufficiency using abatacept and sirolimus. Blood 2018;132:2409.

73. Kiykim A, Ogulur I, Dursun E, et al. Abatacept as a long-term targeted therapy for LRBA deficiency. J Allergy Clin Immunol Pract 2019. https://doi.org/10.1016/j.jaip.2019.06.011.

74. De Bruyne M, Bogaert DJ, Venken K, et al. A novel LPS-responsive beige-like anchor protein (LRBA) mutation presents with normal cytotoxic T lymphocyte-associated protein 4 (CTLA-4) and overactive TH17 immunity. J Allergy Clin Immunol 2018;142(6):1968–71.

75. Esfahani K, Buhlaiga N, Thebault P, et al. Alemtuzumab for immune-related myocarditis due to PD-1 therapy. N Engl J Med 2019;380(24):2375–6.

76. Salem JE, Allenbach Y, Vozy A, et al. Abatacept for severe immune checkpoint inhibitor-associated myocarditis. N Engl J Med 2019;380(24):2377–9.

77. Kumar B, Ballas Z. Adverse events associated with immune checkpoint blockade. N Engl J Med 2018;378(12):1164 [Letter to the editor].

78. Stroud CR, Hegde A, Cherry C, et al. Tocilizumab for the management of immune mediated adverse events secondary to PD-1 blockade. J Oncol Pharm Pract 2019;25(3):551–7.

79. Samson M, Audia S, Janikashvili N, et al. Brief report: inhibition of interleukin-6 function corrects Th17/Treg cell imbalance in patients with rheumatoid arthritis. Arthritis Rheum 2012;64(8):2499–503.

80. Kikuchi J, Hashizume M, Kaneko Y, et al. Peripheral blood CD4(+)CD25(+) CD127(low) regulatory T cells are significantly increased by tocilizumab treatment in patients with rheumatoid arthritis: increase in regulatory T cells correlates with clinical response. Arthritis Res Ther 2015;17:10.

81. Furiati SC, Catarino JS, Silva MV, et al. Th1, Th17, and Treg responses are differently modulated by TNF-alpha inhibitors and methotrexate in psoriasis patients. Sci Rep 2019;9(1):7526.

82. Martins F, Sykiotis GP, Maillard M, et al. New therapeutic perspectives to manage refractory immune checkpoint-related toxicities. Lancet Oncol 2019;20(1): e54–64.

83. Toussirot E, Aubin F. Paradoxical reactions under TNF-alpha blocking agents and other biological agents given for chronic immune-mediated diseases: an analytical and comprehensive overview. RMD Open 2016;2(2):e000239.

84. Calzascia T, Pellegrini M, Hall H, et al. TNF-alpha is critical for antitumor but not antiviral T cell immunity in mice. J Clin Invest 2007;117(12):3833–45.

85. Tsukamoto H, Fujieda K, Senju S, et al. Immune-suppressive effects of interleukin-6 on T-cell-mediated anti-tumor immunity. Cancer Sci 2018;109(3):523–30.

86. Vainer N, Dehlendorff C, Johansen JS. Systematic literature review of IL-6 as a biomarker or treatment target in patients with gastric, bile duct, pancreatic and colorectal cancer. Oncotarget 2018;9(51):29820–41.

87. Abu-Sbeih H, Ali FS, Alsaadi D, et al. Outcomes of vedolizumab therapy in patients with immune checkpoint inhibitor-induced colitis: a multi-center study. J Immunother Cancer 2018;6(1):142.

88. Wang Y, Wiesnoski DH, Helmink BA, et al. Fecal microbiota transplantation for refractory immune checkpoint-associated colitis. Nat Med 2018;24(12): 1804–8.

Molecular Diagnosis of Inherited Immune Disorders

Jocelyn R. Farmer, MD, PhD[a,b,c,]*, Vinay S. Mahajan, MD, PhD[b,c]

KEYWORDS

- Molecular diagnostics • Primary immunodeficiency • Newborn screening
- TREC assay • Next-generation sequencing • Exome sequencing
- Severe combined immune deficiency (SCID)
- Common variable immune deficiency (CVID)

KEY POINTS

- The field of primary immunodeficiency diagnostics has been revolutionized by 2 major molecular advancements: (1) newborn screening and (2) next-generation sequencing.
- PCR-based newborn screening for severe combined immune deficiency (SCID) is cost-effective and reduces SCID morbidity and mortality in the United States.
- Next-generation sequencing has led to an exponential increase in ascribed monogenic causes of primary immunodeficiencies and the opportunity for molecularly targeted therapeutic interventions.

NEWBORN SCREENING

Severe combined immune deficiency (SCID) is a model disease for newborn screening.[1] Patients with SCID are at risk for life-threatening infections starting at birth. Knowledge of an SCID diagnosis in a newborn dramatically alters recommendations for patient care, including avoidance of live viral vaccinations and definitive early management, which have been shown to significantly decrease overall patient mortality.[2] In addition to being life-saving, early intervention for SCID has been shown to be cost-effective.[3] Despite these data, newborn screening for SCID lagged behind testing for inborn errors of metabolism by more than 4 decades.[1] This was due in part to the knowledge base required to develop a successful molecular diagnostic assay to detect intact lymphocyte development in peripheral blood.[4]

Disclosure Statement: This work was supported by the National Institutes of Health (T32-HL116275 to J.R. Farmer and K08-AI113163 to V.S. Mahajan).
[a] Division of Rheumatology, Allergy and Immunology, Massachusetts General Hospital, Boston, MA, USA; [b] Ragon Institute of MGH, MIT and Harvard, Cambridge, MA, USA; [c] Center for Advanced Molecular Diagnostics, Brigham and Women's Hospital, Boston, MA, USA
* Corresponding author. COX 201, MGH, 55 Fruit Street, Boston, MA 02114.
E-mail address: jrfarmer@partners.org

Technical Concepts in T Cell Receptor Excision Circle Testing

In the course of their development in the thymus, all T cells must generate a functional T cell receptor (TCR) to survive. Each TCR gene is encoded by a cluster of V, J, or D gene segments. Through a process called V(D)J rearrangement, randomly chosen V, J, or D gene segments are assembled into a single contiguous TCR gene (**Fig. 1**). During this rearrangement event, which brings together 2 distal gene segments, the intervening stretch of DNA is excised as a circular molecule by the RAG recombinase, and the exposed breaks at the ends (coding joints) of the 2 DNA segments are joined together by DNA repair enzymes. The excised DNA is called a T cell receptor excision circle (TREC). TRECs themselves do not replicate during cell division, and the number of TRECs per cell is diluted as T cells divide. Thus, the number of TRECs in the peripheral blood can be used as a biomarker to approximate naive T cell production.[5,6]

T cells are divided into 2 subtypes based on their TCR gene usage, alpha/beta and gamma/delta. The TCR delta locus is embedded within the TCR alpha locus and is deleted during TCR alpha-chain rearrangement. The human TCR delta locus is flanked by delta-deleting elements, δRec and ψJα. Recombination of the delta-deleting elements results in the removal of the TCR delta locus accompanied by the formation of a TREC, which includes the signal joints of δRec and ψJα. This TREC is called a δRec-ψJα or signal-joint TREC and is produced by about 70% of

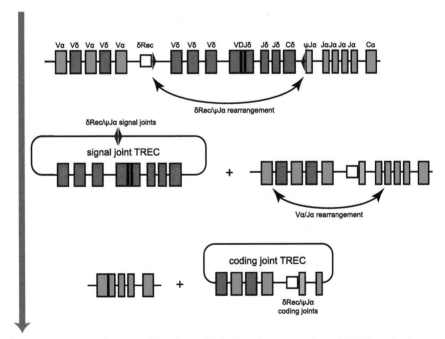

Fig. 1. Generation of TRECs. This schematic depicts the generation of TRECs at the human TCR alpha locus. Please note that the TCR alpha locus is not drawn to scale, and a greatly reduced number of gene segments are depicted for the sake of simplicity. Following TCR gamma, delta, and beta rearrangement, the TCR delta locus is nearly eliminated on recombination of the TCR delta-deleting elements, δRec and ψJα. This is accompanied by the generation of a signal-joint TREC containing the signal joints of δRec and ψJα. Subsequent Vα/Jα rearrangement results in the formation of a coding-joint TREC containing the coding ends of δRec and ψJα.

all T cells. The TRECs generated by subsequent TCR alpha-chain rearrangement contain the coding joints of the δRec and ψJα segments and are referred to as coding-joint TRECs. Clinically used TREC assays specifically detect and quantify the δRec-ψJα TREC using a real-time quantitative polymerase chain reaction (qPCR) approach. In 2005, this technique was first shown to be capable of identifying SCID, regardless of underlying monogenic mutation, in a cohort of 23 infants using DNA extracted from dried blood spots.[7]

Implementation

Newborn screening for SCID by TREC assay was first introduced in the United States in Wisconsin in 2008.[8] By 2014, there were 11 newborn screening programs underway in the United States with more than 3,030,083 newborns screened using the TREC assay.[9] By 2018, newborn screening had been implemented in most of the United States and its territories, with an estimated 92% of American infants undergoing screening for SCID.[10] Data from these newborn screening programs to date have identified SCID at a rate of 1 in 58,000 to 65,000 live births, with major causes including typical SCID, leaky SCID, and Omenn syndrome.[9,11] In addition, newborn screening by TREC assay has identified non-SCID T cell lymphopenia. In a 2014 review, 33% of all cases of non-SCID T cell lymphopenia had a recognized congenital syndrome associated with T cell impairment (majority DiGeorge syndrome/chromosome 22q11.2 deletion), 28% were attributable to other medical conditions (majority congenital heart disease), and idiopathic T cell lymphopenia (infants who did not meet the diagnostic criteria for leaky SCID but had persistent T cell lymphopenia and immune dysfunction without defects in known SCID genes) was a rare cause of non-SCID T cell lymphopenia at only 3%.[9]

Clinical Applications

Severe combined immune deficiency

Early recognition of SCID and prompt therapeutic intervention are essential. Data from the Primary Immune Deficiency Treatment Consortium previously demonstrated an SCID survival rate of 94% for those patients who received hematopoietic stem cell transplantation before 3.5 months of age, compared with only 50% for those transplanted after 3.5 months of age with active infections.[2] Results from the first 7 years of newborn screening by TREC assay in California were recently published, demonstrating an overall SCID survival rate of 94%, thus achieving the goal of improved patient outcome from early therapeutic intervention.[11] Moreover, newborn screening has been shown to be cost-effective, reducing medical care costs from frequent admissions and loss of work productivity for parents.[3,12,13]

Non-severe combined immune deficiency T cell lymphopenias

DiGeorge syndrome/chromosome 22q11.2 deletion is the most common congenital syndrome associated with T cell impairment that has been identified on newborn screening to date.[9] Complete DiGeorge syndrome is a highly morbid condition of absent thymic function, which prevents the further development of T cells in the periphery.[14] Thymic transplant has been shown to be curative in this condition, including in 4 patients with complete DiGeorge syndrome recently identified on newborn screening in California who underwent subsequent successful thymus transplants.[11] For congenital syndromes associated with T cell impairment for which no definitive cure can be offered, early diagnosis may still provide opportunity to protect against early-onset infections or provide disease-specific counseling, such as avoidance of ionizing radiation in the case of ataxia telangiectasia. Finally, hematopoietic stem cell transplantation has been offered in the context of idiopathic T cell lymphopenia identified on newborn screening given the underlying degree of immune impairment in the patient despite the lack of a definitive diagnosis.[9] Together, these data suggest that the benefits of newborn screening by TREC assay will extend beyond patients with SCID, however, given the rare nature of these disorders, long-term follow-up of larger patient cohorts is required.

Long-term Follow-up

All infants identified with SCID or a known congenital syndrome associated with T cell impairment should receive appropriate immunologic follow-up as per the recommended international consensus guidelines for that condition.[15] In contrast, it is unclear how the long-term follow-up of patients otherwise identified on TREC screening as having non-SCID T cell lymphopenia, specifically idiopathic T cell lymphopenia, should proceed.[16] Currently, the United States immunologic societies have efforts underway to prospectively follow the cohort of patients identified with idiopathic T cell lymphopenia on newborn screening to address this deficit in the field.

Pitfalls

TREC screening was implemented in the United States as a state-by-state initiative, therefore interstate variability, both in the reference ranges used to define the pathology and in algorithms for diagnostic confirmation and care referral, still exist.[9] Efforts are underway to develop qPCR standards for the TREC assay that can help to ensure a higher degree of precision and reproducibility between laboratories. Moreover, SCID outcomes will continue to be influenced by geographic access to large nationally renowned referral centers with expertise in the complex care of primary immunodeficiency disorders.[9] In addition, patients with leaky SCID who have significant breakthrough naive T cell production are at increased risk of being missed by TREC assay. In California, 2 such patients were recently described during a 7-year follow-up period of newborn screening, who presented to clinical attention at 7 and 23 months of age.[11] The TREC assay, being T cell centric, also fails to detect newborns with severe forms of B cell predominant primary immunodeficiencies, such as agammaglobulinemia, who would also benefit from early clinical interventions, including immunoglobulin replacement therapy. Finally, TRECs can be low due to secondary causes, including congenital heart disease and pre-term birth.[9] Follow-up serial TREC screening at a 2-week interval has been recommended in the context of acute illness or prematurity until TREC normalization[16]; however, this intervention is inherently cost and time intensive for all parties: the newborn screening program, the managing physician, and the patient's family.

Future Directions

Because the TREC assay can miss selective deficiencies in B cell development, an analogous assay has been developed for B cells. This exploits the fact that developing B cells, which normally fail to productively rearrange the *IGK* gene, excise the constant Kappa gene segment by recombination of the Kappa-deleting element (Kde) and an upstream intronic recombination signal sequence (RSS). This results in the generation of a Kappa receptor excision circle (KREC) comprising the Kde and RSS signal joint, which can also be quantified using real-time qPCR approaches. To date, the KREC assay has shown diagnostic usefulness in identifying patients with B cell predominant primary immunodeficiencies,[17] and the KREC assay (for use in combination with the TREC assay) is currently under pilot investigation for newborn screening in some nations.[18]

NEXT-GENERATION SEQUENCING

Historically, genetic discoveries in primary immunodeficiency disorders centered around techniques, including classic linkage analysis and association mapping, which importantly identified, among many others, the role of *Btk* in X-linked agammaglobulinemia.[19,20] More recently, genome-wide association studies (GWAS) were conducted on common variable immune deficiency (CVID) and selective IgA deficiency, specifically, to address the potential for multi-genetic variants, which elucidated both known and novel gene associations with humoral immune dysfunction and risk for autoimmune disease co-occurrence.[21,22] However, with the onset of next-generation sequencing (NGS), the field of primary immunodeficiency disease diagnostics has seen an exponential increase in ascribed monogenic causes of primary immunodeficiencies in humans.[23]

Technical Concepts in Next-Generation Sequencing

The term NGS refers to any one of the high-throughput sequencing platforms that can sequence a library of millions of DNA molecules in parallel (eg, Illumina, Ion Torrent, Roche 454). Individual DNA molecules in the sequencing library are typically subjected to a spatially localized amplification step on the NGS instrument using a proprietary instrument-specific method to achieve an acceptable signal-to-noise ratio for subsequent sequencing. To facilitate this amplification step on the NGS instrument, the sequencing library is flanked by platform-specific sequencing adapters. On the widely used Illumina platform, the localized amplicons originating from individual DNA molecules in the sequencing library are referred to as "clusters." Millions of such clusters of locally amplified DNA molecules are then sequenced in parallel one base at a time by synthesis (i.e., using a DNA polymerase) using various platform-dependent nucleotide labeling and detection strategies. This requires that the sequencing library also includes sequencing primer binding sites, which are typically incorporated into the flanking sequencing adapters. In NGS parlance, the sequence of nucleotides that is read out from a cluster is called a "read," and it corresponds to a single DNA molecule in the sequencing library. In a single run, a typical NGS sequencing instrument can generate millions of reads, which are a few hundred bases long, and can be either paired-end or single-end, depending on whether the library was sequenced from one or both ends.

In a patient with a suspected genetic cause of immunodeficiency, the pathogenic genetic variant is typically identified by sequencing genomic DNA extracted from a peripheral blood specimen. To sequence genomic DNA, it first needs to be converted into a sequencing library. There are numerous methods for preparing sequencing libraries that depend on the sequencing platform. In the most general sense, sequencing library preparation involves fragmentation of the genomic DNA followed by the addition of sequencing adapters at the ends. Instead of sequencing the whole genome, the library is generally enriched for regions encoding protein-coding genes, which contain most known causal genetic variants linked to disease.[24] Target enrichment can be performed either before or after the addition of sequencing adapters. Enrichment and sequencing of all exons is referred to as exome sequencing. Alternatively, immunodeficiency gene sequencing panels offer a more focused approach restricted to a smaller set of immune-related genes that are known to be mutated in this disorder. NGS technologies are rapidly evolving, and newer platforms for single-molecule sequencing that do not require the pre-amplification or cluster generation step are in the offing. They are currently limited by a high sequencing error rate, but that is declining rapidly. These newer approaches (eg, nanopore technologies,

PacBio SMRT sequencing) will open a new era in molecular genetics diagnostics because they have the potential to sequence extremely long contiguous stretches of DNA and to identify epigenetically modified DNA bases.

Next-Generation Sequencing Pipelines and Analysis

Sequencing is followed by alignment of the reads to a chosen reference genome. Sequence features that differ from the reference genome are called variants. The proportion of reads bearing a variant provides an estimate of the allele fraction of the variant. Inherited variants are typically either homozygous or heterozygous and are thus present at an allele fraction of ~100% or ~50%, respectively. Sequencing depth refers to the number of reads that are aligned to a given region. Sufficient sequencing depth is required to confidently determine the presence of a genetic variant. Artifacts can be encountered in NGS sequencing data; they range from errors arising during library preparation, sequencing errors, as well as analysis errors such as read-mapping artifacts. Excluding such sequencing artifacts and assuring sequencing quality requires a team of bioinformatics specialists. A typical exome sequencing run yields thousands of variants, most of which are polymorphisms that are found in healthy individuals. Fortunately, there are numerous single nucleotide polymorphism (SNP) databases that can be used to help filter commonly occurring polymorphisms (eg, the ExAC and gnomAD databases from the Broad Institute[25]). Some pathogenic variants are present in SNP databases, however, so caution must be exercised in using this as a sole exclusion criterion.[26] Of the remaining variants, those that are predicted to alter the protein sequence, such as missense, frameshift, nonsense, or splice-site variants, are prioritized for detailed review. Confirmatory PCR for pathogenic variants and sequencing by an alternate method such as Sanger sequencing used to be the norm in some laboratories, but this practice has dwindled with growing confidence in the accuracy of NGS methods.

A heterozygous variant can be pathogenic if it causes an autosomal dominant form of immunodeficiency (eg, an activating mutation in *PIK3CD* that results in a constitutively active PI3K-delta,[27,28] or an inactivating mutation in *NFKB1* that results in haploinsufficiency[29]). Although there are algorithms (eg, PolyPhen[30]) that can predict the possible functional impact of a variant on protein structure based on sequence conservation and structural constraints, in practice, determining if a heterozygous missense variant is pathogenic can be challenging, especially if it has not been previously reported or studied.[31] The direct experimental confirmation of the pathogenicity of a novel missense variant that does not obviously have an impact on protein function (eg, a frameshift variant) is now possible with the advent of CRISPR/Cas9 gene-editing technologies, but these approaches still remain outside the scope of most clinical laboratories. Databases that document human genetic variants as well as the disease context in which they were identified are especially helpful (eg, ClinVar[32]). In the absence of a history of consanguinity, it is unusual to encounter rare pathogenic variants in the homozygous state, and compound heterozygosity is far more common. If 2 variants are present in the same gene, it may be necessary to determine if both maternal and paternal copies of the gene are altered. This is particularly important when inactivation of both gene copies is necessary to disrupt cellular function (eg, *RAG* genes[33]). If the distance between the 2 variants is less than the length of the sequencing reads, it may be possible to determining if they are in *cis* or *trans*. If not, excluding the presence of an unaffected allele will require testing of family members. Identification of a variant that is likely to alter protein structure in a gene that has been previously linked to the clinical phenotype may be regarded as suspicious; if immune dysfunction or immunodeficiency is apparent in the family, testing of close relatives may help determine if the suspicious variant is pathogenic by assessing if it segregates with the immunophenotype.[31]

Implementation

Targeted gene sequencing panels

Gene panel testing is commercially available for a wide variety of primary immunodeficiency disorders, from combined immunodeficiencies (eg, SCID) to B cell predominant disorders (eg, CVID) to conditions of immune dysregulation (eg, periodic fever syndromes). There are clear benefits to gene panel testing, specifically time and cost efficiency.[34,35] However, drawbacks exist. First, this type of targeted gene testing is best suited for patients who fit a well-defined clinical phenotype captured by the panel. For example, a patient with B-T-SCID due to null *RAG* mutations would be well captured on an SCID panel, whereas a patient presenting with autoinflammation and intact lymphocyte counts due to leaky *RAG* mutations may not be similarly selected for this genetic analysis and consequently missed. Second, panel testing inherently lags behind newly discovered causal genes in the field.[34] In the fast-paced world of primary immunodeficiency diseases, with more than 300 monogenic causes discovered by 2017,[36] panel testing risks missing both recently discovered and novel genotype-immunophenotype relationships.

Whole-exome sequencing

In contrast to panel testing, whole-exome sequencing (WES) targets all protein-coding regions of the human genome. Whereas WES assays only ~1% of the human genome in total, it is a rational approach in the clinical application of genetic sequencing in that 85% of disease-causing variants have been localized to exons.[24] In clinical application, WES has shown utility in the diagnosis of a broad range of primary immunodeficiency diseases.[36] In CVID specifically, WES has been shown capable of identifying "probable disease-causing mutations" at a rate of 15% to 30%, including novel and unanticipated genotype-immunophenotype correlations.[37,38]

Clinical Applications

Severe combined immune deficiency

Newborn screening by TREC assay identifies SCID by immunophenotype, making all monogenic causes indistinguishable.[7] Yet, care of an infant with SCID can vary according to the exact underlying mutation that is identified. For example, enzyme replacement therapy is a unique consideration in patients with adenosine deaminase (ADA) deficiency,[39] ionizing radiation should be empirically avoided in patients with radiosensitive SCID, such as Artemis deficiency,[40] and gene therapy is a potential therapeutic consideration in only a subset of SCID (eg, ADA deficiency[41] and X-linked disease due to null *IL2RG* mutations[42]). Sequencing of all SCID-causing genes has been proposed in the diagnostic algorithm of a newborn with low TRECs who has a confirmed SCID immunophenotype.[16] It seems that this recommendation is being followed in clinical practice. In a review of 52 cases of SCID identified by newborn screening in 2014, more than 92% of cases had subsequent genetic testing performed.[9] Finally, untargeted WES has shown usefulness in the diagnosis of SCID identified outside the confines of newborn screening.[36] Together, these data suggest that NGS will continue to be integral to SCID diagnostics with direct implications for patient care.

Common variable immune deficiency

CVID is the most common symptomatic primary immunodeficiency disease in the world.[43] Risk loci for CVID were appreciated previously through mechanisms including linkage mapping[44,45] and GWAS.[21] With the onset of NGS in 2010, the genetic basis for CVID has been rewritten, from a disease of polygenic inheritance almost by definition to a disease of monogenic inheritance in up to 30% of patients.[37,46–48] Importantly, elucidating single gene defects in CVID has directly affected patient care. For example, identifying patients with CTLA4 haploinsufficiency has allowed for the directed use of abatacept, CTLA4-Ig, as a form of replacement therapy.[49,50] Similarly, elucidating a role for *PIK3CD* activating mutations in CVID pathophysiology has allowed for the directed use of PI3K-delta inhibitors for therapeutic intervention.[27,28,51] As CVID patient selection in WES cohort studies previously was often biased toward severe clinical presentations (eg, autoimmunity, low B cell counts, or a familial pattern of disease[37]), the practicality and cost-effectiveness of untargeted NGS in all forms of CVID remain to be determined. NGS may prove most beneficial in a defined CVID subset, particularly as immunophenotypes that correlate with increased risk for autoinflammation and poor prognosis, including low class-switched memory B cells and loss of naive T cells, have already been defined.[52–54]

Inherited immune dysregulation syndromes

Atypical presentations of primary immunodeficiency, including autoimmunity and autoinflammation, are becoming increasingly recognized.[55–57] Moreover, many patients fall between the classic definitions of primary immunodeficiency disorders such as SCID and CVID. NGS may still be warranted in these clinical contexts. Across all forms of primary immunodeficiency disorders (including patients with autoimmunity or autoinflammation as primary clinical presentations), WES was recently shown to elucidate a likely molecular diagnosis in 40% of unrelated probands.[36] Moreover, single immune gene defects are being elucidated in severe forms of primary autoinflammatory disease, such as very early-onset inflammatory bowel disease.[58,59] These data suggest a potential usefulness for NGS beyond the clinical context of classic primary immunodeficiency. However, larger cohort studies are required to determine the cost-effectiveness of NGS in these broader immune dysregulatory syndromes.

Pitfalls

Both targeted and untargeted NGS have some shared limitations. First, gene coverage varies widely and can result in false negatives. To firmly exclude a potential gene candidate, coverage should reach 100% of the targeted nucleotides at a minimum depth of 20 reads.[23] Second, the usefulness of NGS in primary immunodeficiency disease diagnostics is inherently tied to an accurate method for variant calling. Although established techniques exist in the field,[36,60] there is no current standard of practice. Even when rare variants of interest are correctly identified and flagged for consideration, there can be misinterpretation of genotype-immunophenotype correlations in the context of heterozygous mutations; for example, compound heterozygosity that is missed either due to low gene coverage of a second coding variant or a copy number variant.[61] Moreover, novel variants of unknown significance (VUS) must undergo careful in silico and wet laboratory validation to demonstrate causality,[31] which is technically impractical in most clinical laboratory settings. Thus, a careful cost-benefit analysis must be considered in each clinical context before pursuing NGS. This includes educating both patient and family members on the potential for ambiguity should a VUS be identified.[62,63] For now, in patients in whom a causal variant cannot be identified, efforts are underway to develop a syndromal classification approach using detailed immunophenotypic and functional characterization of affected immune cell subsets that can be used to guide therapy.[53]

Future Directions

Clinically used NGS approaches focus predominantly on coding regions. It remains possible that a significant proportion of monogenic disease-causing variants are present in noncoding regions of the genome. Such variants may have an impact on the function of regulatory elements (eg, promoters, enhancers, UTRs) or noncoding genes such as microRNAs that regulate the expression of protein-coding genes linked to immunodeficiencies. Case examples of rare variants identified in noncoding genomic regions, functionally validated as causal for immune dysregulation in the patient, have been described.[64,65] Whole-genome sequencing (WGS) has also been examined at a population level for CVID[66,67] and for primary immunodeficiencies more globally.[61] However, reliable approaches to identify pathogenic noncoding variants are still under investigation, and the benefit of WGS in clinical practice has not been validated to date.[63] These approaches may require parallel analysis of the genome, transcriptome, proteome, or epigenome. Recently, use of WGS in combination with RNA sequencing to explore rare genetic variants in parallel with the transcriptome for component functional validation was described in a CVID cohort.[66] With the growing potential for single-cell analysis techniques, the ability to connect germline DNA variants to unique immune profiles will likely only deepen.[68] Finally, our understanding of epigenetic complexity in primary immunodeficiency disorders is in its infancy. However, as recently demonstrated in a study of monozygotic twins with discordant immunophenotypes,[69] epigenetics will certainly play an overarching role in dictating the ultimate degree of immune system impairment in the patient.

REFERENCES

1. Kelly N, Makarem DC, Wasserstein MP. Screening of newborns for disorders with high benefit-risk ratios should be mandatory. J Law Med Ethics 2016;44(2):231–40.
2. Pai SY, Logan BR, Griffith LM, et al. Transplantation outcomes for severe combined immunodeficiency, 2000-2009. N Engl J Med 2014;371(5):434–46.
3. Ding Y, Thompson JD, Kobrynski L, et al. Cost-effectiveness/cost-benefit analysis of newborn screening for severe combined immune deficiency in Washington State. J Pediatr 2016;172:127–35.
4. Puck JM. Laboratory technology for population-based screening for severe combined immunodeficiency in neonates: the winner is T-cell receptor excision circles. J Allergy Clin Immunol 2012;129(3):607–16.
5. Hazenberg MD, Verschuren MC, Hamann D, et al. T cell receptor excision circles as markers for recent thymic emigrants: basic aspects, technical approach, and guidelines for interpretation. J Mol Med (Berl) 2001;79(11):631–40.
6. Douek DC, McFarland RD, Keiser PH, et al. Changes in thymic function with age and during the treatment of HIV infection. Nature 1998;396(6712):690–5.
7. Chan K, Puck JM. Development of population-based newborn screening for severe combined immunodeficiency. J Allergy Clin Immunol 2005;115(2):391–8.
8. Routes JM, Grossman WJ, Verbsky J, et al. Statewide newborn screening for severe T-cell lymphopenia. JAMA 2009;302(22):2465–70.
9. Kwan A, Abraham RS, Currier R, et al. Newborn screening for severe combined immunodeficiency in 11 screening programs in the United States. JAMA 2014;312(7):729–38.
10. King JR, Hammarstrom L. Newborn screening for primary immunodeficiency diseases: history, current and future practice. J Clin Immunol 2018;38(1):56–66.

11. Amatuni GS, Currier RJ, Church JA, et al. Newborn screening for severe combined immunodeficiency and T-cell lymphopenia in California, 2010-2017. Pediatrics 2019;143(2) [pii:e20182300].

12. Clement MC, Mahlaoui N, Mignot C, et al. Systematic neonatal screening for severe combined immunodeficiency and severe T-cell lymphopenia: analysis of cost-effectiveness based on French real field data. J Allergy Clin Immunol 2015;135(6):1589–93.

13. Chan K, Davis J, Pai SY, et al. A Markov model to analyze cost-effectiveness of screening for severe combined immunodeficiency (SCID). Mol Genet Metab 2011;104(3):383–9.

14. Sullivan KE. DiGeorge syndrome/chromosome 22q11.2 deletion syndrome. Curr Allergy Asthma Rep 2001;1(5):438–44.

15. Bonilla FA, Khan DA, Ballas ZK, et al. Practice parameter for the diagnosis and management of primary immunodeficiency. J Allergy Clin Immunol 2015;136(5): 1186–205.e1-78.

16. Thakar MS, Hintermeyer MK, Gries MG, et al. A practical approach to newborn screening for severe combined immunodeficiency using the T cell receptor excision circle assay. Front Immunol 2017;8:1470.

17. Nakagawa N, Imai K, Kanegane H, et al. Quantification of kappa-deleting recombination excision circles in Guthrie cards for the identification of early B-cell maturation defects. J Allergy Clin Immunol 2011;128(1):223–225 e222.

18. Kanegae MPP, Barreiros LA, Sousa JL, et al. Newborn screening for severe combined immunodeficiencies using trecs and krecs: second pilot study in Brazil. Rev Paul Pediatr 2017;35(1):25–32.

19. Thomas JD, Sideras P, Smith CI, et al. Colocalization of X-linked agammaglobulinemia and X-linked immunodeficiency genes. Science 1993;261(5119):355–8.

20. Rawlings DJ, Saffran DC, Tsukada S, et al. Mutation of unique region of Bruton's tyrosine kinase in immunodeficient XID mice. Science 1993;261(5119):358–61.

21. Orange JS, Glessner JT, Resnick E, et al. Genome-wide association identifies diverse causes of common variable immunodeficiency. J Allergy Clin Immunol 2011;127(6):1360–7.e6.

22. Ferreira RC, Pan-Hammarstrom Q, Graham RR, et al. Association of IFIH1 and other autoimmunity risk alleles with selective IgA deficiency. Nat Genet 2010; 42(9):777–80.

23. Meyts I, Bosch B, Bolze A, et al. Exome and genome sequencing for inborn errors of immunity. J Allergy Clin Immunol 2016;138(4):957–69.

24. Hodges E, Xuan Z, Balija V, et al. Genome-wide in situ exon capture for selective resequencing. Nat Genet 2007;39(12):1522–7.

25. Lek M, Karczewski KJ, Minikel EV, et al. Analysis of protein-coding genetic variation in 60,706 humans. Nature 2016;536(7616):285–91.

26. Kobayashi Y, Yang S, Nykamp K, et al. Pathogenic variant burden in the ExAC database: an empirical approach to evaluating population data for clinical variant interpretation. Genome Med 2017;9(1):13.

27. Lucas CL, Kuehn HS, Zhao F, et al. Dominant-activating germline mutations in the gene encoding the PI(3)K catalytic subunit p110delta result in T cell senescence and human immunodeficiency. Nat Immunol 2014;15(1):88–97.

28. Angulo I, Vadas O, Garcon F, et al. Phosphoinositide 3-kinase delta gene mutation predisposes to respiratory infection and airway damage. Science 2013; 342(6160):866–71.

29. Fliegauf M, Bryant VL, Frede N, et al. Haploinsufficiency of the NF-kappaB1 sub-unit p50 in common variable immunodeficiency. Am J Hum Genet 2015;97(3): 389–403.

30. Adzhubei I, Jordan DM, Sunyaev SR. Predicting functional effect of human missense mutations using PolyPhen-2. Curr Protoc Hum Genet 2013. Chapter 7:Unit7 20.

31. Casanova JL, Conley ME, Seligman SJ, et al. Guidelines for genetic studies in single patients: lessons from primary immunodeficiencies. J Exp Med 2014; 211(11):2137–49.

32. Harrison SM, Riggs ER, Maglott DR, et al. Using ClinVar as a resource to support variant interpretation. Curr Protoc Hum Genet 2016;89. 8.16.1-18.16.23.

33. Villa A, Sobacchi C, Notarangelo LD, et al. V(D)J recombination defects in lym-phocytes due to RAG mutations: severe immunodeficiency with a spectrum of clinical presentations. Blood 2001;97(1):81–8.

34. Rae W, Ward D, Mattocks C, et al. Clinical efficacy of a next-generation sequencing gene panel for primary immunodeficiency diagnostics. Clin Genet 2018;93(3):647–55.

35. Bisgin A, Boga I, Yilmaz M, et al. The utility of next-generation sequencing for pri-mary immunodeficiency disorders: experience from a clinical diagnostic labora-tory. Biomed Res Int 2018;2018:9647253.

36. Stray-Pedersen A, Sorte HS, Samarakoon P, et al. Primary immunodeficiency dis-eases: genomic approaches delineate heterogeneous Mendelian disorders. J Al-lergy Clin Immunol 2017;139(1):232–45.

37. Maffucci P, Filion CA, Boisson B, et al. Genetic diagnosis using whole exome sequencing in common variable immunodeficiency. Front Immunol 2016;7:220.

38. de Valles-Ibanez G, Esteve-Sole A, Piquer M, et al. Evaluating the genetics of common variable immunodeficiency: monogenetic model and beyond. Front Im-munol 2018;9:636.

39. Chan B, Wara D, Bastian J, et al. Long-term efficacy of enzyme replacement ther-apy for adenosine deaminase (ADA)-deficient severe combined immunodefi-ciency (SCID). Clin Immunol 2005;117(2):133–43.

40. Dvorak CC, Cowan MJ. Radiosensitive severe combined immunodeficiency dis-ease. Immunol Allergy Clin North Am 2010;30(1):125–42.

41. Ferrua F, Brigida I, Aiuti A. Update on gene therapy for adenosine deaminase-deficient severe combined immunodeficiency. Curr Opin Allergy Clin Immunol 2010;10(6):551–6.

42. Mamcarz E, Zhou S, Lockey T, et al. Lentiviral gene therapy combined with low-dose Busulfan in infants with SCID-X1. N Engl J Med 2019;380(16):1525–34.

43. Bonilla FA, Barlan I, Chapel H, et al. International consensus document (ICON): common variable immunodeficiency disorders. J Allergy Clin Immunol Pract 2016;4(1):38–59.

44. Finck A, Van der Meer JW, Schaffer AA, et al. Linkage of autosomal-dominant common variable immunodeficiency to chromosome 4q. Eur J Hum Genet 2006;14(7):867–75.

45. Schaffer AA, Pfannstiel J, Webster AD, et al. Analysis of families with common variable immunodeficiency (CVID) and IgA deficiency suggests linkage of CVID to chromosome 16q. Hum Genet 2006;118(6):725–9.

46. Ameratunga R, Lehnert K, Woon ST, et al. Review: diagnosing common variable immunodeficiency disorder in the era of genome sequencing. Clin Rev Allergy Immunol 2018;54(2):261–8.

47. Bogaert DJ, Dullaers M, Lambrecht BN, et al. Genes associated with common variable immunodeficiency: one diagnosis to rule them all? J Med Genet 2016; 53(9):575–90.
48. Li R, Zheng Y, Li Y, et al. Common variable immunodeficiency with genetic defects identified by whole exome sequencing. Biomed Res Int 2018;2018: 3724630.
49. Lee S, Moon JS, Lee CR, et al. Abatacept alleviates severe autoimmune symptoms in a patient carrying a de novo variant in CTLA-4. J Allergy Clin Immunol 2016;137(1):327–30.
50. Schubert D, Bode C, Kenefeck R, et al. Autosomal dominant immune dysregulation syndrome in humans with CTLA4 mutations. Nat Med 2014;20(12):1410–6.
51. Rao VK, Webster S, Dalm V, et al. Effective "activated PI3Kdelta syndrome"-targeted therapy with the PI3Kdelta inhibitor leniolisib. Blood 2017;130(21): 2307–16.
52. Wehr C, Kivioja T, Schmitt C, et al. The EUROclass trial: defining subgroups in common variable immunodeficiency. Blood 2008;111(1):77–85.
53. Farmer JR, Ong MS, Barmettler S, et al. Common variable immunodeficiency non-infectious disease endotypes redefined using unbiased network clustering in large electronic datasets. Front Immunol 2017;8:1740.
54. Resnick ES, Moshier EL, Godbold JH, et al. Morbidity and mortality in common variable immune deficiency over 4 decades. Blood 2012;119(7):1650–7.
55. Haas OA. Primary immunodeficiency and cancer predisposition revisited: embedding two closely related concepts into an integrative conceptual framework. Front Immunol 2018;9:3136.
56. Bussone G, Mouthon L. Autoimmune manifestations in primary immune deficiencies. Autoimmun Rev 2009;8(4):332–6.
57. Sokol K, Milner JD. The overlap between allergy and immunodeficiency. Curr Opin Pediatr 2018;30(6):848–54.
58. Conrad MA, Kelsen JR. Genomic and immunologic drivers of very early-onset inflammatory bowel disease. Pediatr Dev Pathol 2019;22(3):183–93.
59. Martorana D, Bonatti F, Mozzoni P, et al. Monogenic autoinflammatory diseases with mendelian inheritance: genes, mutations, and genotype/phenotype correlations. Front Immunol 2017;8:344.
60. McKenna A, Hanna M, Banks E, et al. The Genome Analysis Toolkit: a MapReduce framework for analyzing next-generation DNA sequencing data. Genome Res 2010;20(9):1297–303.
61. Mousallem T, Urban TJ, McSweeney KM, et al. Clinical application of whole-genome sequencing in patients with primary immunodeficiency. J Allergy Clin Immunol 2015;136(2):476–479 e476.
62. Hoffman-Andrews L. The known unknown: the challenges of genetic variants of uncertain significance in clinical practice. J Law Biosci 2017;4(3):648–57.
63. Schwarze K, Buchanan J, Taylor JC, et al. Are whole-exome and whole-genome sequencing approaches cost-effective? A systematic review of the literature. Genet Med 2018;20(10):1122–30.
64. Hsu AP, Johnson KD, Falcone EL, et al. GATA2 haploinsufficiency caused by mutations in a conserved intronic element leads to MonoMAC syndrome. Blood 2013;121(19):3830–7. S3831–7.
65. Mooster JL, Cancrini C, Simonetti A, et al. Immune deficiency caused by impaired expression of nuclear factor-kappaB essential modifier (NEMO) because of a mutation in the 5' untranslated region of the NEMO gene. J Allergy Clin Immunol 2010;126(1):127–32.e7.

66. van Schouwenburg PA, Davenport EE, Kienzler AK, et al. Application of whole genome and RNA sequencing to investigate the genomic landscape of common variable immunodeficiency disorders. Clin Immunol 2015;160(2):301–14.

67. Tuijnenburg P, Lango Allen H, Burns SO, et al. Loss-of-function nuclear factor kappaB subunit 1 (NFKB1) variants are the most common monogenic cause of common variable immunodeficiency in Europeans. J Allergy Clin Immunol 2018;142(4):1285–96.

68. Stubbington MJT, Rozenblatt-Rosen O, Regev A, et al. Single-cell transcriptomics to explore the immune system in health and disease. Science 2017;358(6359): 58–63.

69. Rodriguez-Cortez VC, Del Pino-Molina L, Rodriguez-Ubreva J, et al. Monozygotic twins discordant for common variable immunodeficiency reveal impaired DNA demethylation during naive-to-memory B-cell transition. Nat Commun 2015;6: 7335.

The Future of Clinical Immunology Laboratory Testing

Hugues Allard-Chamard, MD, PhD, FRCPC[a,b,c,d],*,
Vinay S. Mahajan, MD, PhD[a,e],*

KEYWORDS

- Transcriptomics • Repertoire • Immune function testing
- Next-generation sequencing • High-dimensional analysis

KEY POINTS

- Deep immune profiling is a constellation of high-dimensional analysis technologies, encompassing but not limited to genomic, transcriptomic, epigenomic profiling, next-generation flow cytometry, single-cell transcriptomics, and repertoire analysis.
- Deep immune profiling has greatly improved knowledge of human immunologic disorders and has the potential to provide a holistic picture of immune dysfunction with clinical ramifications.
- Broad clinical adoption of deep immune profiling requires the development of automated specimen processing and analysis methods, assay standardization, and prospective validation in clinical cohorts.
- Assay automation and miniaturization will also lead to the development of a wide range of point-of-care immunodiagnostics.

TECHNOLOGICAL ADVANCES IN MULTIPLEXED PROTEIN DETECTION

Measuring an autoantibody with clinically acceptable sensitivity and precision is critical, but the need for testing a rapidly growing number of autoantibody specificities for

The authors contributed equally to this work.

Disclosure: The authors have nothing to disclose.

[a] Ragon Institute of MGH, MIT and Harvard, 400 Technology Square, Cambridge, MA 02139, USA; [b] Division of Rheumatology, Faculty of Medicine and Health Sciences, Université de Sherbrooke; [c] Centre de Recherche Clinique du Centre Hospitalier Universitaire de Sherbrooke, Sherbrooke, Québec, Canada; [d] Division of Rheumatology, Centre intégré universitaire de santé et de service sociaux de l'Estrie – Centre hospitalier universitaire de Sherbrooke (CIUSSS de l'Estrie-CHUS), 3001, 12th Avenue North, Room 3853, Sherbrooke, Québec J1H 5N4, Canada; [e] Department of Pathology, Brigham and Women's Hospital, 75 Francis Street, Armory 3, Boston, MA 02115, USA

* Corresponding authors. Ragon Institute of MGH, MIT and Harvard, 400 Technology Square, Cambridge, MA 02139, USA

E-mail addresses: hugues.allard-chamard@USherbrooke.ca (H.A.-C.); Vinay.Mahajan@mgh.harvard.edu (V.S.M.)

Clin Lab Med 39 (2019) 699–708
https://doi.org/10.1016/j.cll.2019.07.014
0272-2712/19/© 2019 Elsevier Inc. All rights reserved.

a particular clinical indication poses a new problem, that is, the need for immunoassay multiplexing, often in the form of disease-specific autoantibody panels (**Fig. 1**). Similarly, there is growing demand for multiplexed detection of immune mediators, such as cytokines and chemokines. This challenge is being addressed using microfluidic assay miniaturization with patterned antigen arrays or barcoded capture antibodies and the adoption of label-free techniques.[1,2] Patterned antigen arrays are used to multiplex detection in a manner that is easily amenable to automation and artificial intelligence–assisted diagnosis. An alternative to patterned antigen arrays is addressable laser bead immunoassays in which beads are optically barcoded using fluorescence or light-scattering properties and subsequently coated with distinct capture reagents.[3] Analyte quantification and demultiplexing is simultaneously performed on a flow cytometer that can read the optical bead barcodes and the signal from a fluorophore-coupled detection antibody. These micron-scale beads are manufactured with quantized combinations of fluorescent markers that allows easy multiplexing of 100 to 200 analytes. The availability of new generation of multispectral detectors that allows the deconvolution of fluorescent dyes with minor differences in their fluorescent spectra will expand the capabilities of conventional fluorescent reagents and allow further multiplexing of immunoassays. In addition, antibodies are barcoded by an arbitrary number of distinct nucleic acid sequences such that signals from individual antibody reagents are demultiplexed by high-throughput sequencing. An added advantage of such an approach is that the DNA barcodes may be amenable to signal amplification by polymerase chain reaction, an approach sometimes called immunopolymerase chain reaction.[4] Microscopic polymeric hydrogels, which are uniquely

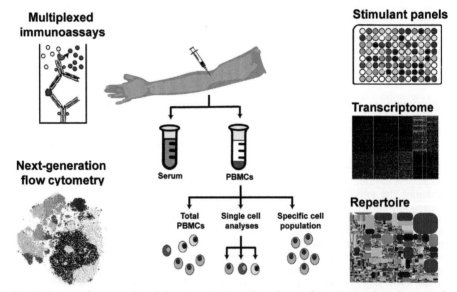

Fig. 1. Future of immunology laboratory testing. The advent of "omics" tools and nanotechnologies has led to the development of high-throughput and multiplexed methods that are becoming increasingly common in immunology research laboratories. These techniques rapidly allow for the simultaneous extraction of transcriptional and proteomic information from a large number of cells, and continue to grow in their complexity and potential. Machine learning approaches that can be used to derive clinically useful interpretive scores and signatures from high dimensional data are being developed, and it will not be long before they are used to guide clinical decision making. PBMCs, peripheral blood mononuclear cells.

suited for use as a solid support in sandwich immunoassays because of their biophysical characteristics, are manufactured with arbitrary optical or shape characteristics in microfluidic devices.[5] Such optical and graphical characteristics are used to encode and multiplex immunosandwich probes, resulting in a high degree of multiplexing; this technology has been commercialized in a manner that is compatible with the use of a conventional flow cytometer or a laser scanner as a detector (FirePlex immunoassays, AbCam, Cambridge, UK). Improvements in mass spectrometry methods have led to a revival of plasma proteomics, allowing the quantitative analysis of approximately 3000 plasma proteins.[6]

Although assay miniaturization can lower costs significantly, because of the potential for reduced reagent consumption and greater automation, it often necessitates the use of techniques with greater analytical sensitivity to capture and detect targets from greatly reduced sample volumes. The twenty-first century will be the age of nanotechnology, and commercial nanotechnology products are already beginning to enter the diagnostic laboratory and change its practice. The discoveries of unexpected optical, mechanical, and electrical properties of nanomaterials, often influenced by quantum phenomena, have resulted in the development of highly sensitive biosensors that can recognize very small molecular perturbations, such as protein binding.[7] One such technology that is close to commercialization relies on multiplexed optical ring resonators.[8] The previously mentioned technologies have the potential to lower detection limits while allowing for greater degree of multiplexing. Furthermore, these approaches are made even more efficient as they are miniaturized and automated using microfluidic platforms.

Sandwich enzyme-linked immunosorbent assay (ELISA) for autoantibodies generally requires tethering of an antigen to a solid support, which has the potential to mask autoreactive epitopes. The tethering approach that offers the least steric hindrance is a polymeric linker. However, even third-generation antineutrophil cytoplasmic antibody ELISA assays for proteinase-3/myeloperoxidase that use such linkers are unable to fully match performance of indirect immunofluorescence assays. In some cases, the antineutrophil cytoplasmic antibody may simply target other possible antigens, such as elastase, cathepsin G, lactoferrin, or epitopes that span the interface of protein complexes containing proteinase-3/myeloperoxidase, which may be picked up by indirect immunofluorescence. Additional innovations in polymer chemistry used for tethering antigens that can reduce antigen masking, or the adoption of label-free approaches, may be needed to further improve these assays.[9,10]

NEXT-GENERATION FLOW CYTOMETRY AND SINGLE-CELL APPROACHES

Immune cells have been classified into a large number of subsets that perform highly specialized functions. Multiplexed analysis of proteins or genes expression at the single cell level is leading to a further expansion in the understanding of specialized innate and adaptive immune cell subsets. For instance, activated or memory CD4 T cells are divided into Th1, Th2, Th17, Tfh, and cytotoxic CD4 T cells, to name a few.[11] There is now an extensive literature on the pathogenic expansion of characteristic T-cell subsets in immune disorders, which has already led to the development of targeted therapies (eg, anti-interleukin-17 in psoriasis, CTLA4-Ig in rheumatoid arthritis [RA], and anti-p40 antibody used to target interleukin-12 and -23 in Crohn's disease). Single-cell approaches are likely to play a key role in realizing the diagnostic and prognostic potential of these findings.

Assessing the quantitative and qualitative dynamics in serologic parameters may predict immune behavior and help monitor the development of autoimmunity. The production of specific high-affinity antibodies in response to pathogens and vaccines is a hallmark of a healthy immune system and is used in the clinic to identify patients with common variable immune deficiency. In addition to the affinity, antibody function dictated by antibody isotype or other modifications, such as glycosylation, is now recognized as especially important and can dramatically impact antibody effector functions.[12] Analyzing Fc function using biochemical means or functional assays can help provide a better indicator of immune dysfunction. For instance, the immune privileged anterior chamber is generally associated with the production of a strong Th2 biased immune response with an antibody response that lacks the ability to activate complement. This protects the ocular microenvironment from deleterious inflammation that could result in blindness, but also prevents an efficient cytotoxic T-cell response, Antibody-dependent cell-mediated cytotoxicity, and the production of complement-fixing antibodies that may be necessary for the control of intraocular tumors. However, deep-seated ocular antigens can gain access to the lymphatics following ocular trauma and be transported to the lymph node, triggering a flagrant immune response that is not typical of the otherwise immune-privileged anterior chamber, which manifests as sympathetic ophthalmia, often leading to blindness.[13] The ability to detect such a shift in immune activity following ocular trauma, by monitoring antibody function and CD4 T-cell polarization, may help provide an early warning for a pathogenic shift in immune bias resulting in destructive ocular inflammation.

Immunophenotypic characterization of immune cell subsets defined by cell surface markers is one of the mainstays of clinical immunology diagnostics. The incorporation of highly sensitive multispectral detectors allows the latest generation of flow cytometers to simultaneously detect several dozen fluorescently labeled antibodies. A similar degree of multiplexing is achieved using antibodies tethered to isotopic mass labels and a CyTOF instrument.[14] These approaches allow the delineation of hundreds of distinct immune cell subsets. Such high dimensional analysis has led to the identification of several novel lymphoid and myeloid lineage subsets that are specifically involved in various immune-mediated diseases. Although not yet used in the clinical setting, "omics" platforms that combine transcriptomic and proteomic information are emerging with incredible diagnostic potential (**Fig. 1**). For example, parallel detection of single-cell transcriptomes with cell surface proteins marked by DNA-barcoded antibodies combines the best of flow cytometry and whole transcriptomics. Similarly, DNA-barcoded peptide-Major Histocompatibility Complex tetramers enable high-throughput screening of T-cell antigen specificity and function. These powerful methods can reveal discrepancies in the expression of mRNA and protein level caused by post-transcriptional regulation thus paving the way for an even more extensive characterization of dysfunctional cells. Integrating T-cell receptor (TCR) antigen specificity, TCR clonality, and T-cell functional status at the single-cell level can provide comprehensive T-cell profiling for T-cell-dependent cancer immunotherapy and monitoring immune-mediated disorders.

Resting lymphocytes are metabolically quiescent, and antigen-induced activation is coincident with a dramatic alteration in their metabolism, a proliferative burst, and the acquisition of specialized functions, such as cytotoxicity, or the ability to secrete specific effector molecules, such as cytokines. In the diagnostic immunology laboratory, in vitro testing of lymphocyte function usually takes the form of measuring activation-induced cell surface markers, cytokine production, cell proliferation, or cytotoxic function. These in vitro approaches are especially relevant to the diagnosis of inherited immunodeficiencies, and are often complemented with in vivo testing of immune function, such as analysis of the humoral response by eliciting a vaccine response in suspected cases of immunodeficiency or identification of sensitized allergens using skin prick tests. In the diagnostic immunology laboratory setting, analysis of immune cell function in response to a stimulant typically involves read-outs based on flow cytometry, ELISA, or ELISPOT; more complex "omics" immune profiling readouts are likely to become the norm in the future. Unlike conventional approaches, which generally require the elicitation of a response to a stimulant, newer immune profiling approaches have the potential to capture the functional state of the immune system without any additional in vitro stimulation. This is possible because cells already carry transcriptomic and epigenetic marks at genes that enable the antigen-induced response, which is measured by conventional immune function assays.

DEEP IMMUNE PHENOTYPING: ANALYSIS OF THE GENOME, TRANSCRIPTOME, AND EPIGENOME

The use of optically barcoded beads, hydrogels, or DNA barcoding techniques has increased the range of multiplexing to the midplex (20–1000) scale, superseding conventional ELISAs or flow cytometry, which operate at a low-plex (<20) scale. However, modern next-generation sequencing (NGS) technologies have ushered in an extremely high-plex (>1000) "omics" era where the simultaneous characterization of thousands of transcripts or genomic variants is routinely possible. The clinical adoption of NGS techniques is growing at an exponential pace, and its application to the diagnosis of inherited immune diseases is described in an accompanying article, "Molecular Diagnosis of Inherited Immune Disorders," in this issue. NGS approaches are already widely used to detect inherited and acquired genetic variants in the context of inherited disease or tumor sequencing, respectively. Effective use of NGS methods requires advanced knowledge of bioinformatics and computational biology, necessitating an interdisciplinary approach to complex diagnostics. The application of NGS is likely to continue to grow at a steady pace. However, automated library preparation methods and the adoption of standardized validated bioinformatic pipelines is critical for the widespread adoption of NGS techniques.

NGS is also prying open the doors of preventive medicine. Although dozens of disease-linked polymorphisms have been identified in genome-wide association studies of immune-mediated disorders, they have had limited clinical utility in the context of an individual patient. Fortunately, recent human genetics research suggests that the presence of a combination of disease-linked loci in the form of a polygenic risk score can be used to estimate the risk of developing disease. Genome-wide single-nucleotide polymorphism analysis techniques have become commonplace driven by and widely adopted in the recreational genetics sector. At the moment, even if one can reliably identify a patient with a significant risk of developing RA, this information is not directly actionable because there are no prospectively validated preventive therapies, other than perhaps smoking avoidance. However, once it becomes possible to make reliable predictions of disease development, it will be only a matter of time before preventive medications or interventions are developed and commercialized. Once genetic information becomes actionable, it will provide an additional impetus for genetic testing.

It is conceivable but impractical to develop individual tests of immune cell function for each clinical scenario. For instance, Pleximmune is a test that examines CD154 levels on cells in a mixed culture of lymphocytes from the recipient and the transplant donor, and can predict the risk of acute rejection in children with liver or small bowel transplants. Other studies suggest that the occurrence of secondary infection in critically ill patients is predicted using simple flow cytometry–derived parameters, such as neutrophil CD88, HLA-DR, and the percentage of T regulatory cells. Instead of developing tests of immune function for specific scenarios, global transcriptomic profiling of immune cells could serve as an attractive approach in the management of immune-mediated diseases.[15] Automated transcriptomic profiling of immune-related genes using platforms, such as NanoString, have made their foray into the clinic in the context of tumor immunology to help identify which patients can benefit from immunotherapy. These may also help predict autoimmune risk or monitor the development of autoimmunity in the context of checkpoint inhibitor therapy. Gene signatures derived from transcriptomic data have proved to be highly predictive of rejection in some studies.[16] Immune cell signature deconvolution techniques have been developed to estimate the immune cell subset composition present in whole blood transcriptomes. However, before these approaches are incorporated into clinical practice these results need to be prospectively validated in independent research cohorts.

Despite the proven utility of consensus diagnostic criteria for classification of rheumatologic diseases, the clinical evolution of many rheumatologic conditions still remains highly variable. This likely reflects unaccounted for heterogeneity in patient background and a gap in fundamental understanding of underlying pathogenic processes. Most autoimmune disorders are multifactorial and arise from a combination of multiple disease-linked genetic loci and environmental factors, most notably the microbiome. High-dimensional data-driven approaches may be well suited to address this challenge. For instance, patients with juvenile idiopathic arthritis from the REACCH OUT and BBOP consortia were enrolled in a study aiming at agnostically classifying juvenile idiopathic arthritis using clinical and proteomic data. Probabilistic principal components analysis was able to resolve five granular categories that strongly predicted disease evolution.[17]

To consider another example, the treatment of systemic lupus erythematosus (SLE) is especially challenging given the intrinsic heterogeneous nature of the disease and current biomarkers simply do not capture the complexity and heterogeneity of this disease. Despite intensive research and a well-stocked pipeline, only one drug has been approved by the Food and Drug Administration since 1997, namely belimumab (a humanized anti-BAFF antibody). All other trials failed to meet their primary end points. The lack of treatments making their way to clinic is perhaps best understood as a direct reflection of incomplete understanding of the pathogenesis of SLE and the heterogeneity in this disease, which has limited the ability to design effective clinical trials. However newer transcriptomic and epigenomic approaches promise to offer a more comprehensive view of the disease. For instance, transcriptomic analysis of a cohort of 158 pediatric patients with SLE was able to stratify patients into seven distinct subsets with different clinical states and response to treatment.[18] Moreover, it is well established that African-Americans patients with SLE present with more active disease then their Hispanic or white counterparts. The observed molecular signature of SLE was significantly different in African-American patients, who exhibited an enrichment for functional module of plasmablast, erythropoiesis, and cell cycle as opposed to enrichment for neutrophil, myeloid lineage, and inflammation-related modules in the rest of the cohort. This study highlights the heterogeneity of the disease and the need for a better classification of lupus, perhaps based on molecular methods, such as transcriptomics, and paves the way to personalized treatment in SLE.

DEEP IMMUNE PROFILING: ANALYSIS OF T-, B-, OR NATURAL KILLER–CELL REPERTOIRE

The capacity of the immune system to target nearly any antigen is caused by the immense diversity of the repertoire of B-cell receptors and TCR. In a healthy individual, the antigen receptor repertoire is highly diverse in naive cells, becoming more constricted among subsets of lymphocytes that selectively proliferate in response to an antigen. This is the hallmark of a targeted immune response to an antigen. NGS techniques have now enabled the analysis of the nucleotide sequences of the antigen receptors from lymphocytes in a single specimen. Single cell approaches now allow the determination of paired heavy/light chain immunoglobulin or α/β TCR genes in combination with the single-cell transcriptomics. Although the development of high-throughput repertoire analysis technique was initially driven by the strong interest in the analyzing tumor-infiltrating lymphocytes, these methods have enormous potential in the context of infectious or autoimmune disease, and in the monitoring of repertoire evolution following bone-marrow transplantation and vaccination.[19]

Any adaptive immune response is characterized by changes in the antigen receptor repertoire. In patients at high risk of developing RA, the presence of five or more dominant BCR clones heralds the development of RA.[20] On the development of arthritis the expanded clones initially disappear from the circulation and are found infiltrating the joints. With the progression of RA, further changes are also noted in the circulating T-cell compartment characterized by a contraction of the TCR repertoire. Repertoire analysis is therefore likely to provide important information. CD4+ T cells reactive to commensal gut bacteria are normally present in the blood at frequencies of 40 to 500 per millions of total CD4+ T cells. During gut dysbiosis inflammatory bowel disease the proportion of circulating T cells harboring TCR reactive to microbiota increase and on stimulation they produce more TH17 cytokines.[21] Such studies use in vitro stimulation to determine antigenic specificity, because determining the antigenic specificity from the sequence of the antigen receptor alone is not currently feasible, but the application of novel computational approaches to rapidly expanding databases of TCR sequences with known specificities is likely to help improve the ability to computationally predict their specificity. The ability of single-cell transcriptomics and repertoire analysis to reveal the functional state of clonally expanded lymphocyte populations is likely to yield useful information of an ongoing immune response; this area has exploded given the emergence of commercially available automated platforms for single cell transcriptomics and is mainly limited by sequencing bandwidth.[22] Natural killer cells express varying combinations of activating and inhibitory receptors, and the analysis of the natural killer cell repertoire is still in its infancy. Nonetheless, it is speculated that it is an untapped metric of immune history and function that may be clinically useful in forecasting the outcomes of infection and malignancy.

CHALLENGES IN THE CLINICAL ADOPTION OF DEEP IMMUNE PROFILING APPROACHES

Using modern immune profiling techniques to develop global metrics of immune dysfunction is a daunting task. In order for widespread clinical adoption of such assays, the concurrent development of automated sequencing library preparation and automated bioinformatic analysis pipelines is critical. This is a feasible goal given the advances in lab-on-chip technologies. Although whole blood assays of transcriptome and epigenome are likely to be the most widely applicable, variations in immune cell composition can limit their utility. Cell composition may need to be inferred by computational deconvolution. When dealing with a rare cell population, cell sorting approaches become necessary. Isolation of specific immune cell types using microfluidic approaches that offer reliable cell separation with minimal handling stress and toxicity may enable more advanced interrogation of particular immune subsets. Such assays need prospective validation in clinical cohorts.

High-dimensional analysis of immune cell function in response to an in vitro stimulus will herald a new generation of immune function tests. Again, automated procedures for specimen or cell handling with a controlled duration of stimulus and a standardized readout may be necessary to avoid operator effects. Laboratory professionals will need to work together to harmonize the assays with standard stimulants, develop standard benchmarks, define normal ranges, and develop standardized computational analysis pipelines for interpretation. It is likely that due consideration of patient factors, such as age, microbiome, or other clinical parameters that have a significant impact on immune function, will also need to be incorporated into the standardized analysis pipelines.

POINT-OF-CARE IMMUNODIAGNOSTICS

The need to deliver care closer to the patient will result in an increase in the volume of testing performed outside the conventional laboratory setting. Point-of-care testing has matured into a field of its own, and numerous technologies and designs have been proposed to address unmet challenges in laboratory testing. These range from low-cost lateral flow assays to fully integrated miniaturized lab-on-chip devices, which have been enabled by advances in semiconductors and nanotechnology. In principle, any sandwich immunoassay can be implemented as a lateral flow assay. In the past two decades, the ability to rapidly develop high-quality monoclonal antibodies with increased affinity, improved techniques for reagent stabilization, and the availability of optimized membranes and filters have together allowed the commercialization of low-cost lateral flow assays against a broad range of analytes. Further improvements in the detection modalities using nanoparticles and optical enhancements or electronic measurements have made these assays more sensitive and quantitative but lateral flow assays still remain limited in the degree of multiplexing. Moreover, the past two decades have witnessed an explosion of publications on lab-on-chip concepts that use a variety of novel immunoassay formats but they have yet to achieve widespread commercial success. However, their compact design, potential for automation, capacity for multiplexing, reduced risk of operator-dependent errors, automated interpretation, and continued improvements in analytical performance makes it inevitable that they will enter the clinic realm. Nonetheless, it is unlikely that there will be a one-size-fits-all solution. Rather, the lab-on-chip approaches will be optimized for the particular clinical setting, or a specific clinical situation, such as a physician's office in a community practice setting, a remote area without access to laboratory testing, a hospital ward, a surgical operating room, and diagnostic work-up of undifferentiated small vessel vasculitis.

SUMMARY

Recent technological and conceptual advances in genomic, transcriptomic, and epigenomic profiling methods have allowed researchers to apply advanced immunologic methods to interrogate small numbers of immune cells obtained from peripheral blood specimens, leading to novel insights into the pathogenesis of immune-mediated diseases. Given a steady reduction in sequencing costs, it is only a matter of time before these techniques emerge in clinical settings and become recognized as a new class of clinical immunology assays because of their added diagnostic or prognostic potential. A concurrent demand for interpretive guidance on immunological tests that continue to grow in their complexity will also call for clinical laboratory immunologists with a strong background in basic immunology to interface with physicians. Furthermore, with the refinement of the lab-on-chip technologies several novel bioassays will become available for testing at the bedside and in resource-constrained settings.

ACKNOWLEDGMENTS

This work was supported by the National Institutes of Health (K08-AI113163 to V.S.M.).

REFERENCES

1. Balboni I, Chan SM, Kattah M, et al. Multiplexed protein array platforms for analysis of autoimmune diseases. Annu Rev Immunol 2006;24:391–418.
2. Ellmark P, Woolfson A, Belov L, et al. The applicability of a cluster of differentiation monoclonal antibody microarray to the diagnosis of human disease. Methods Mol Biol 2008;439:199–209.
3. Hanly JG, Su L, Farewell V, et al. Comparison between multiplex assays for autoantibody detection in systemic lupus erythematosus. J Immunol Methods 2010; 358:75–80.
4. Lundberg M, Eriksson A, Tran B, et al. Homogeneous antibody-based proximity extension assays provide sensitive and specific detection of low-abundant proteins in human blood. Nucleic Acids Res 2011;39:e102.
5. Dendukuri D, Pregibon DC, Collins J, et al. Continuous-flow lithography for high-throughput microparticle synthesis. Nat Mater 2006;5:365–9.
6. Pernemalm M, Lehtiö J. Mass spectrometry-based plasma proteomics: state of the art and future outlook. Expert Rev Proteomics 2014;11:431–48.
7. Zhu C, Yang G, Li H, et al. Electrochemical sensors and biosensors based on nanomaterials and nanostructures. Anal Chem 2015;87:230–49.
8. Sun Y, Fan X. Optical ring resonators for biochemical and chemical sensing. Anal Bioanal Chem 2011;399:205–11.
9. Stern E, Klemic JF, Routenberg DA, et al. Label-free immunodetection with CMOS-compatible semiconducting nanowires. Nature 2007;445:519–22.
10. Ray S, Mehta G, Srivastava S. Label-free detection techniques for protein microarrays: prospects, merits and challenges. Proteomics 2010;10:731–48.
11. Nakayamada S, Takahashi H, Kanno Y, et al. Helper T cell diversity and plasticity. Curr Opin Immunol 2012;24:297–302.
12. Seeling M, Brückner C, Nimmerjahn F. Differential antibody glycosylation in autoimmunity: sweet biomarker or modulator of disease activity? Nat Rev Rheumatol 2017;13:621–30.
13. Caspi RR. Ocular autoimmunity: the price of privilege? Immunol Rev 2006;213: 23–35.
14. Behbehani GK. Applications of mass cytometry in clinical medicine: the promise and perils of clinical CyTOF. Clin Lab Med 2017;37:945–64.
15. Ermann J, Rao DA, Teslovich NC, et al. Immune cell profiling to guide therapeutic decisions in rheumatic diseases. Nat Rev Rheumatol 2015;11:541–51.
16. Famulski KS, Reeve J, de Freitas DG, et al. Kidney transplants with progressing chronic diseases express high levels of acute kidney injury transcripts. Am J Transplant 2013;13:634–44.
17. Eng SWM, Duong TT, Rosenberg AM, et al, REACCH OUT and BBOP Research Consortia. The biologic basis of clinical heterogeneity in juvenile idiopathic arthritis. Arthritis Rheumatol 2014;66:3463–75.
18. Banchereau R, Hong S, Cantarel B, et al. Personalized immunomonitoring uncovers molecular networks that stratify lupus patients. Cell 2016;165:551–65.

19. Robins H. Immunosequencing: applications of immune repertoire deep sequencing. Curr Opin Immunol 2013;25:646–52.

20. Tak PP, Doorenspleet ME, de Hair MJH, et al. Dominant B cell receptor clones in peripheral blood predict onset of arthritis in individuals at risk for rheumatoid arthritis. Ann Rheum Dis 2017;76:1924–30.

21. Hegazy AN, West NR, Stubbington MJT, et al. Circulating and tissue-resident CD4+ T cells with reactivity to intestinal microbiota are abundant in healthy individuals and function is altered during inflammation. Gastroenterology 2017;153: 1320–37.e16.

22. Papalexi E, Satija R. Single-cell RNA sequencing to explore immune cell heterogeneity. Nat Rev Immunol 2018;18:35–45.

![UNITED STATES POSTAL SERVICE] **Statement of Ownership, Management, and Circulation**
(All Periodicals Publications Except Requester Publications)

1. Publication Title	2. Publication Number	3. Filing Date
CLINICS IN LABORATORY MEDICINE	000 – 713	9/18/2019

4. Issue Frequency	5. Number of Issues Published Annually	6. Annual Subscription Price
MAR, JUN, SEP, DEC	4	$274.00

7. Complete Mailing Address of Known Office of Publication (Not printer) (Street, city, county, state, and ZIP+4®)

ELSEVIER INC.
230 Park Avenue, Suite 800
New York, NY 10169

Contact Person
STEPHEN R. BUSHING
Telephone (Include area code)
215-239-3688

8. Complete Mailing Address of Headquarters or General Business Office of Publisher (Not printer)

ELSEVIER INC.
230 Park Avenue, Suite 800
New York, NY 10169

9. Full Names and Complete Mailing Addresses of Publisher, Editor, and Managing Editor (Do not leave blank)

Publisher (Name and complete mailing address)

TAYLOR BALL, ELSEVIER INC.
1600 JOHN F KENNEDY BLVD. SUITE 1800
PHILADELPHIA, PA 19103-2899

Editor (Name and complete mailing address)

STACY EASTMAN, ELSEVIER INC.
1600 JOHN F KENNEDY BLVD. SUITE 1800
PHILADELPHIA, PA 19103-2899

Managing Editor (Name and complete mailing address)

PATRICK MANLEY, ELSEVIER INC.
1600 JOHN F KENNEDY BLVD. SUITE 1800
PHILADELPHIA, PA 19103-2899

10. Owner (Do not leave blank. If the publication is owned by a corporation, give the name and address of the corporation immediately followed by the names and addresses of all stockholders owning or holding 1 percent or more of the total amount of stock. If not owned by a corporation, give the names and addresses of the individual owners. If owned by a partnership or other unincorporated firm, give its name and address as well as those of each individual owner. If the publication is published by a nonprofit organization, give its name and address.)

Full Name	Complete Mailing Address
WHOLLY OWNED SUBSIDIARY OF REED/ELSEVIER, US HOLDINGS	1600 JOHN F KENNEDY BLVD. SUITE 1800 PHILADELPHIA, PA 19103-2899

11. Known Bondholders, Mortgagees, and Other Security Holders Owning or Holding 1 Percent or More of Total Amount of Bonds, Mortgages, or Other Securities. If none, check box. ☑ None

Full Name	Complete Mailing Address
N/A	

12. Tax Status (For completion by nonprofit organizations authorized to mail at nonprofit rates) (Check one)
The purpose, function, and nonprofit status of this organization and the exempt status for federal income tax purposes:
☑ Has Not Changed During Preceding 12 Months
☐ Has Changed During Preceding 12 Months (Publisher must submit explanation of change with this statement)

PS Form **3526**, July 2014 (Page 1 of 4 (see instructions page 4)) PSN: 7530-01-000-9931 PRIVACY NOTICE: See our privacy policy on www.usps.com.

---

13. Publication Title			14. Issue Date for Circulation Data Below
CLINICS IN LABORATORY MEDICINE			JUNE 2019

15. Extent and Nature of Circulation			Average No. Copies Each Issue During Preceding 12 Months	No. Copies of Single Issue Published Nearest to Filing Date
a. Total Number of Copies (Net press run)			98	84
b. Paid Circulation (By Mail and Outside the Mail)	(1)	Mailed Outside-County Paid Subscriptions Stated on PS Form 3541 (Include paid distribution above nominal rate, advertiser's proof copies, and exchange copies)	31	34
	(2)	Mailed In-County Paid Subscriptions Stated on PS Form 3541 (Include paid distribution above nominal rate, advertiser's proof copies, and exchange copies)	0	0
	(3)	Paid Distribution Outside the Mails Including Sales Through Dealers and Carriers, Street Vendors, Counter Sales, and Other Paid Distribution Outside USPS®	17	18
	(4)	Paid Distribution by Other Classes of Mail Through the USPS (e.g., First-Class Mail®)	0	0
c. Total Paid Distribution (Sum of 15b (1), (2), (3), and (4))		▶	48	52
d. Free or Nominal Rate Distribution (By Mail and Outside the Mail)	(1)	Free or Nominal Rate Outside-County Copies included on PS Form 3541	39	18
	(2)	Free or Nominal Rate In-County Copies Included on PS Form 3541	0	0
	(3)	Free or Nominal Rate Copies Mailed at Other Classes Through the USPS (e.g. First-Class Mail)	0	0
	(4)	Free or Nominal Rate Distribution Outside the Mail (Carriers or other means)	0	0
e. Total Free or Nominal Rate Distribution (Sum of 15d (1), (2), (3) and (4))		▶	39	18
f. Total Distribution (Sum of 15c and 15e)		▶	87	70
g. Copies not Distributed (See Instructions to Publishers #4 (page #3))		▶	11	14
h. Total (Sum of 15f and g)		▶	98	84
i. Percent Paid (15c divided by 15f times 100)		▶	55.17%	74.29%

* If you are claiming electronic copies, go to line 16 on page 3. If you are not claiming electronic copies, skip to line 17 on page 3.

PS Form **3526**, July 2014 (Page 2 of 4)

16. Electronic Copy Circulation	Average No. Copies Each Issue During Preceding 12 Months	No. Copies of Single Issue Published Nearest to Filing Date
a. Paid Electronic Copies	▶	
b. Total Paid Print Copies (Line 15c) + Paid Electronic Copies (Line 16a)	▶	
c. Total Print Distribution (Line 15f) + Paid Electronic Copies (Line 16a)	▶	
d. Percent Paid (Both Print & Electronic Copies) (16b divided by 16c × 100)	▶	

☑ I certify that 50% of all my distributed copies (electronic and print) are paid above a nominal price.

17. Publication of Statement of Ownership

☑ If the publication is a general publication, publication of this statement is required. Will be printed
in the DECEMBER 2019 issue of this publication.

☐ Publication not required.

18. Signature and Title of Editor, Publisher, Business Manager, or Owner

STEPHEN R. BUSHING - INVENTORY DISTRIBUTION CONTROL MANAGER

Date 9/18/2019

I certify that all information furnished on this form is true and complete. I understand that anyone who furnishes false or misleading information on this form or who omits material or information requested on the form may be subject to criminal sanctions (including fines and imprisonment) and/or civil sanctions (including civil penalties).

PS Form **3526**, July 2014 (Page 3 of 4) PRIVACY NOTICE: See our privacy policy on www.usps.com

Moving?

Make sure your subscription moves with you!

To notify us of your new address, find your **Clinics Account Number** (located on your mailing label above your name), and contact customer service at:

Email: journalscustomerservice-usa@elsevier.com

800-654-2452 (subscribers in the U.S. & Canada)
314-447-8871 (subscribers outside of the U.S. & Canada)

Fax number: 314-447-8029

Elsevier Health Sciences Division
Subscription Customer Service
3251 Riverport Lane
Maryland Heights, MO 63043

*To ensure uninterrupted delivery of your subscription, please notify us at least 4 weeks in advance of move.